Women's Reproductive Mental Health
Across the Lifespan

Diana Lynn Barnes
Editor

Women's Reproductive Mental Health Across the Lifespan

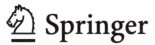

Editor
Diana Lynn Barnes
The Center for Postpartum Health
Sherman Oaks, CA, USA

ISBN 978-3-319-05115-4 (hardcover) ISBN 978-3-319-05116-1 (eBook)
ISBN 978-3-319-21685-0 (softcover)
DOI 10.1007/978-3-319-05116-1
Springer Cham Heidelberg New York Dordrecht London

Library of Congress Control Number: 2014939381

© Springer International Publishing Switzerland 2014, First softcover printing 2015
This work is subject to copyright. All rights are reserved by the Publisher, whether the whole or part of the material is concerned, specifically the rights of translation, reprinting, reuse of illustrations, recitation, broadcasting, reproduction on microfilms or in any other physical way, and transmission or information storage and retrieval, electronic adaptation, computer software, or by similar or dissimilar methodology now known or hereafter developed. Exempted from this legal reservation are brief excerpts in connection with reviews or scholarly analysis or material supplied specifically for the purpose of being entered and executed on a computer system, for exclusive use by the purchaser of the work. Duplication of this publication or parts thereof is permitted only under the provisions of the Copyright Law of the Publisher's location, in its current version, and permission for use must always be obtained from Springer. Permissions for use may be obtained through RightsLink at the Copyright Clearance Center. Violations are liable to prosecution under the respective Copyright Law.

The use of general descriptive names, registered names, trademarks, service marks, etc. in this publication does not imply, even in the absence of a specific statement, that such names are exempt from the relevant protective laws and regulations and therefore free for general use.

While the advice and information in this book are believed to be true and accurate at the date of publication, neither the authors nor the editors nor the publisher can accept any legal responsibility for any errors or omissions that may be made. The publisher makes no warranty, express or implied, with respect to the material contained herein.

Printed on acid-free paper

Springer is part of Springer Science+Business Media (www.springer.com)

TO MY MOTHER
Who gave me life

Foreword

This book is about women's mental health across the reproductive lifespan. It covers puberty, the menstrual cycle, pregnancy and postpartum, and the menopause, as well as contraception, infertility, miscarriage and birth trauma, eating disorders, and other relevant topics. It is both interesting and unusual to examine all these together. Many of the same themes reappear. The biological bases, the importance of the social environment and social support, as well as the role of health professionals are rightly recurring themes.

In Genesis, Eve was told, "In sorrow you will bear children" (as Diana Lynn Barnes quotes in her chapter), and sadly, for too many women, this is still true. About 10–15 % of women experience anxiety and depression either during pregnancy or in the postnatal period, and often during both. Women in general have double the rate of depression than men, with the increase starting in puberty and continuing until the menopause. They also have increased rates of almost all the anxiety disorders when compared with men. Except for psychosis, women's mental health problems across the reproductive lifespan are common. Some women suffer especially in the premenstrual period, and this has been shown to occur worldwide. Many women have increased irritability, anxiety or depression, or mood lability during the menopause. Nearly a quarter of women in the USA in their 40s and 50s take an antidepressant. The peak time for a woman's admission as an inpatient to a psychiatric ward is immediately after childbirth, when she is much more likely to need hospital treatment for psychosis than at any other time in her life. All this suggests that there are periods in a woman's life, associated with reproduction, which make her especially vulnerable to mood changes and mental illness.

There is good evidence that levels of the reproductive hormones, estrogen and progesterone, as well as others, such as the stress hormone cortisol, change during these reproductive periods; their rise, and especially their withdrawal, can cause changes in mood in certain vulnerable women. However, it is clear that not all women are affected. For example, the interesting studies of Rubinow and his colleagues have shown that when high doses of estrogen and progesterone are withdrawn in nonpregnant women who have been given these hormones, some women become depressed, but only women who have a history of postnatal depression, but it is only women who have a history of postnatal depression (Bloch, Daly, & Rubinow, 2003). Other women are not affected. This shows that reproductive hormone withdrawal can affect mood, but only in susceptible people. Some women are more sensitive to the withdrawal of these hormones than others, presumably at least in part due to their genetic makeup. Recent research is showing how complex the genetics of diseases such as schizophrenia and bipolar disorder are. More than 120 susceptibility genes have now been identified for schizophrenia, each contributing a very small part of the variance. The genetic component of sensitivity to reproductive hormone withdrawal is likely to be complex also.

The social and psychological environments are clearly very important too. The very early environment can affect susceptibility to the hormonal changes that occur later during a woman's life. Biological studies are showing the molecular basis of some of the long-lasting effects of the early environment in altered epigenetic profiles. Epigenetics means "on top of genetics." Epigenetic changes do not change the base sequence of the genes in the DNA, but control how much of each gene is turned on or off. Studies of early mothering, or early childhood trauma, have been shown to change the epigenetic makeup of the future child. This, in turn, may contribute to women's mood changes at particular times in their lives, such as during the premenstrual or postpartum period. Thus a women's early experience of how she was mothered or of early abuse or trauma can affect how she responds to hormonal or environmental changes for the rest of her life.

Indeed the environment which can predispose a woman to later affective disorders such as anxiety and depression can start in the womb. There is increasing evidence that if a mother is stressed, anxious, or depressed while she is pregnant, this increases the risk of her child suffering from a range of problems, including anxiety and depression, in later life. There is evidence from animal studies, as well as from studies allowing for a wide range of possible confounders, that this association is, at least in part, causal. Both animal and human studies are uncovering some of the underlying mechanisms, and show the importance of epigenetic changes here too. They show that if a woman is anxious or depressed while she is pregnant, this can alter the filtering capacity of the placenta with a reduction, for example, in the enzyme which breaks down cortisol. Thus the environmental contribution to a woman's vulnerability to mood problems throughout the lifespan starts before she is born.

As many of these chapters show, although her biology contributes to these mood disorders in women, the immediate emotional and social environments are very important too. The subject of this book is certainly one that demonstrates the interaction of genetics, hormonal fluctuations, and the social environment. A recurring theme is how protective social support can be, especially that of the partner. Social support has been shown to be important in protection against both prenatal and postnatal depression, as well as during the menopause. It is likely to be a protective factor in the prevention of affective disorders throughout the lifespan.

All this rightly raises questions about what should be done to help. Mental health care is still the poor relation of physical health care. And mental health care for women is very neglected. Health professionals need to be more aware of the themes covered in this book. A history of depression at any time is a risk factor for depression during times of reproductive hormone fluctuation, and a history of emotional disturbance associated with one reproductive event can increase the risk for it to be associated with another, such as during the menopause.

A time when most women come into contact with health professionals is when they are pregnant. This should be a time for taking both a detailed history of their emotional problems associated with reproductive events, and a detailed examination of their current emotional state. Appropriate screening instruments, such as the Edinburgh Depression Scale, could be used more widely. Several studies have shown that both prenatal and postnatal depression are very under recognized by health professionals, and even when recognized are often not treated appropriately. Women themselves may not realize that they need help, and if they do, they can be scared of the attached stigma, or even of having their baby taken away. For severe depression, antidepressants are the most appropriate treatment, and there is now evidence that most of them do not harm the fetus, or the future child, when taken in pregnancy. Health professionals need to have up-to-date knowledge of this and to know which are safe to use in different situations. However, understandably, many women would rather have non-pharmacological treatments at this time, and more research needs to be carried out on these topics. As well as various talking therapies, we need to have more research on how effective other interventions can be, such as transcranial stimulation or music therapy.

As a society, we need much more public education about mental illness in general, and women's mental health problems across the lifespan, in particular. We need to try to reduce the stigma and fear of mental illness. Partners, relations, friends, and employers all need to know how they can assist by providing extra social support. A greater knowledge of the themes covered in this book will help.

London, UK   Vivette Glover

Reference

Bloch, M., Daly, R. C., & Rubinow, D. R. (2003). Endocrine factors in the etiology of postpartum depression. *Comprehensive Psychiatry, 44*(3), 234–246.

Preface

In the last several decades, the subject of women's mental health, particularly as it relates to women's reproductive lives, has garnered substantial interest. There has been growing recognition and concern that especially during their childbearing years women are even more vulnerable to significant changes in mood. Perinatal mood and anxiety disorders have become the focus of numerous studies, and current statistics estimate that as many as 800,000 to 1 million women each year will experience some mood-related disorders in regard to their pregnancies and births. Research findings indicate a greater increase in psychiatric admissions during this period of a woman's reproductive life than at any other time in the female life cycle. Women with chronic mental illnesses, such as bipolar disorder or schizophrenia, are at even greater risk of complications regarding their mental health during pregnancy and the postpartum period.

There is growing confirmation that a mother's depression during pregnancy impacts the fetus in utero, disrupting the growing attachment relationship between mother and infant which, in turn, often compromises a mother's capacity and desire to provide sensitive and attuned caregiving during the postpartum period. Furthermore, women's mood disorders around childbearing often create discord in partner relationships and a decline in marital satisfaction with potentially adverse consequences for the stability of the marital relationships and the larger family. Maternal depression reverberates throughout the family system with potentially serious repercussions for the cognitive, social-emotional, and psychological health of the developing child across her lifespan.

In response to the evolving body of scientific and clinical literature that continues to substantiate the realities about women's psychological and emotional vulnerabilities around pregnancy and childbirth, legislation is being enacted at both the state and federal level with a push towards learning more about women's reproductive mental health and providing a structure by which women's risks can be identified. Consequently, the study of perinatal mood disorders has been a catalyst for research around other aspects of women's reproductive lives along with a much deeper understanding that the foundation of women's reproductive mental health begins many years before a pregnancy is even contemplated. In fact, a woman's risks for mood and anxiety disorders around the childbearing years originate in a psychological and biological process that occurs as early as her own experience in utero.

My own interest in women's reproductive mental health dates back more than 21 years ago after my second child, my daughter, was born. Within hours of her birth, I suffered anxiety that became intolerable and paralyzing; within the first year of her life, I was hospitalized four different times and never even heard the word postpartum depression until the day of her first birthday. By that time I was in such a fragile emotional and physiological state that I continued to relapse and was continually in and out of the hospital for the next 2 years. In 1992 when my daughter was born, the idea of a woman's risks and her vulnerability to mood-related illness in the peripartum was never discussed or even considered, and certainly never mentioned during pregnancy, which at that time was believed to be protective against depression and anxiety. Upon my recovery from illness that proved to be life threatening, I began to delve into the field of women's mental health, perhaps out of a curiosity to understand more deeply what had happened to me and probably because of my growing fascination with the breadth of this field. It wasn't until many years later that I came to recognize how my own early reproductive history bore a significant connection to my later vulnerability to changes in mood around my childbearing years, first with the birth of my son and more critically with the birth of my daughter. Postpartum depression also laid the groundwork for heightening my vulnerability to fluctuations in mood, given some reproductive events that followed.

The psychological experience of womanhood is embedded in the fabric of a woman's reproductive life and exists not as a series of isolated events, but as a psychological continuum across her lifespan. The quality of women's mental health around reproductive issues and events that begin in the earliest years of their lives is inextricably linked to emotional well-being throughout their years. A woman's experience of her changing body as she approaches puberty, the advent of menstruation, her predisposition to conditions like premenstrual dysphoric disorder, or the impact of body image perceptions on eating disorders have a significant impact on her vulnerability to later episodic depression and anxiety. Even after the childbearing years come to a close, women's concerns about their reproductive health as it influences their mental health continue into the later years of their lives.

Divided into four parts, the following chapters look at the intersection between reproductive health and mental health across the continuum of women's lives. Because a woman's body and psyche are so delicately intertwined, *Women's Reproductive Mental Health Across the Lifespan* looks at the female experience through a biopsychosocial lens. The researchers and clinicians who have gathered throughout the pages of this book to share their wisdom are some of the top experts in their related fields. I hope you will take a closer look not only at their writings in this work, but also at the remarkable contributions each of these authors has made to their respective areas of study.

The conventional wisdom of the early to middle twentieth century accepted women's changes in mood as just a fact of life because after all, "we are women." The 1990s gradually saw the emergence of a profoundly different perspective about the origins of women's mental health. Part 1, *The Early Years*, begins at the very beginning as Drs. Marcy Axness and Joel Evans, experts in perinatal psychology, discuss how a woman's own experience as a fetus in utero creates a psychological roadmap for the future of her reproductive mental health. Along with this increasingly important recognition that we all need "a good psychological head start," Dr. Melissa J. Johnson, founder of The Institute for Girls' Development, explains in chapter "Girls In-Between: Social, Emotional, Physical, and Sexual Development In Context" that the social, emotional, and physical experiences of girls as they move into womanhood continue to provide the context for stable psychological health as their bodies and psyches mature. A fundamental milestone for young women is the advent of menstruation. A known rite of passage, both physiologically and emotionally, the onset of menses can be a tenuous time of adjustment for many women; for those who are most at risk, menstruation can be a source of monthly emotional turmoil. Dr. Neil Epperson has written extensively on the subject of premenstrual dysphoric disorder and along with her coauthor Lisa Hantsoo explains in great detail both the science and the psychology of these extreme monthly changes in mood.

Part 2, *The Reproductive Years*, addresses the psychological experiences and vulnerabilities of women around pregnancy and the childbearing years, which have much broader dimensions than just the logistics of prenatal care, labor, and delivery. A woman's longing for a child and her wish to become a mother often begins many years before conception and eventually becomes an essential part of the outline of her life. Along with these plans, however, are her seemingly nonnegotiable expectations that becoming pregnant, staying pregnant, and giving birth will be automatic and seamless. When unanticipated events like infertility, pregnancy loss, or birth trauma disrupt this vision, it can be psychologically devastating. These experiences stand in stark contrast with what most women expect from their bodies—that they can create life, carry to term without pause, and deliver without incident.

In chapter 4 "The Psychological Gestation of Motherhood," I write about the trans- formation of a woman's psychological self as she steps into the unchartered emotional territory of new motherhood. The psychological gestation that accompanies the physiologic changes of pregnancy sets the stage for a woman's mental health during the peripartum period. Researcher Carol Henshaw has written numerous papers and books about the critical importance of risk assessment and screening. In chapter 5, "Screening and Risk Assessment for Perinatal Mood Disorders." she outlines the protocols for identifying a woman's risks for a perinatal mood or anxiety disorder so that treatment plans can be implemented in an effort to prevent the onset of a depression during the perinatal period. In the chapter "Postpartum Adjustment: What's Normal and What's Not," well-known reproductive psychiatrist, Lucy J. Puryear, distinguishes between the normal and not-so-normal anxieties of the postpartum period while in their chapter "Chronic Mental Illness in Pregnancy and Postpartum," Drs. Melissa L. Nau and Alissa M. Peterson discuss the impact of chronic and severe mental illness on women's experiences of pregnancy and childbirth. With the striking advances in reproductive technology, many women who struggle with infertility are now able to realize their capacity to conceive and bear children. Alongside the newfound physical possibilities also lie any numbers of psychological and emotional challenges as Dr. Dorette Noorhasan describes in chapter "Does Psychiatric Diagnosis Affect Fertility Outcomes?" Does a psychiatric history affect fertility outcomes and/or do fertility treatments have a definitive impact on women's mental health? In chapter "The Reproductive Story: Dealing with Miscarriage, Stillbirth, or Other Perinatal Demise" Janet Jaffe, PhD takes a clinical look at the pain of pregnancy loss and the ways in which it disrupts women's stories about their reproductive lives. Part 2 ends with a chapter on birth trauma and post-traumatic stress, articulately explained by Dr. Kathleen Kendall-Tackett, a health psychologist, prolific writer, and a foremost expert on the varied experiences of women around childbearing and the potentially serious repercussions of these events on their psychological health.

Part 3 addresses the *Later Years* of women's reproductive lives and its connection to their experience of emotional and psychological stability. Born into a generation in which women routinely had babies in their twenties and a mom over 30 was considered "old," I am continually amazed by the gifts that reproductive technologies are able to provide in terms of extending the childbearing years well into a woman's 40s. Does that mean, however, that we can prolong reproduction indefinitely, a question that fertility specialist Dr. Nurit Winkler answers in her chapter on the ticking of the biological clock. As women move into the final chapter of their reproductive lives, they are especially vulnerable to fluctuations in mood. In chapter "Risk Factors for Depression During Perimenopause," Dr. Zoe Gibbs and Dr. Jayrashi Kulkharni identify those risk factors that predispose women to mood disorders around perimenopause, drawing specific connections between earlier reproductive mental health concerns, like premenstrual dysphoric disorder, PMDD, or perinatal depression and heightened risks for depression as they transition into menopause.

Although this work establishes a timeline for the reproductive events that can compromise women's mental health as they age, there are also those issues that affect women across the lifespan as delineated in the chapters of Part 4. Stephanie Zerwas, PhD and Elizabeth Claydon, MPH discuss the potentially grave impact of body image issues and eating disorders on women's mental health from menstruation through menopause. Choosing hormonal contraception is a concern for many women at varying junctures across the lifespan, such as when they become sexually active or after giving birth. There has been ongoing discussion in the scientific and psychological communities about whether hormonal contraception has any direct impact on women's moods, as obstetrician Dr. Lauren Schiff outlines in chapter "The Use of Hormonal Contraception and Its Impact on Women's Moods." In addition to addressing this question, Dr. Schiff discusses the current biological basis for mood fluctuations, and describes in depth the current contraception options available to women in the USA, highlighting the indications, risks, and common side effects of these contraceptives. She presents several case scenarios, and outlines treatment recommendations that consider a woman's unique mental health history in concert with the available scientific literature. Any conversation about women's moods in relation to their reproductive lives would not be sufficient without a chapter on the impact of cancer on a woman's mental health. Current statistics estimate that in 2014, there will be approximately 14 million cancer survivors, and 30 % of those who survive will be women with breast and other gynecological cancers. The word cancer is infused with a range of emotions that exist independently of any woman's preexisting mental health history. However, a previous history of trauma often exacerbates the shock already associated with the word cancer. With an emphasis on the psychosocial impact of a cancer diagnosis, oncology expert Dr. Doreen L. Wiggins along with her co-authors Dr. Carmen Monzon and researcher Beth R. Hott address the physiologic implications of cancer treatments and surgery on a woman's psychological health. They look at the psychological ramifications for women at any age. In chapter "The Impact of Reproductive Cancers on Women's Mental Health," they also examine the emotional impact of genetic testing as markers of heightened risk for breast and ovarian cancers and speak to the literature on posttraumatic growth as a potentially positive outcome for a woman with cancer. Reproductive psychiatry is an emerging and evolving medical specialty that often plays a critical role in managing women's mental health across the lifespan. Reproductive and perinatal psychiatrist Dr. Emily C. Dossett discusses the significant partnership between pharmacology and psychology in treating women's mood disorders. In chapter "The Role of Reproductive Psychiatry in Women's Mental Health," she takes a look at this growing specialty with an emphasis on case examples as a way of understanding current symptoms within the context of women's mental health history and the overall impact on the complexities of clinical decision-making.

Women's emotional lives are shaped by the relationship between biology, culture, and psychology. *Women's Reproductive Mental Health Across the Lifespan* brings current research and clinical application together through the varied perspectives of prominent experts in the field of women's reproductive mental health. Because this text intends to deepen the understanding of the indelible link between women's psychology and their reproductive timeline, it has interdisciplinary relevance to all health care practitioners who treat women.

Sherman Oaks, CA   Diana Lynn Barnes

Acknowledgments

This book would not have come to life without the extraordinary contributions of the distinguished authors whose insight, knowledge, and vast experience in the field of women's reproductive mental health fill the pages of this work. I offer each of you my deepest appreciation for your enthusiasm about this project, your availability, and your patience in moving around your incredibly packed schedules in order to meet the requirements of mine.

I also want to recognize my friends and colleagues in maternal mental health who have devoted a lifetime of their energies to increasing awareness about women's mental health and changing perception about the emotional challenges women face around the childbearing years. To the members of the Los Angeles County Perinatal Mental Health Task Force, the statewide Maternal Mental Health Collaborative and 2020 Moms, and Postpartum Support International—over the years we have worked together, your passion continues to inspire me and the remarkable inroads you have made have helped shape the direction and course of my own thinking about women's mental health.

I am forever grateful to my dear friend and colleague Sonia Murdock of the Postpartum Resource Center of New York who has been an ongoing source of support and encouragement since the day we met at a Marcé Society Conference in Iowa City and to Dr. Margaret Spinelli who has mentored my work in ways she could not possibly imagine.

My heartfelt appreciation and thanks to Jennifer Hadley at Springer who understood the importance of a book on women's reproductive mental health and honored my vision to help make it a reality. I also want to acknowledge Cheryl Barnett who read and re-read countless pages of manuscript copy.

To my partners in life, my children David and Danielle, and my husband Jerry Cohen, you have always been my cheerleaders, voicing your pride, continually motivating me to learn more and to follow the paths that move me.

Contents

Part I The Early Years

Pre- and Perinatal Influences on Female Mental Health 3
Marcy Axness and Joel Evans

**Girls In-Between: Social, Emotional, Physical,
and Sexual Development in Context**... 27
Melissa J. Johnson

**Menstruation and Premenstrual Dysphoric Disorder:
Its Impact on Mood**... 49
C. Neill Epperson and Liisa Hantsoo

Part II The Reproductive Years

The Psychological Gestation of Motherhood.. 75
Diana Lynn Barnes

Screening and Risk Assessment for Perinatal Mood Disorders................. 91
Carol Henshaw

Postpartum Adjustment: What Is Normal and What Is Not..................... 109
Lucy J. Puryear

Chronic Mental Illness in Pregnancy and Postpartum 123
Melissa L. Nau and Alissa M. Peterson

Does Psychiatric Diagnosis Affect Fertility Outcomes? 141
Dorette Noorhasan

**The Reproductive Story: Dealing with Miscarriage,
Stillbirth, or Other Perinatal Demise**... 159
Janet Jaffe

**Birth Trauma: The Causes and Consequences
of Childbirth-Related Trauma and PTSD** 177
Kathleen Kendall-Tackett

Part III The Later Years

Babies After 40: Is the "Biological Clock" Really Ticking? 195
Nurit Winkler

Risk Factors for Depression During Perimenopause 215
Zoe Gibbs and Jayashri Kulkarni

Part IV Across the Lifespan

**Eating Disorders Across the Life-Span:
From Menstruation to Menopause** 237
Stephanie Zerwas and Elizabeth Claydon

**The Use of Hormonal Contraception and Its Impact
on Women's Moods** 263
Lauren Schiff

The Impact of Reproductive Cancers on Women's Mental Health 283
Doreen L. Wiggins, Carmen Monzon, and Beth R. Hott

The Role of Reproductive Psychiatry in Women's Mental Health 301
Emily C. Dossett

Index 329

Author Biographies

Marcy Axness, Ph.D. is internationally recognized for her work on prenatal development and is the author of *Parenting for peace: Raising the next generation of peacemakers*. A member of *Mothering* Magazine's expert panel, Dr. Axness has been featured in several documentary films as an expert in adoption, prenatal development, and Waldorf education.

Elizabeth Claydon, M.P.H. has her degree in Social and Behavioral Sciences from Yale School of Public Health. Her primary research interests include the simultaneous prevention of obesity and eating disorders in children and adolescents as well as the role that eating disorders play in maternal health and parenting.

Emily C. Dossett, M.D., M.T.S. is the founder and director of the Maternal Wellness Clinic at Los Angeles County University of Southern California Medical Center. In addition to a private practice in Pasadena, California specializing in reproductive psychiatry, Dr. Dossett is an Assistant Clinical Professor of Psychiatry at USC's Keck School of Medicine. She has served on the Executive Committee of the Los Angeles County Perinatal Mental Health Task Force, a consortium of over 30 individuals and agencies dedicated to policy change and service improvement for perinatal mood and anxiety disorders.

C. Neill Epperson, M.D. is Associate Professor of Psychiatry and Obstetrics and Gynecology and the Director of the Penn Center for Women's Behavioral Wellness at the Perelman School of Medicine of the University of Pennsylvania. Dr. Epperson's research interests are in the neuroendocrine basis for mood, behavior, and cognitive changes across the female lifespan. As the Co-Director for the Penn Center for the Study of Sex and Gender in Behavioral Health, Dr. Epperson also investigates the contribution of sex to the pathogenesis and treatment of psychiatric and substance use disorders and cognitive aging.

Joel Evans, M.D. is the founder and director of The Center for Women's Health in Stamford, Connecticut. The author of *The whole pregnancy handbook* (Gotham, 2005), Dr. Evans is Assistant Clinical Professor in the Department of Obstetrics, Gynecology and Women's Health at the Albert Einstein College of Medicine and the Founding Diplomate of the American Board of Holistic Medicine. He serves on the editorial advisory board of Bottom Line/Women's Health and as a peer reviewer for the Journals *Alternative Therapies in Health and Medicine* and *Global Advances in Health and Medicine.*

Zoe Gibbs, Psy.D. specializes in the impact of perimenopause on women's moods and her research has been published in a number of journals, including the *Archives of Women's Mental Health*. In addition to her work as a researcher in women's mental health, Dr. Gibbs is a practicing clinician in Melbourne, Australia.

Vivette Glover, M.A., Ph.D., D.Sc. is a Professor of Perinatal Psychobiology on the faculty of medicine at Imperial College in London, England. She has a long-standing interest in biological psychiatry, including the impact of perinatal depression on fetal development. An honorary Senior Lecturer at the Institute of Psychiatry at King's College in London, Dr. Glover has authored over 400 papers, over 200 of which are in peer-reviewed journals. She is the Director of the Fetal and Neonatal Stress Research Group, a multidisciplinary center which aims to study fetal and neonatal stress responses, methods to reduce them and their long-term effects.

Liisa Hantsoo, Ph.D. is a postdoctoral fellow in the Perelman School of Medicine of the University of Pennsylvania, Penn Center for Women's Behavioral Wellness. She completed her undergraduate degree in neuroscience at the Johns Hopkins University, and her doctorate in clinical psychology at Ohio State University. Dr. Hantsoo's research interests lie in stress biology across the female lifespan, genetics, and immune function.

Carol Henshaw, M.B., Ch.B., M.D., F.R.C.Psych. is a consultant in perinatal mental health at Liverpool Women's Hospital and an honorary visiting fellow at Staffordshire University in the UK. A former president of the International Marcé Society, Dr. Henshaw is internationally recognized for her contributions to the field of perinatal mental illness and women's reproductive mental health. She has authored a number of papers and books, including *Screening for perinatal depression* (Jessica Kingsley, 2009).

Beth R. Hott, B.A. has worked in the academic research field for 20 years with a special focus on psychiatry, pregnancy, and women's health. She has coauthored several articles and prepared numerous presentations for national and international medical conferences. She is currently working alongside Dr. Doreen L. Wiggins at the Women's Medicine Collaborative at the Miriam Hospital in Providence, Rhode Island.

Janet Jaffe, Ph.D. is the co-founder and co-director of the Center for Reproductive Psychology in San Diego, California. Her clinical practice focuses on issues of loss and bereavement related to miscarriage, infertility, and other reproductive trauma. Dr. Jaffe is the coauthor of two books on the subject of reproductive loss—*Unsung lullabies: Understand and coping with infertility* and *Reproductive trauma: Psychotherapy with infertility and pregnancy loss clients.*

Melissa J. Johnson, Ph.D. is the founder of the Institute for Girls' Development in Pasadena, California. An expert on child and teen development, she has served on the faculty of the University of LaVerne and the University of Southern California. Her articles on raising strong girls have been published in a number of academic journals, including *The Journal of Humanistic Psychology and Professional Psychology* and *Professional Psychology*.

Kathleen Kendall-Tackett, Ph.D., I.B.C.L.C., F.A.P.A. is a health psychologist and an International Board Certified Lactation Consultant. Dr. Kendall-Tackett is a Clinical Associate Professor of Pediatrics at Texas Tech University School of Medicine in Amarillo, Texas. She is a Fellow of the American Psychological Association in both the Divisions of Health and Trauma Psychology and is President-Elect of the APA Division of Trauma Psychology. Dr. Kendall-Tackett has authored more than 320 journal articles and book chapters and is the author or editor of 22 books in the fields of trauma, women's health, depression, and breastfeeding, including *The hidden feelings of motherhood: Coping with stress, depression and burnout* (New Harbinger, 2001), and *Depression in new mothers, 2nd Edition* (Routledge, 2010).

Jayashri Kulkarni, M.D. is a Professor of Psychiatry at The Alfred and Monash University in Australia where she directs a large psychiatric research group, the Monash Alfred Psychiatry Research Center with approximately 150 staff and students. Before deciding to specialize in psychiatry, Dr. Kulkarni worked in Emergency Medicine. In 1989, she became a Fellow for the Royal Australian and New Zealand College of Psychiatrists. Dr. Kulkarni has pioneered the novel use of estrogen as a treatment for schizophrenia and is internationally acknowledged as a leader in the field of reproductive hormones and their impact on mental health.

Carmen Monzon, M.D. is a psychiatrist in Women's Behavioral Medicine at the Women's Medicine Collaborative in Providence, Rhode Island. A Clinical Assistant Professor of Psychiatry and Human Behavior at The Warren Alpert Medical School of Brown University in Providence, Dr. Monzon received a medical degree from National University Pedro Henriquez Urena in Santo Domingo, Dominican Republic, and completed a residency at Yale University School of Medicine in New Haven, Connecticut. Dr. Monzon is board certified in psychiatry and psychosomatic medicine. She is the 2013 recipient of the Dean's Excellence in Teaching Award at Alpert Medical School. Her clinical interests include perinatal psychiatry, oncology, and consultation-liaison psychiatry.

Melissa L. Nau, M.D. is a graduate of the Columbia College of Physicians and Surgeons and completed her residency in psychiatry at the University of California, San Francisco where she served as chief resident in 2009. She also completed a fellowship in Forensic Psychiatry at the University of California, San Francisco in 2011. Dr Nau is recognized as a national expert on violence and mental illness and is a frequent presenter on this topic. Her recent publications include Postpartum Psychosis and the Courts published in the *Journal of the American Academy of*

Psychiatry and the Law, a book chapter on Risk Assessment published in the *Encyclopedia of Neurological Sciences*, and an article on Substance-induced Psychosis published in the DSM V casebook. Dr. Nau has also worked in international mental health, helping to develop a mental health program in Sierra Leone in 2010.

Dorette Noorhasan, M.D. is Board Certified in both Obstetrics and Gynecology and Reproductive Endocrinology and Infertility. She is a physician at the Fertility Specialists of Texas. She earned her Doctorate in Medicine from Boston University School of Medicine. Dr. Noorhasan subsequently completed her Obstetrics and Gynecology residency at University of Texas—Houston, and her subspecialty training in Reproductive Endocrinology and Infertility at New Jersey Medical School—University of Medicine and Dentistry of New Jersey. While in medical school, Dr. Noorhasan participated in medical missions to Guatemala and Mexico and is conversant in Spanish. She has received numerous awards including the David Rothbaum, M.D. Award in Obstetrics and Gynecology, the Southern Medical Association Research Grant Award, and the George Schneider Second Prize presented by the American College of Obstetrics and Gynecology. Dr. Noorhasan has published several articles in *Human Reproduction*, *Fertility and Sterility*, and *Women's Health Issues*. She is a member of the American Society of Reproductive Medicine, and the Society for Reproductive Endocrinology and Infertility.

Alissa M. Peterson, M.D. is an Assistant Clinical Professor of Psychiatry at the University of California, San Francisco. A graduate of UCSF medical school and psychiatry residency training program, Dr. Peterson has worked in a variety of settings including primary care, psychiatric jail units, and in the legal system testifying in conservatorship hearings. In 2009, she returned to academic medicine as the attending physician for the women's focus inpatient psychiatry team at San Francisco General Hospital. She is currently one of the primary educators for UCSF medical students and residents on the topic of women's mental health.

Lucy J. Puryear, M.D. known nationally for her testimony in the Andrea Yates trial and re-trial is a psychiatrist in private practice and specializes in women's reproductive mental health. The Maureen Hackett Endowed Chair in Reproductive Psychiatry, Dr. Puryear is also Associate Professor of Psychiatry at Baylor College of Medicine in Houston, Texas. The author of *Understanding your emotions when you're expecting: Emotions, mental health and happiness—before, during and after pregnancy*, Dr. Puryear received her BS in Nursing from Baylor University and her MD from Baylor College of Medicine.

Lauren Schiff, M.D. received her medical degree from Mount Sinai Medical School in New York City and completed her Obstetrics and Gynecology residency at the Boston Medical Center of Boston University. She is a current fellow at Henry Ford Hospital in Detroit where she specializes in minimally invasive gynecologic surgery. Her research focuses on improvement in patient safety and quality of care in gynecologic surgery.

Author Biographies

Doreen L. Wiggins, M.D., F.A.C.O.G., F.A.C.S. received her medical degree from Brown University where she currently is an Assistant Clinical Professor. In 1999, she founded the Center for Obstetrics & Gynecology at the University. In 2003, she was chosen to be 1 of 26 cyclists in the Tour of Hope, a transcontinental bicycling relay with Lance Armstrong to promote cancer research and clinical trials. Dr. Wiggins has continued her relationship with the Lance Armstrong Foundation serving as a delegate to meet with members of Congress to support cancer research. She has published numerous books and journal articles in her areas of expertise that include breast cancer surgery, gynecologic surgery, female cancer genetics, female sexuality, and cancer survivorship.

Nurit Winkler, M.D. is Board Certified in Obstetrics and Gynecology as well as Reproductive Endocrinology and Infertility and is in practice at the Center for Fertility and Gynecology in Tarzana, California. She completed her residency in obstetrics and gynecology at Brown University School of Medicine and a fellowship in Reproductive Endocrinology from the University of Texas Southwestern Medical Center in Dallas. Dr. Winkler has authored numerous papers in the field of reproductive medicine and is the recipient of a number of awards, including *Excellence in teaching Medical Students* Award from both Brown University School of Medicine and the Sackler School of Medicine at Tel Aviv University in Israel. She is a member of the American College of Obstetrics and Gynecology and the American Society of Reproductive Medicine.

Stephanie Zerwas, Ph.D. is a nationally recognized researcher in the developmental psychopathology of eating disorders and disordered eating. Assistant Professor and Associate Research Director of the UNC Center of Excellence for Eating Disorders housed in the Department of Psychiatry, School of Medicine at the University of North Carolina at Chapel Hill, Dr. Zerwas has published numerous articles on prognostic factors for the course of eating disorders across the lifespan. In addition to clinical practice which focuses on the family-based treatment of eating disorders, she serves on the social media committee for the Academy for Eating Disorders. Dr. Zerwas' work on maternal eating disorders and infant temperament has been honored by the *International Journal of Eating Disorders* and she is the recipient of a ridging Interdisciplinary Research Careers in Women's Health Award given by the National Institute of Child Health and Human Development.

Editor's Biography

Diana Lynn Barnes, Psy.D., L.M.F.T. is an internationally recognized expert in women's reproductive mental health. A past president of Postpartum Support International, she currently sits on the President's Advisory Council for that organization. She is a member of the Los Angeles County Perinatal Mental Health Task Force, a core faculty member of their training institute, as well as a member of the statewide California Maternal Mental Health Collaborative. In 2009, she co-founded "The Motherhood Consortium," an interdisciplinary network of professionals working with mothers, infants, and young families.

In addition to private practice, Dr. Barnes is often called upon by defense counsel to consult and testify on criminal cases involving infanticide, pregnancy denial, neonaticide, child abuse, and neglect. Coauthor of *The Journey to Parenthood— Myths, Reality and What Really Matters*, Dr. Barnes is a fellow of the American Psychotherapy Association, and a clinical fellow of the California Association of Marriage and Family Therapists and the American Association of Marriage and Family Therapists. She is also a member of the Marcé Society and the North American Society of Psychosocial Obstetrics and Gynecology. In 2007, she received an award from Postpartum Support International for her work in maternal mental health and in 2009, she was the recipient of a Lifetime Achievement Award presented by the Eli Lilly Foundation for her outstanding contributions to the field of mood disorders and childbearing illness.

Part I
The Early Years

Pre- and Perinatal Influences on Female Mental Health

Marcy Axness and Joel Evans

Introduction

The human being is a story whose beginnings foretell countless later chapters. Just as the womb serves as the point of origin for the physical body—where it develops from a single fertilized ovum into a human in infant form—it is clear that the womb is also ground zero for myriad developmental trajectories related to both physiological and psychosocial health. Female mental and psychological well-being is shaped through a dynamic interplay of multiple factors beginning in utero.

The fetal origins of adult physiological health and disease are well established, as are the fetal origins of psychosocial well-being. A fetus's in utero experiences can foreshadow her gestational age, birth outcome, and her behavior as a neonate, infant, toddler, and beyond. It is therefore essential to consider pre- and perinatal experiences and exposures when exploring female mental health. Attachment, one of the most potent agents on lifelong mental health, is also theorized to begin in the womb.

We are in the midst of a historic sea change of expanding role and scope of obstetric care. No longer are the obstetrician's or midwife's[1] primary goals a vigorous baby (defined by a high Apgar score) and a mother free from prolonged pregnancy or birth complications. With a wide array of literature accumulating in the areas of "Developmental Origin of Adult Disease" (Barker, 2007) and "Environmental Influences on Fetal Development" (Swanson, Entringer, Buss, & Wadhwa, 2009),

---

[1] To avoid the cumbersome dual reference throughout, whenever we refer to "obstetrician" we include midwives as obstetrical care professionals.

M. Axness, Ph.D. (✉)
Los Angeles, CA, USA
e-mail: marcy@marcyaxness.com

J. Evans, M.D.
The Center for Women's Health, Stamford, CT, USA

Department of Obstetrics, Gynecology and Women's Health, Albert Einstein College of Medicine, Bronx, NY, USA obstetricians are becoming aware of the impact of the totality of the prenatal experience on myriad downstream physical, mental, and emotional effects.

A direct and comprehensive call for a wider understanding of the importance of the prenatal period comes from Michael Gravett and Craig Rubens, who state in a prominent obstetric journal, "Today, mothers and their children around the world pay an immense toll in terms of mortality and morbidity due to a lack of knowledge about pregnancy, childbirth, and early life" (Gravett, Rubens, & Global Alliance to Prevent Prematurity and Stillbirth Technical Team, 2012). A fetus's in utero experiences are inextricably tied to her pregnant mother's experiences; what the mother offers, the baby learns. Both Marcy Axness (Axness, 2012) and Bruce Lipton (Kamrath, 2013) have referred to pregnancy as Nature's Head Start program: the mother downloads lessons to her growing baby about the kind of world she needs to prepare for.

Our goal in this chapter is to help answer the call of Gravett and Rubens by:

(a) Surveying the pre- and perinatal influences on female mental morbidity.
(b) Offering avenues by which to optimize the pre- and perinatal experience in order to reduce female mental health morbidity in future generations.

Fetal Programming of Lifelong Health

The groundbreaking "fetal programming hypothesis" connecting in utero conditions to adult disease was first introduced over 20 years ago when British epidemiologist David Barker linked fetal weight at birth to adult death from ischemic heart disease (Barker, Osmond, Winter, Margetts, & Simmonds, 1989). His initial use of the term "fetal programming" referred to the process whereby a fetus, as early as the first trimester, responds to environmental signals—in these cases, caloric and nutrient availability—by making adaptations in its development. These adaptations affect cardiovascular, metabolic, or endocrine function and growth; can permanently change the structure and function of the body for its lifetime; and can determine later disease.

For example, if the mother is severely undernourished early in the pregnancy, or if, as in the case of teenage pregnancy, the mother is still growing herself, the fetus will "grow" a relatively larger placenta to compensate for the shortage—similar to hoarding for the winter famine (Nathanielsz, 1992). It appears that the result is smaller, less developed fetal organs, and a later-in-life vulnerability to myriad degenerative diseases related to those organs: cardiovascular disease due to a smaller, less efficient liver to process out cholesterol; diabetes, due to a less efficient pancreas and glucose metabolism; and hypertension, due to fetal circulatory adaptation and altered arterial function and perhaps also to kidneys inadequate to the task of regulating blood pressure. Indeed, large placental weight and a high ratio of placental to birth weight are known predictors of adult blood pressure (Barker, 1992).

The theory that Barker and his colleagues put forth regarding diabetes is a particularly good example of the fetal adaptation notion, and one that paves the way for a discussion of fetal programming of mental health. Barker maintains that a baby responds to undernutrition with slowed growth, an adaptive response enabling it to survive (Barker & Thornburg, 2013). Consumption of limited resources is allotted by hierarchal need, prioritizing the brain over skeletal, muscle, and organ growth. This includes impaired development and function of the β cells of the islet of Langerhans in the pancreas, predisposing the individual to later type II diabetes. They suggest that poor fetal and early postnatal nutrition "imposes mechanisms of nutritional thrift on the growing individual" (Hales & Barker, 1992), and further, as long as nutritional circumstances persist for the individual, problems do not arise, since the need for insulin is low. But if food becomes abundant—i.e., discordant with the maternal/fetal "instruction" about scarcity—impaired glucose tolerance or type II diabetes will result when the insulin demand exceeds the supply.

We can see a mental health fetal programming correlate in the case of, for example, maternal stress during pregnancy predisposing offspring to more hypersensitive, hyperreactive temperaments (Grizenko et al., 2012)—i.e., more suited to a threatening environment than to a safe one. Here again, after persistent in utero maternal-fetal "instruction" that the world is dangerous, not only is the fetus prepared to survive in adverse conditions, it is *not* prepared to survive—much less thrive—in optimal conditions! Barker himself has been quoted as saying, "When a fetus adapts to conditions in the womb, that adaptation tends to be permanent" (Begley, 1999).

Fetal development can be modified either as an adjustment in response to adversity, including hypoxemia and nutritional compromise, or as a result of fetal exposure to excess glucocorticoids, where these adaptations serve to prepare the fetus for the anticipated postnatal environment. In cases where the prediction and the actual environment mismatch, these developmental modifications become maladaptive, and the maladaptation is often exhibited in impaired mental health.

Fetal Programming of Mental Health

In addition to many physical disorders, there is a growing literature tracing mental health issues back to the prenatal experience (Schlotz & Phillips, 2009). We use the term "challenging fetal environment" (CFE) to refer to prenatal circumstances that comprise environmental, physical, and/or emotional influences that deviate from the norm, often calling for compensatory in utero fetal developmental adaptations.

A highly instructive example of a CFE occurred during the "Dutch hunger winter" during wartime famine (1944–1945). Fetuses were exposed to extreme caloric, micronutrient and macronutrient deprivation for 3–5 months. As is the case with so many environmental influences on human development, timing makes a difference. Studies of the offspring of the Dutch hunger winter revealed a 25–50 % increase in major affective disorder (Brown, van Os, Driessens, Hoek, & Susser, 2000) and 20 % impairment of cognitive function in middle age (de Rooij, Wouters, Yonker, Painter, & Roseboom, 2010). Alan Brown speculates that there is a continuum of psychiatric disorders, from affective disorder to schizophrenia, and that the clinical picture of an individual was related to the timing of the gestational exposure to the famine. In this paradigm, early gestational famine gives rise to schizophrenia, whereas later gestational famine gives rise to affective disorders (Brown et al., 2000).

The Impact of Stress

One of the most challenging tasks in advising pregnant women is having a discussion on maternal stress in a way that doesn't create additional stress. Every practitioner must find a way to do this because the negative effects of stress are so important and well described that failure to discuss stress levels and stress reduction techniques with pregnant women could almost be called a departure from good prenatal care.

Frances Rice conducted a review and found that gestational stress and poor fetal growth lead to elevated rates of emotional problems as a result of maternal prenatal stress, depression, and anxiety (Rice, Jones, & Thapar, 2007). Her conclusion, that there is increasing and replicated evidence of associations between gestational stress, low birth weight (corrected for gestational age), and emotional problems in adolescents and adults, is based on a thorough literature review and the biologic mechanisms discussed above.

There is strong evidence that prenatal stress exposure can negatively impact mental and motor development (Huizink, Robles de Medina, Mulder, Visser, & Buitelaar, 2003) and can increase the risk for later psychopathology (Glover, 2011; Wadhwa, Sandman, & Garite, 2001); the association between maternal prenatal stress and such psychosocial symptoms as attention deficit hyperactivity disorder, conduct disorder, aggression, or anxiety in offspring is well established (Glover, 2011). Some investigators assert that only pregnancy-specific stress (e.g., fears about or negative appraisals of pregnancy) is associated with these negative outcomes, and that nonspecific anxiety, stress, and depression have actually been associated with motor development gains (DiPietro, 2010). This issue is a breathtakingly complex causal/correlational tapestry; for instance, maternal prenatal stress predicts premature birth (Sandman, Davis, & Glynn, 2012; Wadhwa et al., 2001) and therefore low birth weight, which itself is associated with offspring mental health challenges (Bohnert & Breslau, 2008; Fullmer, 2006). Despite the growing literature, the mechanisms at work here remain poorly understood. Of particular relevance to this volume—in accordance with several examples in the animal and human literature suggesting that many prenatal insults produce sexually dimorphic developmental sequelae—is the finding of higher anxiety levels in prenatally stressed females as compared to males (Bowman et al., 2004).

Recent findings include the impact of stress on the developing amygdala, a brain structure associated with fear processing, stress reactivity, and affect regulation. The association between high maternal cortisol concentrations and higher prevalence of child affective problems is partially mediated by greater amygdala volume in the offspring of mothers chronically stressed in pregnancy (Buss, Entringer, & Wadhwa, 2012). Breaking research as this volume goes to press reveals a significant association between prenatal maternal depression and changes in the neonatal microstructure of the right amygdala, findings the authors suggest "establish evidence for the transgenerational transmission of vulnerability for affective disorders during prenatal development" (Rifkin-Graboi et al., 2013).

Another significant mechanism at work in the connection between maternal stress in pregnancy and mental health issues in offspring is the effect of stress on the fetal hypothalamic–pituitary–adrenal (HPA) axis.

Stress and the HPA Axis

When a stressful situation is perceived, whether real or imagined, cortisol is called for: the hypothalamus secretes corticotropin-releasing hormone (CRH), which stimulates the pituitary gland to secrete adenocorticotropin-releasing hormone (ACTH), which stimulates the adrenal glands to release cortisol. Negative feedback occurs as the cortisol in the blood is sensed by the pituitary and hypothalamus, which decrease the secretion of CRH and ACTH. This is the normal functioning of the HPA axis; in this case, negative feedback is a good thing.

It is critical to understand that this feedback loop is reversed in the fetus; cortisol produced by the mother stimulates the placenta to produce CRH, leading to both the production of cortisol by the fetal adrenals and the stimulation of the maternal pituitary to secrete more ACTH. The maternal ACTH in turn further stimulates the maternal adrenal to make more cortisol, and so on and so on; a positive feedback loop leads to increased cortisol in both the mother and fetus (Wadhwa, 2005).

Prenatal maternal mood, specifically anxiety and depression, impacts the HPA axis of adolescent children by inducing a reduced cortisol awakening response and a flatter diurnal slope. These changes in the HPA axis, considered to be a blunted response to stress, are seen to be potential markers for psychopathology (O'Donnell, 2013). When a fetus is continually exposed to maternal cortisol, its distress is expressed with an accelerated fetal heartbeat and hyperactivity (Sandman et al., 2003), while its developing HPA set points (i.e., capacity to effectively manage stress) are being permanently downregulated (Davis et al., 2007). The feedback system designed to keep its experience of stress within normal levels is damped, leading to lifelong hypersensitivity to what would normally be benign stimuli (Barbazanges, Piazza, Le Moal, & Maccari, 1996; Green et al., 2011). Along with this hypersensitivity to minor environmental stimuli that is hardwired into the baby's brain by prenatal stress, there is also impairment of the baby's opioid system (Huizink, Mulder, & Buitelaar, 2004; Insel, Kinsley, Mann, & Bridges, 1990; Sandman & Yessaian, 1986); in other words, the brain-based ability to experience pleasure and contentment, or what Peter Kramer calls "hedonic capacity," is corrupted.

So, as O'Donnell's study illuminated, not only will this daughter's hypersensitive HPA axis render her more prone to experiencing the environment as stressful, she will get little relief from the action of her brain's pleasure axis, which would normally help mediate the effects of stress by engendering feelings of satisfaction, reward, and contentment. She loses mental well-being from both ends, so to speak—feeling hammered by distressing stimuli while never quite able to feel much at ease or gratified. No wonder the downregulation of these fundamental neurochemical receptors has been implicated in depression and other mood disorders (Vollmayr & Henn, 2003).

Nature in her wisdom has decreed that while a daughter is in the womb, her brain develops in direct response to her mother's experience of the world. If a pregnant mother's thoughts and emotions are *persistently* negative, if she is under *unrelenting* stress, the internal message delivered to her developing baby is, "It's a dangerous world out there," regardless of whether this is objectively true. In an evolutionary bid for survival, her baby's neural cells and nervous system development will adapt to prepare for the unsafe environment it perceives being born into (Glover, 2011).

Toxins, Nutrients, and Epigenetics

The mechanisms for the effects of maternal stress in pregnancy on mental health seem to extend beyond the impact of cortisol, CRH, and downregulation of the fetal HPA axis. Recent literature (Zucchi et al., 2013) describes epigenetic changes (altered gene expression) caused by maternal stress in 336 different micro RNAs (miRNA) in rat pups of stressed mothers. This is significant because when miRNA expression is altered, different proteins (such as those involved in neuronal function) are produced. It is well known that miRNA expression is altered in many psychiatric and neurological disorders, such as bipolar disorder, schizophrenia, autism, and depression (Moreau, Bruse, David-Rus, Buyske, & Brzustowicz, 2011). Prenatal stress, particularly during the middle of pregnancy, is known to be associated with adult schizophrenia, depression, and drug abuse (Weinstock, 2005).

In addition to maternal emotional factors, such as stress, anxiety, and depression, and extreme nutritional factors, such as famine or severe malnutrition, impacting mental health in offspring, other nutritional factors play an important role. Maternal obesity leads to a chronic inflammatory state; as such, before and during pregnancy it has been associated with deficits in neurodevelopmental outcomes during both childhood and adulthood, including ADHD in childhood, eating disorders in adolescence, and psychotic disorders in adulthood (Lieshout, Taylor, & Boyle, 2011).

Prenatal maternal depression itself is associated with poorer nutrition and in turn lower child cognitive function (Barker, Kirkham, Ng, & Jensen, 2013). A pregnant mother's intake of choline—one of the B vitamins—has recently been shown to influence her child's stress levels; choline supplementation in pregnancy changes epigenetic expression of genes involved in cortisol production and moderates infants' stress response (Jiang et al., 2012). There is now evidence linking folic acid, as well as vitamin D, and iron deficiency, to schizophrenia (McGrath, Brown, & Clair, 2011). Also, genetic differences in COMT, one of the enzymes that utilize downstream nutrients from folic acid, have been shown to impact how women interpret faces of strangers. Changes in COMT were correlated with both a stronger bias to perceive neutral faces as expressing anger and a reduced bias to perceive neutral faces as expressing happiness, demonstrating that folic acid metabolism has the potential to impact susceptibility to emotional disorders (Gohier et al., 2013).

Prenatal exposure to toxins, including drugs, is another important, yet relatively unacknowledged, under-researched influence on offspring mental health morbidity. In utero exposure to cigarette smoke, including secondhand smoke, is associated with violent behavior (Gibson & Tibbetts, 2000).

Temperament: Bellwether of Mental Health

One aspect of fetal learning related to future mental health involves the maternal heartbeat; brainstem and cerebellum development organizes around the drumbeat of the mother's heart (Sandman, Davis, Cordova, Kemp, & Glynn, 2011). If she is generally centered and peaceful, feeling connected, loved, and happy to be pregnant, her heart will drum a rhythmic, metronomic beat. Renowned child psychiatrist Bruce Perry tells us that this is why people across all cultures instinctively tend to rock a baby at roughly 80 beats per minute—the resting heart rate of a pregnant woman! The baby responds to this familiar rhythm with a sense of, "Ah, I know that," and settles down (Perry, 2003).

If a pregnant mother is chronically stressed or anxious, her heartbeat will be dysrhythmic and irregular, and her baby's primitive brain structures imprint this heart rate variability as their baseline state. Thus, there is no familiar, at-home rhythm with which to rock the baby, and the infant is far more likely to be born with what Perry calls a state-regulation problem: it is irritable, difficult to soothe, and hard to engage. In turn, parents can get frustrated and overwhelmed, and as Perry states, "Instead of having this smooth, synchronous interaction, you have kind of this bad fit. It leads to problems with normal social, emotional development" (Santa Barbara Graduate Institute, 2004). Frequently experienced stimuli become familiar, and familiar, even if it's negative, becomes comforting, so we gravitate to it. This is a reality that keeps many a therapist in business; familiarity comforts us, and we may unconsciously tend to gravitate toward what's familiar even if it is not healthy and constructive. Robust mental health is present when what is familiar and what is healthy are not at opposite poles; healing comprises bringing consciousness and purposefulness to our choices. We all know people who feel at home with chaos, and a pregnant mother's dysrhythmic heartbeat is how early that affinity can begin.

The Seeds of Attachment Disruption

The newborn's brain that has been exposed to a mother's chronic stress in pregnancy—and thus adapted to survive in a dangerous environment—tends to be short of attention and quick to react; has reduced impulse control and a damped capacity to feel calm and content. This temperamental baby can be challenging to parent, and thus the seeds can be sown this early for parents and child to get stuck in a sad but common vicious cycle of disrupted attachment; dealing with the baby is frustrating for Mom and Dad. This generates a spectrum of strong feelings within, which further activates the baby's heightened antennae for threat, makes it even more agitated, which may distance the exhausted, exasperated parents from their baby. With no positive interruption of this negative feedback loop, secure postnatal attachment is endangered. The child has diminished opportunity to internalize the self-regulating capacities developed through the intimate, engaged, face-to-face, and skin-to-skin attachment interactions that foster healthy development of the social brain (Schore & Schore, 2008). Once the toddler is considered "a handful," there are likely to be consequences—punishments whose shame basis further thwarts peace-oriented brain development, hardwiring it instead to thrive in a threatening world (McGregor, Edgerton, & Courtney, 2012). Later, the child's impulsivity gets labeled, and the sense of alienation—from herself, from others, from life—grows. It is in the womb that this insidiously downward-spiraling cycle so often begins.

Perinatal Influences on Mental Health

Labor and Birth

Childbirth is a decisive developmental window for the wiring of neural circuitry; critical systems in the brain and body of both mother and baby organize in ways that will have lifelong effects. Of fundamental importance, as we consider psychosocial function and mental health, is the oxytocin system. Biochemical cascades triggered during an unimpeded mammalian labor and birth, as well as during the postpartum, establish in the baby enduring set points for the brain's self-regulating and social functions (Foureur, 2008). These thresholds appear exquisitely sensitive to downregulation when hormonal cascades designed by nature are supplanted by modern hospital birth protocols and technologies (Morgan, Horn, & Bergman, 2011), and these thresholds will to a great extent forecast how able this child will be to respond to later influences aimed at fostering mental and emotional well-being (MacDonald & MacDonald, 2010).

An investigation by Scandinavian researcher Bertil Jacobson revealed a strong association between the type of distressing birth circumstance someone experienced and the method that person later used in suicide or suicide attempts (Jacobson & Bygdeman, 2000). For instance, asphyxia, such as having the cord tightly around the neck, correlated with hanging, strangulation, drowning, and gas poisoning; mechanical trauma, such as the use of forceps, was associated with suicide attempts using guns or jumping from heights; drug addiction or overdose was associated with opiate and/or barbiturate medication given to the mother during labor.

Physician and primal health researcher Michel Odent has adopted a revealing lens by zeroing in on a central feature of myriad social-emotional impairments, casting it rather lyrically as "an impaired capacity to love." When Odent used this novel perspective from which to survey a wide range of supposedly disparate research on autism, anorexia nervosa, depression, juvenile criminality, suicide, and more, he found something striking: "When researchers explored the backgrounds of people who have expressed some sort of impaired capacity to love, either love of oneself or love of others, they always detected risk factors in the period surrounding birth" (Odent, 2002). It is of particular interest to our discussion of female mental health to note the compelling parallels Odent identifies between autism and anorexia nervosa, such as right hemisphere deficit in brain function and perceptual/behavioral patterns. Odent cites findings of teams of psychiatrists from Kings College in London and Goteborg University in Sweden, which emphasize the importance of autistic traits in anorexia nervosa, supporting his proposal that "anorexia nervosa might be considered a female variant of the autistic spectrum" (Odent, 2013, p. 119). Here again, all roads lead to oxytocin. Oxytocin levels in anorexic women are far lower than in their control or bulimic counterparts, with the timing of risk factors occurring in the window around birth (Favaro, Tenconi, & Santonastaso, 2006; Odent, 2013).

Odent also directs our attention to research demonstrating a precipitous decline in empathy among college students: a 40 % drop in empathy between 1979 and 2009. Many researchers see the foundations for empathy emerging prenatally (Trevarthen & Aitken, 1994), and Odent proposes that birth circumstances have serious implications for the formation of empathy, due in large part to the oxytocin-wiring window (Odent, 2013).

Given the gender gap of depression, and the fact that twice as many women as men suffer from major clinical depression—one in five women experience at least one episode in her lifetime (Mayo Clinic Staff, 2013)—it is relevant to include Odent's observation that the rate of college students reporting they've been diagnosed with depression has risen from 10 to 21 % in just 11 years! Acknowledging the complex causal tapestry involved in depression, he urges us to consider that in that same decade, 2000–2011, "it was a time when the number of women who were able to give birth to their baby and the placenta, thanks only to the release of their natural hormones, dramatically decreased" (Odent, 2012). He reminds us that depression is related to how the aforementioned stress-axis "set points" are established in the pre- and perinatal period, pointing out the myriad brain areas showing altered activity in depressed subjects that have an important phase of development and "set point" adjustment during the period surrounding birth (Odent, 2012).

Postpartum

Indeed, immediately after birth a complex hormonal cocktail orchestrates biochemical exchanges between a mother and her newborn, offering never-to-be-repeated opportunities to set the stage for optimally healthy psychosocial development. Oxytocin levels peak, potentiating important brain circuitry for the baby's social and emotional centers, and fostering the mother's urge toward maternal behavior. Oxytocin elicits a relaxation and growth response, which in turn reduces HPA axis activity and establishes enduring set points (Feng et al., 2011). Beta-endorphins also flow in abundance in the first hours following birth. Essentially, the newborn's brain is biologically primed to imprint, "connecting with Mom feels good" (Perry, 2003).

Research from the Karolinska Institute confirms a highly sensitive period during the first 1–2 h after birth that lays a long-term foundation for robust mental health in both baby and mother. In studying the long-term effects of hospital delivery and maternity practices on mother–infant attachment and interaction, investigators found that close contact, such as skin-to-skin contact and suckling, during the first 2 h after birth led to increased levels of maternal sensitivity, infant self-regulation, and "dyadic mutuality and reciprocity" 1 year after birth, when compared with pairs who were separated at birth. A most striking aspect of their findings was that the negative effect of a 2-h separation after birth was not compensated for by the practice of rooming-in (Bystrova et al., 2009). There is something unique and irreplaceable about those first hours of uninterrupted connection following birth for fostering healthy attachment.

Yet American hospital protocols typically disturb this momentous process through routine separation of mothers from their newborns, who end up in plastic isolettes, raising the clear and present question, Are our obstetrical care conventions impairing the development of our newest citizens' capacity for healthy human rapport and social-emotional well-being? (Axness, 2012).

Attachment and the Foundations of Mental Health

In the past 15 years researchers have been discovering the intricate details behind the pervasive, lifelong implications of the attachment relationship that John Bowlby began studying in the 1950s (Bowlby, 1980; Hrdy, 1999). While its evolutionary origins are in basic physical survival drive, until fairly recently attachment has been viewed primarily as a psychosocial construct: a measure of the intensity and features of proximity-seeking behavior exhibited by the child in relation to its primary caregiver. This primary caregiver will herein usually be referred to as "mother," or sometimes "attachment figure," for ease of language; it is acknowledged that it can certainly be a father, or any other consistently present and responsive adult.

The Reciprocal Genesis of Mental Health

In the last century, attachment styles were seen as relatively static, based on the child's responses to the mother. Post-Bowlby decades brought further research into the range of infant adaptive attachment styles relative to maternal behavior, and have elucidated the "two-way street" aspects of attachment (Green & Piel, 2002):

it is a dynamic, mutually regulating process marked by reciprocal feedback mechanisms—an "open-loop model" of attachment physiology, in which the process of close, connected communications within the attachment relationship is used by social mammals to "tune" each other's physiologic homeostasis through what Lewis' group calls "limbic regulation" (Amini, Lewis, Lannon, & Louie, 1996).

At the dawn of the twenty-first century, a new wave of research reveals attachment as not simply a context for healthy psychosocial growth, but also as a basic mode of psycho-neurological development (e.g., Perry, 2003; Schore & Schore, 2008; Siegel, 2002a). When infants and parents engage in the kind of mutually attuned, face-to-face, gaze-to-gaze, I-laugh-then-you-laugh encounters that optimally come naturally and instinctively, the infant "piggybacks" on her mother's regulating limbic structures to regulate her affect (internal states and external behavioral responses). Her developmental task over the early months and years is to internalize the capacity to regulate her own inner states.

Further, it is now believed that as the immature affect regulatory system of the infant's brain falls in step with that of the adult, over time it wires itself in emulatory fashion. Over the course of the thousands of mother–child "tuning encounters" that occur in the early months and years of a child's life, the circuitry of the child's orbitofrontal cortex, which is fundamental to her social and emotional functioning (i.e., her mental health), is being laid down according to the model provided by the attachment figure. This is a potent contributor to the intergenerational aspect of mental health: the environmental variable of parents' psychosocial neurobiology and attachment behavior is as significant as, and perhaps more impactful than, genetic inheritance (Siegel, 2004; Strathearn, Fonagy, Amico, & Montague, 2009).

An infant with an emotionally available, attuned, self-possessed caregiver develops different neural templates, or patterns of relating (Bowlby's term was *internal working models*), than an infant whose caregiver is emotionally absent, volatile, insecure, anxious, depressed, etc. The latter is accruing neural patterns of relating that feature shame, distrust, loss, and the experience that human connection is not pleasurable, all of which fundamentally erode mental and emotional well-being (e.g., Perry, 1995a, 1995b).

When speaking of optimal mental health, we mustn't focus solely on the importance of soothing a baby's negative affect—being upset, crying, and in distress. Along with helping her manage her negative states, it is just as important for a baby daughter's optimal mental health that parents also attune to, delight in, mirror, and amplify her positive affective states, such as excitement, laughter, and above all, simple contentment.

We now know that secure attachment isn't simply the optimal context for, or even mode of healthy development, it is the content of development! Just as the infant uses the nourishment of her mother's milk to build her tissue and bones, she uses the attachment relationship to build areas of her brain that are critical to her future social-emotional functioning, particularly the orbitofrontal cortex (Siegel, 2002b), and her lifelong patterns of relating. Attachment, then, is a basic kind of developmental nourishment, as critically important for her growing brain as calories, perhaps even more so (Perry, 2003). Its impairment—through maternal depression or narcissism, neglect, abuse, or other forms of relational trauma (Schore, 2002) and chronic misattunement—has been termed by one of this chapter's authors as *malattachment* (Axness, 2004).

Two Fundamental Aspects of Mental Health

At the root of most forms of disordered mental health we find impairments in one or both of two key aspects of healthy psychosocial development: self-differentiation and self-regulation.

Self-regulation—the capacity to moderate attention (shift and focus attention), emotion (downregulate negative emotions such as fear and anger, or optimize positive emotion, such as interest or delight), and behavior (e.g., engage in behaviors that support one's continued well-being and inhibit negative, reactive, or destructive impulses)—develops early in life and is a strong predictor of psychosocial health in adulthood (Skowron & Dendy, 2004). The profound, extensive impact of the capacity for self-regulation upon the very essence and core of an individual's personality is asserted in the title of one of the seminal texts by field pioneer Allan Schore: *Affect Regulation and the Origin of the Self* (Schore, 1999). Absence of or diminished self-regulation marks such mental health conditions as ADD/ADHD, ODD, OCD, bipolar, dysthymic, and major depressive disorders (e.g., Heatherton & Wagner, 2011).

Self-differentiation—the capacity to maintain a clear sense of self, balancing autonomy and connection—also develops early in life and is associated with healthier psychosocial and emotional functioning across a variety of dimensions (Skowron, Wester, & Azen, 2004). Family systems theory asserts that healthy self-differentiation is predicated on the internalization of attachment relationships marked by a balance of both autonomy and connection. Mental health conditions such as anorexia nervosa, borderline and dissociative disorders feature a lack of such balance (Christenson & Wilson, 1985; Middleton, 2005; Weaver, Wuest, & Ciliska, 2005): awareness of "where I end and others begin" is low, with patients veering into either emotional isolation/cut-off or merging/fusion, and in some cases ricocheting painfully between those exaggerated poles.

The roots of self-differentiation and self-regulation are both found deep in the soil of healthy attachment. The capacity to self-regulate emerges over time for a child whose need for external regulation from her attachment figures is consistently met early on; and a healthy, differentiated self who can effortlessly balance autonomy and intimacy emerges over time in a child who is allowed to be *un*differentiated in the earliest weeks and months, and whose budding differentiation is supported by the mother. So in the paradoxical manner that marks so much of human development, it is in the complete, undefended willingness to let her child be utterly merged and dependent upon her when that is developmentally appropriate, and to find pleasure, rather than abandonment or disappointment, in her daughter's budding autonomy while steadfastly remaining her welcoming safe haven for reconnection and refueling (Cooper, Hoffman, & Powell, 2010) that a mother seeds her child's healthiest unfolding differentiation and regulation.

The Malattachment of Postpartum Separation

An extensive literature shows that the early loss of, or separation from, one's biological mother is associated with impaired physical and neuropsychological wellbeing (Feng et al., 2011; Gunnar & Donzella, 2002; Jimenez-Vasquez, Mathe, Thomas, Riley, & Ehlers, 2001; Morgan et al., 2011). Taking a primate away from her mother too soon or subjecting her to lengthy maternal absences will produce an adult with lifelong heightened vulnerability to psychosocial stressors (Kalinichev, Easterling, Plotsky, & Holtzman, 2002; Lewis, Amini, & Lannon, 2000; Tsuda & Ogawa, 2012).

In many studies of prenatal learning and newborn cognitive capacity, newborns have demonstrated their recognition of, and preference for, their mothers over anyone else (DeCasper & Fifer, 1980). Myron Hofer's team has spent decades studying what happens when that preference is not respected; in researching the biology of loss, Hofer has relentlessly pursued the question, "In maternal separation, what exactly is lost?" His work with orphaned rat pups has led to specific, nuanced findings about the effects of separation on infant physiology. His team found that the bond between mother and infant is woven from many physiological strands, each a distinct regulatory pathway in the body: "The elements of the lost interaction…that we had sought…turned out to be *regulators* of the infant's developing neural systems" (Hofer, 1996, pp. 573, italics his).

Simply through her presence, a mother continuously adjusts her infant's physiology in countless healthy ways, including mitigating nervous system arousal (Morgan et al., 2011). As psychiatrist Thomas Lewis and colleagues put it—referring to all mammals, including humans—"When the mother is absent, an infant loses all his organizing channels at once. Like a marionette with its strings cut, his physiology collapses into the huddled heap of despair. Once separated from their attachment figures, mammals spiral down into a somatic disarray that can be measured from the outside and painfully felt on the inside" (Lewis et al., 2000, p. 83).

Clearly, early maternal–infant separation qualifies as trauma, in that it overwhelms the nervous system, leaves the baby unable to regain homeostasis, and leaves the individual unable to regain internal balance, in other words, unable to perform one of the most basic functions of sound mental health, to self-regulate (Levine, 2002; van der Kolk, McFarlane, & Weisaeth, 1996). Moreover, such early loss leaves the individual forever more highly vulnerable to other losses, both real and perceived (Lewis et al., 2000; Solomon, 1989). As recognized in the process of "state-bound learning" and traumatic event memories, the brain and psyche become wired to recognize the shape of that early loss, and any experience that closely enough resembles the same buffeting blow will fire up the same emotional responses. Lynda Share suggests that trauma forms "meaning networks"; trauma becomes an "organizer of experience," whereby "all later developmental events, conflicts, and experiences are drawn into it" (Share, 1994, p. 60). Share poignantly characterizes unconscious memories of loss and trauma as "mentally *unrememberable*, while concurrently somatically and behaviorally *unforgettable*" (Share, 1994, p. 11, italics hers).

Premature Self-Differentiation

The mental health foundation of self-differentiation is steeply compromised by separation. Adoption therapist Nancy Verrier sees that a newborn's separation from its mother forces premature ego development:

> If for some reason the mother cannot be counted on to be the "whole environment" for the infant, he begins to take over that function from her. Rather than a gradual, well-timed developmental process, the child is forced by this wrenching experience of premature separation to be a separate being, to form a separate ego before he should have to do so. …The danger is that we may too readily accept this premature ego development as proof that the child is adjusting well to his environment (Verrier, 1993, pp. 30–31).

Rather than healthy self-differentiation, this abrupt, forced individuation can engender a "pseudoautonomy" thought to be part of the spectrum of narcissistic personality features (Miller, 1981; Watson, Hickman, Morris, & Milliron, 1999). A woman with this history will often be repulsed by and deflect what she needs most and never received at the developmentally appropriate time: someone to really see her, to really connect with her, and to truly love her. Such deflection strategies comprise aspects of suboptimal mental health: defenses to buffer her from the relational losses suffered through trauma. Trauma expert and Harvard professor of psychiatry Judith Herman points out these kinds of traumatic relational losses include a "loss of basic trust. A loss of feeling of mutuality of relatedness. In its stead is emplaced a contempt for self and others" (cited in Jensen, 2000, p. 353). Not the best foundation for mental and emotional well-being.

Prenatal–Postnatal Attachment Continuum

We earlier established that attachment comprises a reciprocal, mutual regulation process as well as a series of lessons internalized by the child/infant as neural patterns of relating. Theories of prenatal attachment (Brandon, Pitts, Denton, Stringer, & Evans, 2009; Doan & Zimmerman, 2004) emphasize the reciprocal aspect through which, for example, a fetus' behavior or developmental status can impact a mother's emotional state and reciprocally, a mother's chronic prenatal stress can wreak such havoc with her daughter's budding lifelong self-regulation capacities.

And decades of clinical research have elucidated many facets of a series of relational lessons a fetus encounters in the womb, which contribute to the prenatal attachment process. There is significant literature detailing impressive fetal responsiveness in the womb to maternal stress (DiPietro, Costigan, & Gurewitsch, 2003) and voice (Hepper, Scott, & Shahldullah, 1993); fetal learning that informs and persists into infancy (Hepper, 2005; James, Spencer, & Stepsis, 2002; Partanen et al., 2013), and the continuity of fetal-to-infant behavioral and temperamental states (DiPietro, Hodgson, Costigan, & Johnston, 1996; Werner et al., 2007). Another stream of literature supporting the existence and persistence of fetal awareness and learning comprises highly detailed in utero and birth memories of older children or adults undergoing regressive experiences, usually within a therapeutic context using hypnosis or directed breathing (Chamberlain, 1999; Ham & Klimo, 2000; Lyman, 2005; Renggli, 2003).

A large clinical literature illustrates the relevance of prenatal awareness, faculties, and memory to the discussion of the foundations of mental health. One study of four suicidal young women found that their suicide attempts were taking place at the same time of the year as their mothers tried to abort them. None of these adolescents had consciously known of their mothers' attempted abortions (Feldmar, cited in Sonne, 2000), which were verified by the mothers when later interviewed. In a case reported by prenatal psychologist David Chamberlain, Shirley came into therapy "desperate and depressed" (Chamberlain, 2012, p. 139). Her third marriage was collapsing, and though intelligent and attractive, Shirley's life was littered with losses and broken relationships. During a hypnotherapy session she slipped into a prenatal memory: "Somebody's missing! It's lonely. Something's pushing against my back. It's dead." Shirley thus joined a growing population of people who have retrieved memories of having lost a twin in utero (Chamberlain, 1998; Hayton, 2008). The heightened developmental and psychological risks that attend so-called vanishing twin syndrome are acutely relevant in today's reproductive technology era, since one in ten IVF-conceived singleton babies originates as a twin (Pinborg, Lidegaard, la Cour Freiesleben, & Andersen, 2005). Shirley's therapy brought to light her lifelong guilt for the loss of her twin, and unconscious neurobehavioral patterns in which she sought ways to punish herself, denying herself healthy relationships, a successful career, and virtually any feelings of satisfaction and joy.

Our learning systems—conscious and preconscious, verbal and preverbal, explicit and implicit—retain an unfortunate feature from our more dangerous evolutionary past: a bad news bias (Amini et al., 1996; Blum, 2002; Burgess, Hartman, & Clements, 1995; Herman, 1997; Levine, 2002). Happy, contented circumstances pass across the neural plains like the faintest breeze, making virtually no impression; they are the default, the way things should be, business as usual. Rather, it is in response to the dangerous, shocking, or frightening experiences or impressions that neurochemicals flood the memory-making system, etching the neural grooves that trace temperament, behavior, and the basis of personality.

Prenatal Malattachment and Self-Differentiation

One kind of prenatal memory involves the malattachment of premature ego development, which is deleterious to burgeoning mental health. While we're being knit together in the womb, our negative experiences indelibly mark us in ways that become acutely felt when the "interchange of satisfactory maternal-fetal emotion, so reliably good as to be scarcely noticed, is interrupted by the influx of maternal distress" (Lake, cited in House, 2000, p. 225); when successive hormonal jolts destroy the "blankness that is the normal state of the womb" (Verny, cited in Wade, 1999, p. 129). Fetal consciousness researcher Jenny Wade notes the general consensus among pre- and perinatal psychology researchers that a chronically stressful situation, or repetition of negative events, gradually reaches "a critical level where it constitutes a rudimentary sense of self, distinct from the mother" (Verny, cited in Wade, 1999, p. 130).

In the face of negative circumstances, particularly those experienced or perceived by the mother, fetal defenses begin to develop, and a premature sense of self, similar to—if more primitive than—that described by Frances Tustin relative to infant trauma, which "create a premature 'not-me' awareness (via severe physical pain, separations from the mother, …sexual abuse, etc.) and prevent the 'illusion of oneness' with the mother, so necessary for the baby's sense of safety, security, and peace of mind. What occurs instead is a premature awareness of a separate bodily self" (Tustin, cited in Share, 1994, p. 240). Ironically, this can result in a fundamental disconnection from her body, which is associated with self-objectification (Daubenmier, 2005). Self-objectification entails the habitual self-surveillance of an observer's perspective rather than a participant's perspective a woman holds toward her own body (Fredrickson & Roberts, 1997), and is associated with a range of female mental health consequences, including depression, disordered eating (Miner-Rubino, Twenge, & Fredrickson, 2002), and self-injury (Croyle & Waltz, 2007).

Of particular relevance to this volume, self-objectification is associated with diminished reproductive mental health (Johnston-Robledo, Sheffield, Voigt, & Wilcox-Constantine, 2007). Many researchers, most notably Daniel Stern, have elucidated the fact that an infant's early emotional experiences, or affects, are sensations experienced through the body (Stern, 1998). Thus an integral aspect of a daughter's primal bargain for survival, when faced with in utero relational trauma, is alienation from her body from the very beginning (Bernhardt, 1992; Levine, 2005; Rosenberg, Rand, & Asay, 1985).

The work of Emerson and other pre- and perinatal psychotherapists (e.g., Grof, 1976; House, 2000; Maret, 1997; Verny, 2002) suggests an existential paradox is posed to the embryo by first trimester traumas such as mistaken conception, tentative implantation journey, difficult or maternally rejecting implantation, and maternally negative or ambivalent pre-discovery and discovery periods. Emerson points out that while the ego begins functioning in the third trimester, and primitive ego defense mechanisms such as splitting and dissociation become functional in the first year, an embryo and fetus during the first two trimesters is totally and completely without any defense against trauma, and has no option but to in essence turn away from herself at the deepest level of self (Emerson, W., personal communication, 1993). Here Reiner's words—coined about infant trauma—ring achingly true that in this process a strange irony occurs: a "psychological death" at the very first moments of physical life (cited in Share, 1994, p. 52).

Thus, some hold that narcissism has its beginnings in utero (Kestenberg & Browitz, 1990); indeed, through his years of pioneering work in primal therapy, Frank Lake determined that the delicate first trimester developmental processes had the most powerful, lasting effects on a person, and that they are "the time and place of origin of the common personality disorders, as well as psychosomatic reactions" (House, 2000, p. 232). In his remarkable clinical portrait "The Pre- and Perinatal Development of a Sense of Self," Jeffrey Von Glahn shares the pre- and perinatal recollections/reconstructions of a woman who experienced this kind of existential dilemma as "a continual assault on her developing sense of a *self*, and which eventually resulted in a dissociation that caused her to not experience herself as a needing, wanting person; or in her words, as not having a *me*" (Von Glahn, 1998, p. 155).

Indeed, in an imprint of fundamental *wrongness* that is common among those who experience first trimester trauma, "Jessica" was "terrified that she had been ...*made up*, with a *flaw* in the basic structure of her humanness," the result of which was:

> You see, I had to give me up. ...This part of me that cared about anything, that loved and needed and wanted, the real human being in me, I had to send "her" away. ...I had to scrape my "human being" out of me and let "her" float off. ...I sent "her" away because "she's" bad and no good (Von Glahn, 1998, p. 164).

Conclusion

We have already covered the severe lifelong derangement of a daughter's self-regulation capacities—her downregulated HPA-axis, her irritable temperament—that can be wrought by her mother's persistent stress during pregnancy. When looked at through the lens of a continuum of attachment beginning in utero, pregnancy is also a series of lessons in which we can appreciate the guiding relevance of neuropsychiatrist Allan Schore's definition of stress as "an asynchrony in an interactional sequence" (Schore, 2001).

So how to bring more synchrony to the infinite series and layers of behavioral, biochemical, and energetic interactional sequences that make up pregnancy, so prenatal attachment doesn't veer toward prenatal malattachment? How to best counsel pregnant women through the stress that is the reality of today's world, in a way that optimizes protective factors? Perhaps my coauthor has forgotten his contribution to my book *Parenting for Peace*, in which he offered this prescription:

> If I was forced to reduce all of the important information I want to share with women as they think about pregnancy and motherhood to one recommendation, it would be to never lose sight of the power of intentionality. Through intention you can give your child the gift of feeling loved, desired, and connected; a gift that easily overcomes whatever challenging circumstances arise that you feel prevent you from being the "perfect" mother (Axness, 2012, pp. 108–109).

If a mother is experiencing a stressful day, month, or entire pregnancy because of outer circumstances, she can take a few deep, cleansing breaths, mindfully connect with her daughter in the womb and reassure her, "This upset is not about you; you are safe; you are loved; you are exactly as you need to be, and you are welcomed into my life." And, as the gifted Laura Huxley, late widow of visionary author Aldous Huxley, suggests:

> If you can take even five minutes a day, to think good thoughts, listen to your favorite music, or nourish yourself in any way you want, your kindness will be multiplied a thousand-fold and become an organic part of a person's being for years to come. Five minutes of care is worth years of wellbeing (Huxley & Ferruci, 1992, p. 49).

By weaving our daughters from the strands (and biochemistry) of our joy, our inspiration, our vision, we will be "practicing evolution," in the manner so compellingly described by cell biologist Bruce Lipton in his latest book *Spontaneous Evolution: Our Positive Future and a Way to Get There from Here*. Through understanding and embracing the extraordinary, paradoxical force of human joy, we "claim our right to become personally empowered co-creators and architects of a brave and loving new world" (Lipton & Bhaerman, 2009, p. 5), and we claim our power to set our daughters on a path of a rich, rewarding life marked by flourishing mental health.

References

Amini, F., Lewis, T., Lannon, R., & Louie, A. (1996). Affect, attachment, memory: Contributions toward psychobiologic integration. *Psychiatry, 59*(3), 213–239.
Axness, M. (2004). Malattachment and the self struggle. *Journal of Prenatal and Perinatal Psychology and Health, 19*(2), 131–147.
Axness, M. (2012). *Parenting for peace: Raising the next generation of peacemakers*. Boulder, CO: Sentient Publications.
Barbazanges, A., Piazza, P., Le Moal, M., & Maccari, S. (1996). Maternal glucocorticoid secretion mediates long-term effects of prenatal stress. *Journal of Neuroscience, 16*(12), 3943–3949.
Barker, D. (Ed.). (1992). *Fetal and Infant Origins of Adult Disease*. London: British Medical Journal.
Barker, D. J. (2007). The origins of the developmental origins theory. *Journal of Internal Medicine, 261*(5), 412–417.
Barker, E., Kirkham, N., Ng, J., & Jensen, S. (2013). Prenatal maternal depression symptoms and nutrition, and child cognitive function. *British Journal of Psychiatry, 203*(6), 417–421.
Barker, D. J., Osmond, C., Winter, P., Margetts, B., & Simmonds, S. (1989). Weight in infancy and death from ischaemic heart disease. *Lancet, 2*, 577–580.
Barker, D. J., & Thornburg, K. (2013). The obstetric origins of health for a lifetime. *Clinical Obstetrics and Gynecology, 56*(3), 511–519.
Begley, S. (1999). Shaped by life in the womb. *Newsweek*.
Bernhardt, P. (1992). Individuation, mutual connection, and the body's resources: An interview with Lisbeth Marcher. *Pre- and Perinatal Psychology Journal, 6*(4), 281–293.
Blum, D. (2002, October 6). Young brains shaped by abuse, *Los Angeles Times*.
Bohnert, K. M., & Breslau, N. (2008). Stability of psychiatric outcomes of low birth weight. *Archives of General Psychiatry, 65*(9), 1080–1086.
Bowlby, J. (1980). *Attachment and loss* (Vol. 3: Loss). New York: Basic Books.
Bowman, R. E., MacLusky, N. J., Sarmiento, Y., Frankfurt, M., Gordon, M., & Luine, V. N. (2004). Sexually dimorphic effects of prenatal stress on cognition, hormonal responses and central neurotransmitters. *Endocrinology, 145*(8), 3778–3787.
Brandon, A. R., Pitts, S., Denton, W. H., Stringer, A., & Evans, H. M. (2009). A history of the theory of prenatal attachment. *Journal of Prenatal and Perinatal Psychology and Health, 23*(4), 201–222.
Brown, A., van Os, J., Driessens, C., Hoek, H., & Susser, E. (2000). Further evidence of relation between prenatal famine and major affective disorder. *American Journal of Psychiatry, 2000*(157), 190–195.
Burgess, A. W., Hartman, C. R., & Clements, P. T., Jr. (1995). Biology of memory and childhood trauma. *Journal of Psychosocial Nursing and Mental Health Services, 33*(3), 16–26.
Buss, C., Entringer, S., & Wadhwa, P. D. (2012). Fetal programming of brain development: Intrauterine stress and susceptibility to psychopathology. *Science Signaling, 5*(245), 1–7.

Bystrova, K., Ivanova, V., Edhborg, M., Matthiesen, A. -S., Ransjö-Arvidson, A. -B., Mukhamedrakhimov, R., ... Widström, A. -M. (2009). Early contact versus separation: Effects on mother-infant interaction one year later. *Birth, 36*(2), 97–109.

Chamberlain, D. B. (1998). Prenatal receptivity and intelligence. *Journal of Prenatal and Perinatal Psychology and Health, 12*(3/4), 95–113.

Chamberlain, D. (1999). Reliability of birth memory: Observations from mother and child pairs in hypnosis. *Journal of Prenatal and Perinatal Psychology and Health, 14*(1–2), 19–30.

Chamberlain, D. B. (2012). *Windows to the womb: Revealing the conscious baby from conception to birth*. Berkeley, CA: North Atlantic Books.

Christenson, R. M., & Wilson, W. P. (1985). Assessing pathology in the separation-individuation process by an inventory: A preliminary report. *Journal of Nervous & Mental Disease, 173*(9), 561–565.

Cooper, G., Hoffman, K., & Powell, B. (2010). *Circle of security*, from http://www.circleofsecurity.net/

Croyle, K. L., & Waltz, J. (2007). Sublinical self-harm: Range of behaviors, extent, and associated characteristics. *American Journal of Orthopsychiatry, 77*(2), 332–342. doi:10.1037/0002-9432.77.2.332.

Daubenmier, J. J. (2005). The relationship of yoga, body awareness, and body responsiveness to self-objectification and disordered eating. *Psychology of Women Quarterly, 29*(2), 207–219.

Davis, E. P., Glynn, L. M., Hobel, C., Schetter, C. D., Chicz-DeMet, A., & Sandman, C. A. (2007). Prenatal exposure to maternal depression and cortisol influences infant temperament. *Journal of the American Academy of Child & Adolescent Psychiatry, 46*(6), 737–746.

de Rooij, S. R., Wouters, H., Yonker, J. E., Painter, R. C., & Roseboom, T. J. (2010). Prenatal undernutrition and cognitive function in late adulthood. *Proceedings of the National Academy of Sciences, 107*(39), 16881–16886.

DeCasper, A. J., & Fifer, W. P. (1980). Of human bonding: Newborns prefer their mothers' voices. *Science, 208*(4448), 1174–1176.

DiPietro, J. A. (2010). Maternal influences on the developing fetus. In A. Zimmerman & S. Connors (Eds.), *Maternal influences on fetal neurodevelopment: Clinical and research aspects*. New York, NY: Spring Science+Business Media.

DiPietro, J. A., Costigan, K. A., & Gurewitsch, E. D. (2003). Fetal response to induced maternal stress. *Early Human Development, 74*(2), 125–138.

DiPietro, J., Hodgson, D., Costigan, K., & Johnston, T. (1996). Fetal antecedents of infant temperament. *Child Development, 67*, 2568–2583.

Doan, H. M., & Zimmerman, A. (2004). Conceptualizing prenatal attachment: Toward a multidimensional view. *Journal of Prenatal and Perinatal Psychology and Health, 18*(2), 109–130.

Favaro, A., Tenconi, E., & Santonastaso, P. (2006). Perinatal factors and the risk of developing anorexia nervosa and bulimia nervosa. *Archives of General Psychiatry, 63*(1), 82–88.

Feng, X., Want, L., Yang, S., Qin, D., Want, J., Li, C., ... Hu, X. (2011). Maternal separation produces lasting changes in cortisol and behavior in rhesus monkeys. *Proceedings of the National Academy of Sciences, 108*(34), 14312–14317. doi: 10.1073/pnas.1010943108

Foureur, M. (2008). Creating birth space to enable undisturbed birth. In K. Fahy, M. Foureur, & C. Hastie (Eds.), *Birth territory and midwifery guardianship: Theory for practice, education and research*. San Diego, CA: Elsevier Health Sciences.

Fredrickson, B. L., & Roberts, T.-A. (1997). Objectification theory: Towards understanding women's lived experiences and mental health risks. *Psychology of Women Quarterly, 21*, 173–206.

Fullmer, M. (2006). The neurological impact of preterm and very preterm birth and influence of IVF pregnancies on developmental outcomes: a literature review and case study. *Journal of Prenatal and Perinatal Psychology and Health, 20*(2), 157–170.

Gibson, C., & Tibbetts, S. (2000). A biosocial interaction in predicting early onset of offending. *Psychological Reports, 5*(5), e101. doi:10.1371/journal.pmed.0050101.

Glover, V. (2011). Prenatal stress and the origins of psychopathology: An evolutionary perspective. *Journal of Child Psychology and Psychiatry, 52*(4), 356–363.

Gohier, B., Senior, C., Radua, J., El-Hage, W., Reichenberg, A., Proitsi, P., ... Surguladze, S. (2013). Genetic modulation of the response bias toward facial displays of anger and happiness. *European Psychiatry*. Eur Psychiatry. 2013 Jun 13. pii: S0924-9338(13)00038-2. doi: 10.1016/j.eurpsy.2013.03.003. [Epub ahead of print].

Gravett, M. G., Rubens, C. E., & Global Alliance to Prevent Prematurity and Stillbirth Technical Team. (2012). A framework for strategic investments in research to reduce the global burden of preterm birth. *American Journal of Obstetrics and Gynecology, 207*(5), 368–373.

Green, M., & Piel, J. A. (2002). *Theories of human development: A comparative approach*. Boston, MA: Allyn and Bacon.

Green, M., Rani, C., Soto-Piña, A., Martinez, P., Frazer, A., Strong, R., & Morilak, D. (2011). Prenatal stress induces long term stress vulnerability, compromising stress response systems in the brain and impairing extinction of conditioned fear after adult stress. *Neuroscience, 192*, 438–451.

Grizenko, N., Fortier, M. -E., Zadorozny, C., Thakur, G., Schmitz, N., Duval, R., & Joober, R. (2012). Maternal stress during pregnancy, ADHD symptomatology in children and genotype: Gene-environment interaction. *Journal of the Canadian Academy of Child and Adolescent Psychiatry, 21*(1), 9–15.

Grof, S. (1976). *Realms of the human unconscious*. New York, NY: Dutton.

Gunnar, M. R., & Donzella, B. (2002). Social regulation of the cortisol levels in early human development. *Psychoneuroendocrinology, 27*(1–2), 199–220.

Hales, C., & Barker, D. (1992). Non-insulin dependent (type II) diabetes mellitus: thrifty phenotype hypothesis. In D. Barker (Ed.), *Fetal and Infant Origins of Adult Disease* (pp. 258–272). London: British Medical Journal.

Ham, J. T., Jr., & Klimo, J. (2000). Fetal awareness of maternal emotional states during pregnancy. *Journal of Prenatal and Perinatal Psychology and Health, 15*(2), 118–145.

Hayton, A. M. (2008). The possible prenatal origins of morbid obesity. *Journal of Prenatal and Perinatal Psychology and Health, 23*(2), 79–89.

Heatherton, T. F., & Wagner, D. D. (2011). Cognitive neuroscience of self-regulation failure. *Trends in Cognitive Sciences, 15*(3), 132–139.

Hepper, P. (2005). Unravelling our beginnings. *The Psychologist, 18*(8), 474–477.

Hepper, P. G., Scott, D., & Shahldullah, S. (1993). Newborn and fetal response to maternal voice. *Journal of Reproductive and Infant Psychology, 11*(3), 147–153. doi:10.1080/02646839308403210.

Herman, J. (1997). *Trauma and recovery*. New York, NY: Basic Books.

Hofer, M. A. (1996). On the nature and consequences of early loss. *Psychosomatic Medicine, 58*, 570–581.

House, S. (2000). Primal integration therapy—School of Lake: Dr. Frank Lake MB, MRC Psych, DPM (1914–1982). *Journal of Prenatal and Perinatal Psychology and Health, 14*(3–4), 213–235.

Hrdy, S. B. (1999). *Mother nature: Maternal instincts and how they shape the human species*. New York, NY: Ballantine.

Huizink, A. C., Mulder, E. J., & Buitelaar, J. K. (2004). Prenatal stress and risk for psychopathology: Specific effects or induction of general susceptibility? *Psychological Bulletin, 130*(1), 115–142.

Huizink, A., Robles de Medina, P., Mulder, E., Visser, G., & Buitelaar, J. (2003). Stress during pregnancy is associated with developmental outcome in infancy. *Journal of Child Psychology and Psychiatry, 44*(6), 810–818.

Huxley, L. A., & Ferruci, P. (1992). *The child of your dreams*. Rochester, VT: Destiny Books.

Insel, T., Kinsley, C., Mann, P., & Bridges, R. (1990). Prenatal stress has long-term effects on brain opiate receptors. *Brain Research, 511*, 93–97.

Jacobson, B., & Bygdeman, M. (2000). Obstetric care and proneness of offspring to suicide as adults: A case-control study. *Journal of Prenatal and Perinatal Psychology and Health, 15*(1), 63–74.

James, D., Spencer, C., & Stepsis, B. (2002). Fetal learning: A prospective randomized controlled study. *Ultrasound in Obstetrics and Gynecology, 20*(5), 431–438. doi:10.1046/j.1469-0705.2002.00845.x.

Jensen, D. (2000). *A language older than words*. New York, NY: Context Books.

Jiang, X., Yan, J., West, A. A., Perry, C. A., Malysheva, O. V., Devapatla, S., ... Caudill, M. A. (2012). Maternal choline intake alters the epigenetic state of fetal cortisol-regulating genes in humans. *FASEB Journal, 26*(8), 3563.

Jimenez-Vasquez, P. A., Mathe, A. A., Thomas, J. D., Riley, E. P., & Ehlers, C. L. (2001). Early maternal separation alters neuropeptide Y concentrations in selected brain regions in adult rats. *Brain Research. Developmental Brain Research, 131*(1–2), 149–152.

Johnston-Robledo, I., Sheffield, K., Voigt, J., & Wilcox-Constantine, J. (2007). Reproductive shame: Self-objectification and young women's attitudes toward their reproductive functioning. *Women's Health, 46*(1), 25–39.

Kalinichev, M., Easterling, K. W., Plotsky, P. M., & Holtzman, S. G. (2002). Long-lasting changes in stress-induced corticosterone response and anxiety-like behaviors as a consequence of neonatal maternal separation in Long-Evans rats. *Pharmacology, Biochemistry, and Behavior, 73*(1), 131–140.

Kamrath, S. (2013). Happy healthy pregnancy. In W. L. Media (Producer), *Happy healthy child*. United States.

Kestenberg, J. S., & Browitz, E. (1990). On narcissism and masochism in the fetus and neonate. *Journal of Prenatal and Perinatal Psychology and Health, 5*(1), 87–94.

Levine, P. (2002, March 2–3). *When biology becomes pathology*. Paper presented at the From Neurons to Neighborhoods: The Effects of Emotional Trauma on the Way We Learn, Feel and Act, Mt. St. Mary's College, Los Angeles.

Levine, P. (2005). *Healing trauma: A pioneering program for restoring the wisdom of your body*. Louisville, CO: Sounds True.

Lewis, T., Amini, F., & Lannon, R. (2000). *A general theory of love*. New York, NY: Random House.

Lieshout, R. J. V., Taylor, V. H., & Boyle, M. H. (2011). Pre-pregnancy and pregnancy and neurodevelopmental outcomes in offspring: A systematic review. *Obesity Reviews, 12*(5), e548–e559.

Lipton, B., & Bhaerman, S. (2009). *Spontaneous evolution*. Carlsbad, CA: Hay House.

Lyman, B. (2005). Prenatal and perinatal psychotherapy with adults: An integrative model for empirical testing. *Journal of Prenatal and Perinatal Psychology and Health, 20*(1), 58–76.

MacDonald, K., & MacDonald, T. M. (2010). The peptide that binds: A systematic review of oxytocin and its prosocial effects in humans. [Review]. *Harvard Review of Psychiatry, 18*(1), 1–21.

Maret, S. (1997). *The prenatal person: Frank Lake's maternal-fetal distress syndrome*. Lanham, MD: University Press of America.

Mayo Clinic Staff. (2013, June 13). *Depression in women: Understanding the gender gap*. Retrieved September 17, 2013, from http://www.mayoclinic.com/health/depression/MH00035

McGrath, J., Brown, A., & Clair, D. S. (2011). Prevention and schizophrenia: The role of dietary factors. *Schizophrenia Bulletin, 37*(2), 272–283.

McGregor, B., Edgerton, J., & Courtney, K. (2012). Reflections on Robin Grille's keynote presentation 'Love, fear and shame in education' [opinion]. *Educating Young Children, 18*(2), 13.

Middleton, W. (2005). Owning the past, claiming the present: Perspectives on the treatment of dissociative patients. *Australasian Psychiatry, 13*(1), 40–49. doi:10.1080/j.1440-1665.2004.02148.x.

Miller, A. (1981). *The drama of the gifted child*. New York, NY: Basic Books.

Miner-Rubino, K., Twenge, J. M., & Fredrickson, B. L. (2002). Trait self-objectification in women: Affective and personality correlates. *Journal of Research in Personality, 36*(2), 147–172.

Moreau, M. P., Bruse, S. E., David-Rus, R., Buyske, S., & Brzustowicz, L. M. (2011). Altered microRNA expression profiles in post-mortem brain samples from individuals with schizophrenia and bipolar disorder. *Biological Psychiatry, 69*(2), 188–193. doi:10.1016/j.biopsych.2010.09.039.

Morgan, B. E., Horn, A. R., & Bergman, N. J. (2011). Should neonates sleep alone? *Biological Psychiatry, 70*(9), 817–825.

Nathanielsz, P. W. (1992). *Life Before Birth: The Challenges of Fetal Development*. New York: W.H. Freeman & Co.

O'Donnell, K. (2013). Prenatal maternal mood is associated with altered diurnal cortisol in adolescence. *Psychoneuroendocrinology, 38*(9), 1630–1638.

Odent, M. (2002). The long term consequences of how we are born. *Journal of Prenatal and Perinatal Psychology and Health, 17*(2), 107–112.

Odent, M. (2012). *The Primal Health Research Database in the age of epigenetics.* Paper presented at the The Mid-Pacific Conference on Birth and Primal Health Research, Honolulu, HI.

Odent, M. (2013). *Childbirth and the future of homo sapiens.* London: Pinter & Martin, Ltd.

Partanen, E., Kujala, T., Näätänen, R., Liitola, A., Sambeth, A., & Huotilainen, M. (2013). Learning-induced neural plasticity of speech processing before birth. *Proceedings of the National Academy of Sciences* (in press). doi: 10.1073/pnas.1302159110. Proc Natl Acad Sci USA. 2013 Sep 10;110(37):15145–50

Perry, B. (1995a). Childhood trauma, the neurobiology of adaptation, and "use-dependent" development of the brain: How "states" become "traits". *Infant Mental Health, 16*(4), 271–291.

Perry, B. (1995b). Incubated in terror: Neurodevelopmental factors in the "cycle of violence". In J. Osofsky (Ed.), *Children, youth and violence: Searching for solutions.* New York, NY: Guilford.

Perry, B. (2003). *Nature and nurture of brain development: How early experience shapes child and culture.* Paper presented at the From Neurons to Neighborhoods: The Neurobiology of Emotional Trauma, Los Angeles.

Pinborg, A., Lidegaard, O., la Cour Freiesleben, N., & Andersen, A. (2005). Consequences of vanishing twins in IVF/ICSI pregnancies. *Human Reproduction, 20*(10), 2821–2829.

Renggli, F. (2003). Tracing the roots of panic to prenatal trauma. *Journal of Prenatal and Perinatal Psychology and Health, 17*(4), 289–300.

Rice, F., Jones, I., & Thapar, A. (2007). The impact of gestational stress and prenatal growth on emotional problems in offspring: a review. *Acta Paediactrica, 115*, 171–183.

Rifkin-Graboi, A., Bai, J., Chen, H., Hameed, W. B., Sim, L. W., Tint, M. T., … Qui, A. (2013). Prenatal maternal depression associates with microstructure of right amygdala in neonates at birth. *Biological Psychiatry, 74*(11), 837–844.

Rosenberg, J., Rand, M., & Asay, D. (1985). *Body, self and soul: Sustaining integration.* Atlanta, GA: Humanics Limited.

Sandman, C. A., Davis, E. P., Cordova, C., Kemp, A., & Glynn, L. M. (2011, September). *What the maternal heart tells the fetal brain.* Paper presented at the Developmental Origins of Health and Disease, Portland, OR.

Sandman, C., Davis, E., & Glynn, L. (2012). Psychobiological stress and preterm birth. In J. C. Morrison (Ed.), *Preterm birth—mother and child* (pp. 95–124). Coatia: InTech.

Sandman, C. A., Glynn, L., Wadhwa, P. D., Chicz-DeMet, A., Porto, M., & Garite, T. (2003). Maternal hypothalamic-pituitary-adrenal disregulation during the third trimester influences human fetal responses. *Developmental Neuroscience, 25*(1), 41–49.

Sandman, C., & Yessaian, N. (1986). Persisting subsensitivity of the striatal dopamine system after fetal exposure to beta-endorphin. *Life Sciences, 39*, 1755–1763.

Santa Barbara Graduate Institute (Producer). (2004). The very first relationship. *Trauma, brain and relationship: helping children heal.* Retrieved from http://www.healingresources.info/emotional_trauma_online_video.htm - 1

Schlotz, W., & Phillips, D. (2009). Fetal origins of mental health: Evidence and mechanisms. *Brain, Behavior, and Immunity, 23*, 905–916.

Schore, A. (1999). *Affect regulation and the origin of the self: The neurobiology of emotional development.* Mahwah, NJ: Lawrence Erlbaum.

Schore, A. (2001, December 6–9). *Attachment and the development of the emotional brain.* Paper presented at the Birth: The Genesis of Health, San Francisco, CA.

Schore, A. N. (2002). Dysregulation of the right brain: A fundamental mechanism of traumatic attachment and the psychopathogenesis of posttraumatic stress disorder. *The Australian and New Zealand Journal of Psychiatry, 36*(1), 9–30.

Schore, J. R., & Schore, A. N. (2008). Modern attachment theory: The central role of affect regulation in development and treatment. *Clinical Social Work Journal, 36*(1), 9–20.

Share, L. (1994). *If someone speaks, it gets lighter: Dreams and the reconstruction of infant trauma.* Hillsdale, NJ: Analytic Press.

Siegel, D. (2002, March 2–3). *Relationships and the developing mind*. Paper presented at the From Neurons to Neighborhoods: The Effects of Emotional Trauma on theWay We Learn, Feel and Act, Los Angeles, CA.

Siegel, D. J. (2002b). *The Developing Mind: How Relationships and the Brain Interact to Shape Who We Are*. New York, NY: Guilford Press.

Siegel, D. J. (2004). Attachment and self-understanding: Parenting with the brain in mind. *Journal of Prenatal and Perinatal Psychology and Health, 18*(4), 273–286.

Skowron, E. A., & Dendy, A. K. (2004). Differentiation of self and attachment in adulthood: Relational correlates of effortful control. *Contemporary Family Therapy, 26*(3), 337–357.

Skowron, E. A., Wester, S. R., & Azen, R. (2004). Differentiation of self mediates college stress and adjustment. *Journal of Counseling and Development, 82*, 69–78.

Solomon, M. F. (1989). *Narcissism and intimacy*. New York, NY: Norton.

Sonne, J. (2000). Abortion survivors at Columbine. *Journal of Prenatal and Perinatal Psychology and Health, 15*(1), 3–22.

Stern, D. N. (1998). *Diary of a baby*. New York, NY: Basic Books.

Strathearn, L., Fonagy, P., Amico, J., & Montague, P. R. (2009). Adult attachment predicts maternal brain and oxytocin response to infant cues. *Neuropsychopharmacology, 34*, 2655–2666. doi:10.1038/npp.2009.103.

Swanson, J., Entringer, S., Buss, C., & Wadhwa, P. (2009). Developmental origins of health and disease: Environmental exposures. *Seminars in Reproductive Medicine, 27*(5), 391–402.

Trevarthen, C., & Aitken, K. J. (1994). Brain development, infant communication, and empathy disorders: Intrinsic factors in child mental health. *Development and Psychopathology, 6*(4), 597–633.

Tsuda, M. C., & Ogawa, S. (2012). Long-lasting consequences of neonatal maternal separation on social behaviors in ovariectomized female mice. *PLoS One, 7*(3), e33028. doi:10.1371/journal.pone.0033028.

van der Kolk, B. A., McFarlane, A. C., & Weisaeth, L. (1996). *Traumatic stress: The effects of overwhelming experience on mind, body, and society*. New York, NY: Guilford Press.

Verny, T. (2002). *Tomorrow's baby: The art and science of parenting from conception through infancy*. New York, NY: Simon & Schuster.

Verrier, N. (1993). *The primal wound: Understanding the adopted child*. Baltimore, MD: Gateway.

Vollmayr, B., & Henn, F. A. (2003). Stress models of depression. *Clinical Neuroscience Research, 3*(4–5), 245–251.

Von Glahn, J. (1998). The pre- and perinatal development of a sense of self. *Journal of Prenatal and Perinatal Psychology and Health, 13*(2), 155–169.

Wade, J. (1999). Two voices from the womb: Evidence for physically transcendent and a cellular source of fetal consciousness. *Journal of Prenatal and Perinatal Psychology and Health, 13*(2), 123–147.

Wadhwa, P. (2005). Psychoneuroendocrine processes in human pregnancy influence fetal development and health. *Psychoneuroendocrinology, 30*, 724–743.

Wadhwa, P. D., Sandman, C. A., & Garite, T. J. (2001). The neurobiology of stress in human pregnancy: Implications for prematurity and development of the fetal central nervous system. *Progress in Brain Research, 133*, 131–142.

Watson, P. J., Hickman, S. E., Morris, R. J., & Milliron, J. T. (1999). Narcissism, self-esteem, and parental nurturance. *Journal of Psychology, 129*(1), 61–73.

Weaver, K., Wuest, J., & Ciliska, D. (2005). Understanding women's journey of recovering from anorexia nervosa. *Qualitative Health Research, 15*(2), 188–206. doi:10.1177/1049732304270819.

Weinstock, W. (2005). The potential influence of maternal stress hormones on development and mental health of the offspring. *Brain, Behavior, and Immunity, 19*, 296–308.

Werner, E. A., Myers, M. M., Fifer, W. A., Cheng, B., Fang, Y., Allen, R., & Monk, C. (2007). Prenatal predictors of infant temperament. *Developmental Psychology, 49*(5), 474–484. doi: 10.1002/dev.20232

Zucchi, F., Yao, Y., Ward, I., Ilnytskyy, Y., Olson, D., Benzies, K., … Metz, G. (2013). Maternal stress induces epigenetic signatures of psychiatric and neurological diseases in the offspring. *PLoS One, 8*(2), e56967. doi: 10.1371/journal.pone.0056967

Girls In-Between: Social, Emotional, Physical, and Sexual Development in Context

Melissa J. Johnson

Introduction

Girls' adolescent journeys are marked by the questions they ask about who they are relationally, physically, intellectually, culturally, and sexually. This search for self-definition, also known as identity work, takes place in a social context that profoundly shapes girls' experiences. Bullying, harassment, violence, and abuse are everyday experiences for many. They grow up in a society in which the media sexualizes women and girls from an early age. Discrimination based on gender, culture, race, ethnicity, class, sexual orientation, religion, and disability is damaging. Access to health care and effective education is uneven at best. Real life role models and mentors are not available to all girls, and for millions of teens, the Internet is the primary source of sexual and relationship information. Closer to home, family members may struggle with mental health issues and family communication may not address some of the most salient issues facing adolescent girls today. Young women themselves may confront the pain of depression, anxiety, substance abuse, body dissatisfaction and eating disorders, trauma, self-injury, suicidal ideation, and other psychological issues while trying to come to terms with who they are and who they are becoming.

A biopsychosocial model of girls' development provides a framework to examine these intersections of intrapersonal, interpersonal, and sociocultural factors. Unfortunately, a comprehensive approach to girls' development is not always considered in programming, education, or policy. The sexuality and reproductive health curricula used in many high schools focuses almost exclusively on biology, offering little guidance and information about the relational and emotional aspects of intimacy, attraction, sexuality, and reproduction (Christopher, 2001; Martinez, Abma, Copen, & National Center for Health Statistics, 2010). Quantitative and qualitative

---

M.J. Johnson, Ph.D. (✉)
The Institute for Girls' Development, A Psychological Corporation, Pasadena, CA, USA
e-mail: MJohnson@Instituteforgirlsdevelopment.com

research reviewed in the following chapter indicates a number of external factors that are detrimental to girls as well as protective factors that help them thrive. The chapter concludes with recommendations for research, family life resources, programming, and policy considerations, which can enhance well-being for teen girls as they engage in their identity work.

Ideal Girlhood and Womanhood

Girlhood and womanhood are socially constructed and continually changing (Adams, 2005; Zaslow, 2009). Over the past 20 years the predominant image of adolescent girlhood has shifted away from that of the passive victim. Popular press books in the early 1990s, like Mary Pipher's *Reviving Ophelia* (1995) and Peggy Orenstein's *Schoolgirls* (1994), documented the damaging effects of society. Today, in the age of girl power media (Zaslow, 2009), the image of normative girlhood is a complex blend of self-determination, individuality, assertiveness, athleticism, sexual subjectivity, physical attractiveness, thinness, and niceness (Adams, 2005; Bettis, Jordan, & Montgomery, 2005; Choate, 2007; Girls, Inc., 2006; Zaslow, 2009). Zaslow (2009) posits that the image of the assertive and in-control girl emerged in part through the girl power movement of the 1990s. The image of the strong and sexy girl was then reinforced by media culture, zeroing in on millions of teen and young women consumers. Today's girls face pressure to meet this super girl image while at the same time fulfilling traditional ideas about being nice and attractive in their real life and online identities.

To further complicate the process, girls and young women must grapple with the culture's idealized notions of motherhood. While most adolescent females will eventually have children, not all will. Some may choose not to; some may be unable to have children. Some may raise children that have been adopted or birthed by others, and some may live in circumstances that make childbearing problematic at best. If teen girls can be provided with relationships, environments, and skills to foster psychological well-being, they will be better equipped to deal with whatever present and future challenges and decisions they must face. They will be more skilled at making decisions about relationships, intimacy, sexuality, reproduction, and motherhood. They will have more tools for communicating about and coping with related stresses, boundary setting, and avenues for seeking help. Girls and young women will have greater capacity for refuting the super girl, superwoman, and super mother myths that impair well-being.

"Who Am I Relationally?"

Relationships foster hardiness, growth, and resilience in girls. Through theory and qualitative research, Relational-Cultural Theory, RCT, provides a fresh understanding of girls' developmental trajectory. Rather than the historic emphasis on adolescence as a time for developing individuality and autonomy, RCT places the nexus of development in relationship and connection. This corresponds with current neurobiological research on relationships and the brain (Siegel, 2007). According to RCT the teen years are a time of redefining connections with peers and parents. Multiple studies identify the best predictor of resistance to high-risk behaviors: having a good relationship with an adult, such as a teacher, coach, mentor, spiritual leader, or parent (Armstrong & Boothroyd, 2007; Jordan, 2005; Resnick et al., 1997).

Relational resilience, according to Jordan (2005), includes the capacity for resistance through which girls can deal with their experience of the sociocultural world. Disempowering messages regarding gender, race, sexuality, and sexual orientation come from many places: home, close to home, the Internet, and the larger society (Collins, 2000; Jordan, 2005; Steiner-Adair & Barker, 2013). Resistance to these messages is vital for psychological well-being. In Ward's (2002) work with African American girls, she identifies four steps for developing healthy resistance to stereotypes, oppression, and discrimination:

1. Read it: examining the subtle and blatant discriminatory messages in their sociocultural worlds is a first step.
2. Name it: learning to name specific stereotypes and oppressions such as racism, sexism, and class bias contributes to agency and strength.
3. Oppose the negative force: countering the internal and external impact of forces like racism means countering the associated self-hatred, hopelessness, and anger.
4. Replace it: empowering girls to develop and affirm a reality that is different from the one presented by the situation or culture can provide hope. For example, girls might resist racism by standing up for fairness and justice. They might oppose the sexual objectification of girls in the media by shining the light on advertisers and programs that represent real girls living empowered lives.

While environments free of discrimination, violence, trauma, and poverty are desired, protective factors include helping girls develop the capacity to connect as allies, creatively critique injustices, and take social action regarding inequities (Jordan, 2005; Lalik & Oliver, 2005; Prettyman, 2005; Ward, 2002). As Jordan (2005) poignantly notes, "Relational resilience involves movement toward mutually empowering, growth-fostering connections in the face of adverse conditions, traumatic experiences, and alienating social-cultural pressures" (p. 83).

Relational Stereotypes and Peer Relationships

How does this research on the centrality of relationships and healthy resistance sync with the stereotype of mean girls? Social aggression does exist in the world of children, appearing on the scene as early as age 3 (Underwood, 2003). Social aggression receives extensive media attention and is a source of concern for schools and families. Social aggression includes behaviors intended to harm friendships, social standing, and social esteem. The behaviors include, but are not limited to, exclusion, gossip, and rumors.

Social aggression is a complex dynamic for girls. Researchers have identified a number of possible reasons for this type of aggression in girls including media glorification of the mean, sassy girl; boredom; the wish to belong; and difficulties with effectively expressing anger or being assertive (Brown, 2003; Orpinas & Horne, 2006; Underwood, 2003).

Without oversimplifying a very complex phenomenon, it is important to observe the clash between two opposing cultural demands. The first, promoted in part by girl-power media culture, is the demand for girls to be in control and assertive. The second, entrenched in centuries of "good girl" messages, is the cultural mantra to be nice and kind, which includes avoiding the direct expression of anger (Bettis et al., 2005; Brown, 2003; Schoenberg, Salmond, & Fleshman, 2008; Simmons, 2009). Granted, kindness is an important pro-social skill. Experience and research show there are great benefits to the capacity for kindness in social relationships (Goleman, 1995; Lyubomirsky, 2008; Siegel, 2007). Being nice and kind becomes problematic when they interfere with girls' capacity to be authentic, assertive, and to express anger effectively. Anger is a natural human emotion, signaling when something is amiss. Assertiveness is a tool that can be used to set things right. When girls are unable to directly and effectively express anger or be assertive, there are consequences. Girls and young women may become silent and isolated, even depressed (Brown & Gilligan, 1992) or they may express indirect anger in socially cruel ways (Simmons, 2009; Underwood, 2003). Brown and Gilligan (1992) aptly refer to this phenomenon as the tyranny of nice and kind. Girls and young women benefit from skills that help them navigate this complicated terrain; developing their capacities for authentic kindness, compassion, and empathy, as well as their ability to lead, be assertive, resolve conflict, and set boundaries. These skills are not only important to teen psychological health; they provide necessary scaffolding for women's mental health.

Kin Relationships

Relational resilience is supported by relationships with at least one caring adult who sees the adolescent girl for who she really is, someone who can listen with heart and mind, and can provide validation and valuing. In some cases, these mentoring adults can provide puberty and sexuality education. Parents and extended family can play an important role in helping teens gain accurate knowledge and evaluate information received elsewhere. Past research shows that teens prefer to gain sexuality and relationship information from parents (Simanski, 1998); however, new research shows that millions of teens today use the Internet as their primary source for this information (Steiner-Adair & Barker, 2013). While the Internet is problematic in that it can sometimes expose children and teens to sexual content for which they are not yet ready, it can also be a safe, private place to gain information difficult to access in other ways. For example, lesbian, bisexual, and questioning teen girls may be encouraged to find supportive interactive Internet communities that serve as a resource during the exploration of their emerging identities (Petrovic & Ballard, 2005; Savin-Williams, 2007; Ward, Day, & Epstein, 2006).

Trauma and Relationships

Child abuse, sexual harassment, rape, and other forms of sexual assault are not uncommon in the lives of teen girls. Teen dating violence is pervasive. While three quarters of high school and college women report being victims of verbal aggression, one-third report physical aggression. Women who are not white, middle class, or heterosexual face particular challenges when admitting violence and getting help. Concerns include distrust of white authority and cultural demands to keep personal lives private. For lesbian teens, getting help may require revealing their sexual orientation (Smith, White, & Holland, 2003). The physical and psychological consequences of trauma can be long lasting, especially without early intervention. Identifying trauma and helping adolescent females to heal from these experiences is imperative for lifelong psychological health (Levine & Kline, 2007).

"Who Am I Physically?"

Preteen and teen girls experience many bodily changes. Biopsychosocial theory considers these changes in the context of girls' social and emotional worlds. In the USA the average age of girls' first menstrual cycle is about 12½ years of age. For most girls, it takes another 2 years before the menstrual cycle is stable and mature (Grumbach & Styne, 1998).

Girls and young women have feelings about these bodily changes. Girls frequently compare themselves to others and find themselves lacking. Girls not only compare themselves to their peers, whom they may see as more attractive and thinner: they compare themselves to media images that have been air brushed and digitally altered, resulting in an impossible standard of beauty. The celebrity culture that abounds adds to the harmful message that appearance is the most important asset for girls and women. In the words of one young woman, "A girl could be anyone—as long as she was pretty" (Lemish, 1998, p. 155).

The convergence of bodily changes, media messages, and intra- and interpersonal factors coincide with a dramatic increase in body dissatisfaction for girls around puberty (Barker & Galambos, 2003). For girls between the ages of 8 and 11, approximately 50 % rated their weight as important and expressed the desire to be thinner (Ricciardelli, McCabe, Holt, & Finemore, 2003). Girls' relational worlds are complicated by these physical changes as well. They must cope with whether these changes come early or later. Early maturing females, for example, may exhibit heightened romantic and sexual interests (Brown, Halpern, & L'Engle, 2005; Pearson, Kholodkov, Henson, & Impett, 2012). Girls must also deal with how their female friends, and boys and men in general, respond to their changing bodies. Experiences with sexual harassment and other forms of objectification may become everyday challenges (Charmaraman, Jones, Stein, & Espelage, 2013; Stein, 1995, 1997).

Navigating environments, like school, takes on a new dimension. With the start of menstruation girls must figure out how to manage their periods at school. They report wondering, "How am I going to change my tampon during a 4 min class change and get to class on time?" "What if my teacher won't let me out of class?" and "What if the boys find out?" (Fingerson, 2005a, 2005b). Girls may feel that their school environment is not a welcoming place for their changing bodies, which adds another dimension to body dissatisfaction.

Hormonal Factors

An extensive discussion of hormonal factors during puberty and adolescence is beyond the scope of this chapter and is discussed in greater in the chapter "Menstruation and Premenstrual Dysphoric Disorder: Its Impact on Mood." However, a comprehensive perspective of girls' development would be inadequate if premenstrual syndrome (PMS) and premenstrual dysphoric disorder (PMDD) were not mentioned. PMS is common in teen girls. In one study of girls 13–18 (mean age 16.5 years), 31 % of the participants met the emotional, physical, and behavioral criteria for PMS (Vichnin, Freeman, Lin, Hillman, & Bui, 2006).

Cultural Messages About Girls' Appearance: The Internet and Other Media

Ubiquitous media messages sustain the culture of dieting and thinness in the USA (Lamb & Brown, 2006). Fredrickson and Roberts (1997) provide objectification theory as a tool for both cultural analysis and research. They posit that a culture that objectifies girls and women can result in girls and women objectifying themselves. They describe a peculiar developmental experience in which girls view themselves from an early age through the eyes of others, looking at themselves from the vantage point of the external world. Media outlets such as fashion magazines and MTV have been shown to decrease girls' moods and increase their body dissatisfaction. Grabe and Hyde (2009) found that self-objectification in adolescent girls mediated a direct relationship between music television consumption and body esteem, dieting, depressive symptoms, anxiety, and interestingly, confidence in math ability. Daniels (2009) looked at how young women respond to images of women in magazines and found that the least body shame was evoked by images of the performance-focused woman athlete. Sexualized images evoked greater levels of shame.

Objectification and self-objectification have been shown to have a negative psychological impact on adolescent girls. For some young women, self-objectification has been associated with shame, anxiety, and self-degradation (Hirschman, Impett, & Schooler, 2006; Slater & Tiggemann, 2002). Further research suggests that exposure to media that objectifies girls and young women may contribute to these common psychological difficulties in girls: depression or depressed mood, eating disorders, and low self-esteem. Kim and her colleagues (2007) underscore that a culture of objectification leads to thinking, feeling, and behaving in ways that sustain stereotyped gender relationships and power inequities. Other research indicates that this sexualized cultural climate can decrease both mental focus and confidence.

Alternatively, ethnic and cultural factors may sometimes play a protective role in girls' levels of self-objectification and body satisfaction (Granberg, Simons, & Simons, 2009). Several studies have postulated that there may be cultural factors in the African American community that contribute to positive self-views of adolescent girls who do not meet the thin-ideal of the dominant white culture. More investigations are needed to understand the nuances of this phenomenon for African American teen girls.

Cultural Messages About Girls' Bodies and Appearance: School, Family, and Peers

The emphasis on girls' appearance takes place in schools and families, as well as in the media. School environments send both subtle and blatant messages to girls about their bodies (Larkin & Rice, 2005). Lalik and Oliver (2005) shine light on one school region's practice of the annual Beauty Walk, female contestants only, as a fundraiser for the Parent Teacher Organizations. Student to student sexual harassment is a far too common experience for teen girls and young women (American Association of University Women & Harris Interactive, 2001; Charmaraman et al., 2013). Even though it is addressed in Federal law Title IX, teachers admit they frequently do not know how to identify sexual harassment when it occurs between students. Due to limited or lack of training, they are often uncertain about effective ways to respond when it does occur (Ali & US Department of Education, Office for Civil Rights, 2010; Stein, 1995, 1997).

Parents also send strong messages to their daughters about appearance. Parents may express concern about their daughter's appearance, grooming, and weight. Physical self-care is a developmental task, one that comes more easily to some girls than others. Parents can be critical of their daughter's appearance, wanting them to meet the cultural standards of thinness and beauty (APA Report on the Sexualization of Girls, 2007). In addition, there is a growing body of research that suggests a primary variable influencing the way a girl feels about her body is the way her mother feels about her own adult body (Tiggemann & Lynch, 2001).

The degree of self-objectification a girl experiences can vary over time and circumstance. Researchers identify specific interventions, which may help girls and young women decrease self-objectification in the face of media messages. For example, Greco and her colleagues (2008) incorporate cognitive behavioral and mindfulness-based approaches to help adolescent girls and young women build skills for mindful media consumption. They teach adolescent girls to identify unhelpful thoughts after viewing magazine images and encourage use of a cognitive diffusion intervention to decrease the power of these thoughts as well as improve mood. Daubenmier (2005) and others (Brown & Gerbarg, 2005) have evaluated the role of ongoing yoga practice as an effective intervention for decreasing self-objectification, stress, anxiety, and depression. In addition, media education can help girls increase their capacity to critique cultural messages and take social action regarding objectification (Lalik & Oliver, 2005; Prettyman, 2005).

"Who Am I Sexually?"

Some researchers question whether the definition of adolescent sexual health should be the same as adult sexual health (Halpern, 2006). The World Health Organization, WHO, defines sexual health as "the integration of the somatic, emotional, intellectual, and social aspects of sexual being, in ways that are positively enriching and that enhance personality, communication, and love" (WHO, 1975, p. 41). The National Commission on Adolescent Sexual Health (Sexuality Information and Education Council of the United States, 1995) supports the idea of applying this perspective to adolescence, since adolescent sexual health includes positive interpersonal relationships, emotional expression, intimacy, and personal body perceptions. In addition, many researchers (Graber & Sontag, 2006; Halpern, 2006; Tolman, Striepe, & Harmon, 2003) support this notion of an "integrated lens that captures biology, behavior, and the cultural, social, and physical aspects of an adolescent's environment" (Halpern, 2006, p. 9). That said, no unique criteria for adolescent sexuality have been identified.

Adolescent girls receive messages about their emerging sexual identities from multiple sources: the media, Internet, school, parents, siblings, and peers (Impett, Schooler, & Tolman, 2006; Steiner-Adair & Barker, 2013; Strahan et al., 2008; Sutton, Brown, Wilson, & Klein, 2002). Some of these messages are imposed, like the ubiquitous sexualization of girls and women in the media. Other information comes to girls accidentally, like walking in on a sibling masturbating, finding a used condom in a parent's bedroom, or unknowingly opening a pornographic YouTube video sent as a prank by a friend. Girls learn at school through both direct and indirect communication, as well as the school infrastructure. For example, a health class may focus on the biological aspects of sexuality, neglecting the relational and emotional aspects. At lunch girls may observe or participate in sexual name calling and conversations about sexual reputations.

In terms of sexual activity, the majority of girls in the USA will have engaged in intercourse by the time they are ages 17–18 (Frost & Alan Guttmacher Institute, 2001). At the same time, girls are strongly discouraged from engaging in intercourse and reproduction during the teen years due to a variety of risk factors. Existing research identifies three categories of messages about sexuality:

1. Messages that objectify and sexualize girls and women and invalidate girls' experiences of sexual development.
2. Messages that emphasize sexual risk.
3. Messages about positive sexual health and identity.

Messages That Sexualize Girls

As the discussion of objectification earlier in this chapter notes, there is reason for concern about the impact of objectification and sexualization on girls in this culture. Criteria that help distinguish between healthy sexuality and sexualization assist in research, education, and policy. Sexualization includes basing a person's value exclusively on his or her sexual appeal or behavior, omitting other characteristics or sexually objectifying an individual, such as imposing adult sexuality on children (APA Task Force on the Sexualization of Girls, 2007).

Hirschman and colleagues (2006) studied self-objectification as it relates specifically to sexuality. The study underscores the variability of self-objectification and sexual development in late adolescent females. Young women who rated higher on the self-objectification survey measure were less comfortable talking about sex and expressed regret about having sex. Lower levels of self-objectification were associated with expressed positive attitudes about sexuality, more comfort talking about sexuality, and engagement in sexual experimentation. Hirschman and colleagues (2006) advocate that teaching skills that decrease self-objectification may enhance girls' greater sexual health, agency, sexual satisfaction, and partner communication.

Messages About Sexual Risk

Teen pregnancy, STDs, and traumatic experiences are all risks of sexual activity. The USA saw a rise in teen pregnancies between 2005 and 2007 for all racial/ethnic groups, except Hispanics (Centers for Disease Control and Prevention, 2010). Poverty has a negative effect on adolescents, and is associated with poorer physical and psychological health and an increased likelihood of teenage pregnancy (Boothroyd and Olufokunbi, 2001; East, Khoo, & Reyes, 2006). Armstrong and Boothroyd (2007) found that having a baby dramatically changed the trajectories of many girls' lives. Teen girls' experiences of parenting were found to be further complicated when the baby had medical issues, families were unsupportive, or teens experienced postpartum mood or anxiety disorders. Pregnancy also altered friendships and access to education.

Teen pregnancy is not the only risk in sexual activity. Another concern for parents and public health officials is sexually transmitted diseases. Rape, dating violence, and other forms of sexual assault and trauma are also on the risk list. Research on parental communication about sexuality has found that parents tend to focus on the physical and emotional dangers of sexuality (Lefkowitz & Espinosa-Hernandez, 2007; Lefkowitz & Stoppa, 2006). Because of these dangers and because of values or religious beliefs, parents may encourage postponing sexual intercourse until marriage or a certain age. However, parents may find direct communication about sexuality and sexual behavior quite uncomfortable. Other factors that interfere with communication in urban households may be limited energy and feelings of overwhelm due to long work hours and chronic stress. In some households it is also difficult to find private, one-on-one time with teens. In some studies, adolescent girls have reported they themselves are more comfortable obtaining sexual information from other kin, like grandparents, aunts, or older siblings.

Messages About Positive Sexual Health and Identity

An integrated lens that allows examination of the intrapersonal, interpersonal, and sociocultural dimensions of normative sexuality in teens is vital and vastly understudied. At least three areas of further study will contribute necessary information:

1. Qualitative research that gives voice to girls' and young women's narratives about their emerging sexual selves. Research like Tolman's (2002) groundbreaking work *Dilemmas of Desire* is a useful model for illuminating girls' subjective experience of their sexuality. Tolman brings to life the voices and lived experiences of urban and suburban teen girls as they attempt to understand and respond to their own sexuality in relation to the contradictory cultural messages that bombard them. Other qualitative studies have provided a window into girls' diverse developmental trajectories by investigating: middle school girls' sexuality narratives told through exploratory photography (Charmaraman & McKamey, 2011); Black American adolescent girls sexual self-definitions constructed through use of the media (Stokes, 2007); and lesbian girls and the role of Internet chat rooms for information, connecting with others, and anonymity (Petrovic & Ballard, 2005).
2. Research that examines parent and teen communication about positive sexual health, including ways in which parents help adolescents interpret messages from outside sources (Lefkowitz & Espinosa-Hernandez, 2007; Lefkowitz & Stoppa, 2006). This parental role is especially relevant today given that teens' information about sexual intimacy and romance comes largely from the Internet (Steiner-Adair & Barker, 2013). Positive sexual development themes to be addressed by parents and daughters might include sexual desire, sexual pleasure, and even orgasm. While this has not yet been widely studied, Rosenthal and Feldman (1999) did find that 94 % of high school girls had never discussed sexual desire with their fathers and 76 % had never discussed desire with their mothers. Discussing desire explicitly may be difficult; however, some parents may approach these topics through more socially acceptable themes, like physical attractiveness (Lefkowitz & Espinosa-Hernandez, 2007).
3. Research to improve the effectiveness of programming in school and community environments through promoting learning about positive sexual well-being (Diamond, 2006; Graber, Nichols, Lynne, Brooks-Gunn, & Botvin, 2006). Curricula with a biological emphasis on reproduction are not as effective as curricula that address the relational contexts of teens' sexual lives (Christopher, 2001; Martinez et al., 2010). Education about love, attraction, dating, and desire may

provide a more holistic and relevant perspective. Further study of the cognitions and experiences influencing sexual self-concept is needed (O'Sullivan, 2005; O'Sullivan, Meyer-Bahlburg, & McKeague, 2006).

"Who Am I Emotionally?" Psychological and Emotional Well-Being

Protective Factors

A number of psychological, public health, and educational investigations have explored the protective factors that appear to help girls thrive in the face of difficulty. Several protective factors like relational resilience and media literacy have been discussed earlier in this chapter. The following list includes protective factors that have emerged in the literature and which are relevant to those working with teens and young women:

- *Relational Resilience and Resistance*: Relationships are vital for girls' psychological well-being and growth (Armstrong & Boothroyd, 2007; Jordan, 2005). Girls also benefit from the capacity to resist damaging stereotypes and negative messages about gender, race, class, and sexual orientation. "To the extent that girls feel they are part of mutually growth-fostering relationships in which they care about others and are cared about as well, they will experience a sense of flexibility, worth, clarity, creativity, zest, and the desire for more connection" (Jordan, 2005, p. 85).
- *Self-Awareness and Self-Management* (*Emotional Regulation*): Emotional regulation skills, particularly mindfulness, help girls and young women cope more effectively with feelings of depression, anxiety, and impulses to self-injure (Goleman, 1995; Greco et al., 2008; Hollander, 2008; Siegel, 2007).
- *Body Satisfaction and Low Levels of Self-Objectification*: Studies show that young women fare better with greater body satisfaction and less self-objectification (Barker & Galambos, 2003).
- *Social Agency and Self-Efficacy*: Developing an internal focus of control and sense of social agency is good for girls (Armstrong & Boothroyd, 2007; Brown, 2003; Ward, 2002).
- *Positive Gender Identification*: Determining ways to help girls feel good about being a girl and providing them with positive role models of womanhood is vital (Taylor, Gilligan, & Sullivan, 1995).
- *Positive Cultural Identity*: Helping girls develop a positive cultural identity has been shown to be important for overall psychological well-being (Fordham, 1993; Fullwood, 2001; Taylor et al., 1995).
- *Self-Esteem, Self-Respect, and Self-Compassion*: Currently, there are interesting discussions in the literature about these three constructs. The research on self-respect and on self-compassion both suggests that these constructs may be more

useful than self-esteem when thinking about girls' development. While that debate continues, it appears clear that one or all of these constructs can function as protective factors in girls' lives (Neff, 2011).
- *Future Orientation*: The capacity to envision a positive future has been considered a long-standing protective factor for girls' psychological health (Fullwood, 2001).
- *Awareness, Accurate Knowledge and Skills Regarding Health, Including Sexual and Reproductive Health*: Access to accurate information and effective skills for self-care and self-determination is important (Fullwood, 2001).

Common Psychological Issues Facing Teen Girls Today

Despite the trend to identify a biological base for all mental health issues, there is extensive research to support the notion that external factors contribute to adolescent girls' psychological challenges. The most common psychological issues for teen girls include:

- *Self-criticism and self-degradation*: Girls can be self-denigrating and confronted with a harsh inner critic. Classic research by Carol Dweck and her colleagues (Dweck and Goetz, 1978; Dweck and Reppucci, 1973) found that girls' expectations of future performances are affected more by past or present failures than by successes. Girls blame themselves more than boys do. While optimism plays an important role in resilience (Lyubomirsky, 2008; Seligman, 1991), girls may have a steeper slope to climb than boys in order to develop this skill.
- *Depression*: Before puberty, the prevalence of mood disorders is about the same in boys and girls—3 to 5 %. By mid-adolescence, girls are more than twice as likely to be diagnosed with a mood disorder (Jack & Ali, 2010; Nolen-Hoeksema & Girgus, 1994; Steingard, 2013). As previously noted, researchers have found correlations between depression or depressed mood and self-objectification (Grabe & Hyde, 2009).
- *Stress*: Life stressors exist on many dimensions, from poverty and lack of adult support to achievement pressure and perfectionism (Cohen-Sandler, 2006; Girls, Inc, 2006). Other common stresses include social cruelty and bullying (Mikami & Hinshaw, 2006; Orpinas & Horne, 2006), sexual harassment, and challenges related to learning disabilities. Stress can exacerbate any number of psychological and physical symptoms, including PMS and depression.
- *Body dissatisfaction and eating disorders*: Research shows that living in a culture that significantly objectifies girls puts them at risk for disliking their bodies and attempting to manipulate their bodies through dysfunctional or disordered eating (Dinsmore & Stormshak, 2003).
- *Anxiety*: One in eight children suffers from anxiety and it often co-occurs with other disorders, like depression and eating disorders. Studies show that girls self-report two to three times more worries than boys, as well as greater fear intensity (Gullone, 2000).

- *Self-injury*: Non-suicidal self-injury includes behavior like cutting, burning, picking, and hitting. It occurs more frequently in female adolescents than in males. In fact, a study of ninth grade boys and girls found that non-suicidal self-injury in girls occurred at a rate three times that of boys at the same age (Barrocas, Hankin, Young, & Abela, 2012; Hollander, 2008).
- *Posttraumatic stress disorder* (*PTSD*): Being female or an ethnic minority increases the risk of trauma and poor outcomes (Briere, 2004). Girls are vulnerable to high-impact trauma like rape, sexual and physical abuse, and dating violence. Women are twice as likely to receive a PTSD diagnosis. Girlhood trauma leads to higher risk of re-victimization and psychological and physical health problems (Worell & Goodheart, 2006).

Early intervention makes a difference in the outcomes for these young women. Prevention programs designed to build protective factors hold promise. Protective factors can help girls and young women be embodied, authentic, empowered, and relationally engaged. Development of these protective factors in adolescence supports girls as they cope with the stresses of their lives and prepares them for the challenges of adulthood.

Relational Resilience and Resistance

Providing opportunities for all girls and young women to be involved in mentorship experiences coincides with Judith Jordan's (2005) work on relational resilience. Schools are an obvious environment for providing mentorship for girls. Teachers, counselors, and older students can help girls develop protective factors and connect with their strengths. However, not all girls and young women will stay in school. This underscores the importance of additional environments, such as community programs and religious communities, that can provide support and life-skill education.

Role Models

Schools and community programs are in the unique position to shine the light on women role models. Speaker events, discussion groups, and other formats can be used to help adolescent girls connect with real women whose lives demonstrate alternatives to the idealized and unrealistic view of womanhood. Discussions of the roles of gender, race, culture, class, sexual orientation, physical ability and disability, and religion can be part of the dialogue, helping young women raise awareness about these powerful external factors that influence their individual and collective stories (American Psychological Association Task Force on the Sexualization of Girls, 2010).

Connecting with Peers

Group experiences reduce isolation, enhance identity development, and provide a place for support, skill building, and cultural critique. Group experiences can also be designed to include embodied activities as diverse as self-defense and yoga. Peer groups provide space for developing knowledge and skills for healthy relationships and dating violence prevention (Taylor, Stein, Mumford, & Woods, 2013).

Media Literacy

School- and community-wide efforts to help teens become media savvy should no longer be considered a luxury. The more education provided for parents, the more active they can be in helping girls become media smart. A positive approach to media literacy, rather than a fear-based one, can be incorporated into school curriculum, especially since research indicates the media's impact on the developing identities of girls. Some teachers and program leaders have effectively used television characters, story plots, and photography projects as springboards for educational discussions in the classroom and at home.

Intellectual training in active cultural criticism is part of effective media literacy and digital citizenship. Girls can be encouraged to creatively critique idealized images of girlhood, boyhood, womanhood, and manhood as well as messages about race and class. Girls can practice resisting the message that appearance is their most valuable commodity. They can learn to appreciate their bodies for their abilities and wisdom (Lamb & Brown, 2006; Steiner-Adair & Sjostrom, 2006). Communities can develop media awards for positive portrayals of girls as strong, competent, and non-sexualized. Communities can also recognize companies that develop gender-free toys and products (APA Task Force on the Sexualization of Girls, 2007; Ward et al., 2006).

Positive School Climate

Evaluate the Environment

A systemic evaluation of the school or program environment may reveal blatant and subtle situations that disempower or objectify girls and young women. Organizations can examine direct and indirect communication and stereotypes about gender, power, sexuality, relationships, and class. Questions to consider include:

- What are the physical resources and campus attitudes regarding menstruation and other body needs of girls?
- How does the school educate in regard to sexual harassment, and how does it respond when incidents occur?
- How does the school provide for and celebrate girls' sports when compared to boys' sports?

- How does the curriculum address the role of women in history, science, and other disciplines?
- What educational opportunities are provided for teen girls who are parenting?

The evaluation process should also consider the available social and emotional learning programs, including mindfulness education, and comprehensive sexuality education.

Comprehensive Social and Emotional Learning

A number of protective factors fall under the rubric of social and emotional learning: self-awareness, self-management of emotions, social awareness, relational skills, and responsible decision-making. Contemporary educational and neuroscience research indicate that mindfulness skills can be a major player in helping youths develop these capacities (Siegel, 2007). As suggested by Jordan (2005), girls will develop these skill sets more effectively when they are taught by those who believe in them and who can listen with heart and mind.

Comprehensive Sexuality Education

Comprehensive sexuality education goes beyond a biological emphasis and considers the relational contexts of sexuality (Martinez et al., 2010). Creative, student-centered, developmentally focused ways of teaching this content need to be encouraged. Appropriate discussions about sex and relationships can incorporate small group breakouts, case studies, role-play, storytelling, visual arts, and performance, providing students and program participants with concrete scenarios. The most effective programming for youth often includes programming for nuclear and extended families (Lefkowitz & Stoppa, 2006). Role-play, skill building, discussion, and support among parents may increase their comfort in, and skills for, talking about tough topics. In addition, some parents may benefit from the opportunity to have conversations that help them become more comfortable with their own sexual selves and to be clear about their sexual values in order to communicate more effectively with their children. Parents might also benefit from more broad-based education about protective factors, the sexualization of girls, digital citizenship, and media literacy. Parents can be encouraged to identify and establish rituals to celebrate girls' changing bodies and developmental markers, like a first period.

Health and Psychological Interventions

Research suggests that physicians, nurse practitioners, and mental health providers benefit from solid training in the following: the biopsychosocial model, confidentiality for teens, positive sexual identity development, the impact of the culture's sexualization of girls, digital life realities, teen dating violence, sexual orientation issues, common psychological challenges, and the latest research on the role of hormonal factors (APA Task Force on the Sexualization of Girls, 2007; Pinto, 2004; Steiner-Adair & Barker, 2013; Tolman, Spencer, Rosen-Reynoso, & Porche, 2003). Training for professionals can help ensure much needed early intervention, which is often neglected. For example, in one investigation (Armstrong & Boothroyd, 2007), 66.7 % of the teen girls studied exceeded the criterion on at least one mental health indicator at some point during the course of the 4-year study, indicating some level of emotional distress. In contrast, not more than 5 % reported receiving a mental health service during any year of the study.

Public Health and Policy Leaders

Policy leaders and public health advocates are in a key position to encourage both universal and selective interventions. Universal interventions apply to all individuals within the school, program, or community. Selected interventions are designed to meet the specific needs of a subgroup, like adolescent girls who self-injure or teens who are pregnant.

It can be valuable to involve youth in the policy-making process. Creating opportunities for dialogue between adolescent girls and policy makers is important. In particular, girls may contribute to conversations about teen dating violence, the sexualization of girls, and digital citizenship—all public health priorities.

Protective factors promote girls' and young women's psychological well-being and relational resilience. In addition, these factors equip girls to cope more effectively with present and future challenges. Research, school and community programming, family life resources, health and psychological interventions, and public policy all have important roles to play in ensuring that teen girls have the relationships and environments needed for positive growth.

Conclusion

Psychological and relational health is profoundly important in the lives of adolescent females. Protective factors not only serve girls during their challenging teen years, but they also fortify young women as they move into adulthood with its inevitable difficulties and stresses. Reproductive mental health in adulthood is enhanced by general psychological well-being in adolescence. In order to promote positive mental health for adolescent girls and young women, society must address intrapersonal, interpersonal, and sociocultural factors.

Research can provide insight into the diverse experiential and developmental trajectories of girls as they grow toward womanhood. It can also increase the understanding of protective factors. However, more research is needed. The literature on both sexualization and positive, healthy sexuality will be enhanced by further investigations into the diverse experiences of girls including girls of color; lesbians, bisexuals, those questioning, and transgendered girls; young women from different cultures, ethnicities, and religions; girls with disabilities; and young women from all socioeconomic groups. In addition, investigations are needed to determine:

- The various ways girls construct their attitudes, beliefs, and ideas about girlhood, womanhood, relationships, attractions, intimacy, sexuality, sexual orientation, and reproductive choices.
- Best practices for social and emotional learning for the development of protective factors.
- Effective media literacy education, including Internet literacy and digital citizenship.
- The needs of the understudied population of pregnant teens and mothers who are still in their adolescent years, including mental health needs, like postpartum mood and anxiety disorders.
- The most effective sexuality and human development education in high school, middle school, and in the elementary school years.

Further research will inform education, community programming, family life resources, health and mental health interventions, and policy in creating a world for healthy girls and women.

Resources

Sites for Teen Girls and Young Adult Women

- http://sexetc.org—This site is designed as a tool for teens and young adults seeking accurate information about sexuality and relationships.
- http://www.iwannaknow.org—Designed for teens and young adults, this website is a project of the American Sexual Health Association.
- http://www.newmoon.com—New Moon is written by, and for, girls ages 8–13 and covers a wide range of relevant and important topics.
- http://www.teenvoices.com—Teen Voices is an online resource that covers empowering topics reflecting the lives of diverse and real teen girls and young women.

Online Resources for Professionals Working with Girls and Young Women

- Girls Inc. Media Literacy (http://www.girlsinc.org/about/programs/media-literacy.html)—Content and programs can be used to enhance media literacy and resistance to damaging media messages.

- Hardy Girls, Healthy Women (http://www.hardygirlshealthywomen.org/)—This organization, founded by Lyn Mikele Brown, offers a wide range of online training resources and tangible products to support those who seek to empower girls.
- Institute for Girls' Development (http://www.instituteforgirlsdevelopment.com)—The Institute was founded by chapter author, Melissa J. Johnson, Ph.D. The articles and videos associated with this link provide information for professionals, parents, and young women on diverse and timely topics.

References

Adams, N. G. (2005). Fighters and cheerleaders: Disrupting the discourse of 'girl power' in the new millennium. In P. Bettis & N. Adams (Eds.), *Geographies of girlhood identities in between. Inquiry and pedagogy across diverse contexts* (pp. 101–114). Mahwah, NJ: Lawrence Erlbaum Associates Publishers.

Ali, R., & US Department of Education, Office for Civil Rights. (2010). *Dear colleague letter: Harassment and bullying*. Retrieved from www2.ed.gov/about/offices/list/ocr/letters/colleague-201010.pdf

American Association of University Women, & Harris Interactive (Firm). (2001). *Hostile hallways: Bullying, teasing, and sexual harassment in school*. Washington, DC: American Association of University Women Educational Foundation.

American Psychological Association, Task Force on the Sexualization of Girls. (2010). *Report of the APA task force on the sexualization of girls*. http://www.apa.org/pi/women/programs/girls/report-full.pdf

Armstrong, M., & Boothroyd, R. (2007). Predictors of emotional well-being in at-risk adolescent girls: Developing preventive intervention strategies. *The Journal of Behavioral Health Services & Research, 35*(4), 435–453.

Barker, E. T., & Galambos, N. L. (2003). Body dissatisfaction of adolescent girls and boys: Risk and resource factors. *Journal of Early Adolescence, 23*(2), 141–165.

Barrocas, A. L., Hankin, B. L., Young, J. F., & Abela, J. R. (2012). Rates of nonsuicidal self-injury in youth: Age, sex, and behavioral methods in a community sample. *Pediatrics, 130*(1), 39–45.

Bettis, P. J., Jordan, D., & Montgomery, D. (2005). Girls in groups: The preps and the sex mob try out for womanhood. In P. Bettis & N. Adams (Eds.), *Geographies of girlhood identities in between. Inquiry and pedagogy across diverse contexts* (pp. 69–84). Mahwah, NJ: Lawrence Erlbaum Associates Publishers.

Boothroyd, R. A., & Olufokunbi, D. (2001). Leaving the welfare rolls: The health and mental health status of current and former welfare recipients. *Mental Health Services Research, 3*(3), 119–128.

Briere, J. (2004). *Psychological assessment of adult posttraumatic states: Phenomenology, diagnosis, and measurement*. Washington, DC: American Psychological Association.

Brown, L. M. (2003). *Girlfighting: Betrayal and rejection among girls*. New York, NY: New York University Press.

Brown, R., & Gerbarg, P. (2005). Sudarshan kriya yogic breathing in the treatment of stress, anxiety, and depression. Part II—clinical applications and guidelines. *Journal of Alternative and Complementary Medicine, 11*(4), 711–717.

Brown, L. M., & Gilligan, C. (1992). *Meeting at the crossroads: Women's psychology and girls' development*. Cambridge, MA: Harvard University Press.

Brown, J. D., Halpern, C. T., & L'Engle, K. L. (2005). Mass media as a sexual super peer for early maturing girls. *Journal of Adolescent Health, 36*(5), 420–427.

Centers for Disease Control and Prevention. (2010). *Teen birth rates rose again in 2001, declined in 2008*. Retrieved from http://www.cdc.gov/Features/dsTeenPregnancy/

Charmaraman, L., Jones, A. E., Stein, N., & Espelage, D. L. (2013). Is it bullying or sexual harassment? Knowledge, attitudes, and professional development experiences of middle school staff. *The Journal of School Health, 83*(6), 438–444.

Charmaraman, L., & McKamey, C. (2011). Urban early adolescent narratives on sexuality: accidental and intentional influences of family, peers, and the media. *Sexuality Research and Social Policy, 8*(4), 253–266.

Choate, L. H. (2007). Counseling adolescent girls for body image resilience: Strategies for school counselors. *Professional School Counseling, 10*(3), 317–324.

Christopher, F. S. (2001). *To dance the dance: A symbolic interactional exploration of premarital sexuality*. Mahwah, NJ: Lawrence Erlbaum.

Cohen-Sandler, R. (2006). *Stressed-out girls: Helping them thrive in the age of pressure*. New York, NY: Viking.

Collins, P. H. (2000). *Black feminist thought: Knowledge, consciousness, and the politics of empowerment*. New York, NY: Routledge.

Daniels, E. A. (2009). Sex objects, athletes, and sexy athletes: How media representations of women athletes can impact adolescent girls and college women. *Journal of Adolescent Research, 24*(4), 399–422. doi:10.1177/0743558409336748.

Daubenmier, J. J. (2005). The relationship of yoga, body awareness, and body responsiveness to self-objectification and disordered eating. *Psychology of Women Quarterly, 29*(2), 207–219.

Diamond, L. M. (2006). *Rethinking positive adolescent female sexual development*. San Francisco, CA: Jossey-Bass.

Dinsmore, B. D., & Stormshak, E. A. (2003). Family functioning and eating attitudes and behaviors in at-risk early adolescent girls: The mediating role of intra personal competencies. *Current Psychology, 22*(2), 100–116.

Dweck, C., & Goetz, T. (1978). Attributions and learned helplessness. In J. H. Harvey, W. Ickes, & R. F. Kidd (Eds.), *New directions in attribution research* (Vol. 2). Hilldale, NJ: Erlbaum.

Dweck, C. S., & Reppucci, N. D. (1973). Learned helplessness and reinforcement responsibility in children. *Journal of Personality and Social Psychology, 25*(1), 109.

East, P. L., Khoo, S. T., & Reyes, B. T. (2006). Risk and protective factors predictive of adolescent pregnancy: A longitudinal, prospective study. *Applied Developmental Science, 10*(4), 188–199.

Fingerson, L. (2005a). Agency and the body in adolescent menstrual talk. *Childhood, 12*(1), 91–110.

Fingerson, L. (2005b). "Only 4 minute passing periods!" Private and public menstrual identities at school. In P. Bettis & N. Adams (Eds.), *Geographies of girlhood identities in between: Inquiry and pedagogy across diverse contexts* (pp. 115–136). Mahwah, NJ: Lawrence Erlbaum Associates Publishers.

Fordham, S. (1993). Those loud black girls: (Black) Women, Silence, and Gender "Passing" in the Academy. *Anthropology & Education Quarterly, 24*(1), 3–32.

Fredrickson, B. L., & Roberts, T. (1997). Objectification theory: Toward understanding women's lived experiences and mental health risks. *Psychology of Women, 21*(2), 173–206.

Frost, J., & Alan Guttmacher Institute. (2001). *Teenage sexual and reproductive behavior in developed countries*. New York, NY: Alan Guttmacher Institute.

Fullwood, C. (2001). *The new girls' movement: Implications for youth programs* (p. 161). New York, NY: Ms Foundation for Women. Carmen Sirianni and Diana Marginean Schor.

Girls Incorporated. (2006). *The supergirl dilemma: Girls grapple with the mounting pressures of expectations: Summary findings*. New York, NY: Girls Incorporated.

Goleman, D. (1995). *Emotional intelligence*. New York, NY: Bantam Books.

Grabe, S., & Hyde, J. S. (2009). Body objectification, MTV, and psychological outcomes among female adolescents. *Journal of Applied Social Psychology, 39*(12), 2840–2858. doi:10.1111/j.15591816.2009.00552.

Graber, J. A., Nichols, T., Lynne, S. D., Brooks-Gunn, J., & Botvin, G. J. (2006). A longitudinal examination of family, friend, and media influences on competent versus problem behaviors among urban minority youth. *Applied Developmental Science, 10*(2), 75–85.

Graber, J. A., & Sontag, L. M. (2006). Puberty and girls' sexuality: Why hormones are not the complete answer. In L. M. Diamond (Ed.), *Rethinking positive adolescent female sexual development* (pp. 23–38). San Francisco: Jossey-Bass.

Granberg, E. M., Simons, L. G., & Simons, R. L. (2009). Body size and social self-image among adolescent African American girls: The moderating influence of family racial socialization. *Youth & Society, 41*(2), 256–277. doi:10.1177/0044118X09338505.

Greco, L. A., Barnett, E. R., Blomquist, K. K., & Gevers, A. (2008). Acceptance, body image, and health in adolescence. In L. A. Greco & S. C. Hayes (Eds.), *Acceptance and mindfulness treatment for children and adolescents: A practitioner's guide*. Oakland, CA: New Harbinger Publications.

Grumbach, M. M., & Styne, D. M. (1998). Puberty: Ontogeny, neuroendocrinology, physiology, and disorders. In J. D. Wilson, D. W. Fostor, H. M. Kronenberg, & P. R. Larsen (Eds.), *Williams textbook of endocrinology* (pp. 1509–1625). Philadelphia, PA: Sanders.

Gullone, E. (2000). The development of normal fear: A century of research. *Clinical Psychology Review, 20*(4), 429–451.

Halpern, C. T. (2006). Integrating hormones and other biological factors into a developmental systems model of adolescent female sexuality. In L. M. Diamond (Ed.), *Rethinking positive adolescent female sexual development* (pp. 9–22). San Francisco: Jossey-Bass.

Hirschman, C., Impett, E. A., & Schooler, D. (2006). Disembodied voices: What late adolescent girls can teach us about objectification and sexuality. *Sexuality Research & Social Policy, 3*(4), 8–20. doi:10.1525/srsp.2006.3.4.8.

Hollander, M. (2008). *Helping teens who cut: Understanding and ending self-injury*. New York, NY: Guilford Press.

Impett, E. A., Schooler, D., & Tolman, D. L. (2006). To be seen and not heard: Femininity, ideology, and adolescent girls' sexual health. *Archives of Sexual Behavior, 35*(2).

Jack, D. C., & Ali, A. (2010). *Silencing the self across cultures: Depression and gender in the social world*. Oxford: Oxford University Press.

Jordan, J. (2005). Relational resilience in girls. In S. Goldstein & R. B. Brooks (Eds.), *Handbook of resilience in children* (pp. 79–90). New York, NY: Kluwer Academic/Plenum Publishers.

Kim, J. L., Lynn, S. C., Collins, K., Zylbergold, B. A., Schooler, D., & Tolman, D. L. (2007). From sex to sexuality: Exposing the heterosexual script on primetime network television. *Journal of Sex Research, 44*(2), 145–157.

Lalik, R., & Oliver, K. L. (2005). "The beauty walk" as a social space for messages about the female body: Toward transformative collaboration. In P. Bettis & N. Adams (Eds.), *Geographies of girlhood identities in between. Inquiry and pedagogy across diverse contexts* (pp. 85–100). Mahwah, NJ: Lawrence Erlbaum Associates Publishers.

Lamb, S., & Brown, L. M. (2006). *Packaging girlhood: Rescuing our daughters from marketers schemes*. New York, NY: Macmillan.

Larkin, J., & Rice, C. (2005). Beyond "healthy eating" and "healthy weights": Harassment and the health curriculum in middle schools. *Body Image, 2*(3), 219–232. doi:10.1016/j.bodyim.2005.07.001.

Lefkowitz, E. S., & Espinosa-Hernandez, G. (2007). Sex-related communication with mothers and close friends during the transition to university. *Journal of Sex Research, 44*(1), 17–27.

Lefkowitz, E. S., & Stoppa, T. M. (2006). Positive sexual communication and socialization in the Parent-Adolescent context. In L. M. Diamond (Ed.), *Rethinking positive adolescent female sexual development* (pp. 39–56). San Francisco: Jossey-Bass.

Lemish, D. (1998). Spice Girls talk: A case study in the development of gendered identity. In S. Inness (Ed.), *Millennium girls: Today's girls around the world*. Lanham, MD: Rowman & Littlefield.

Levine, P. A., & Kline, M. (2007). *Trauma through a child's eyes: Awakening the ordinary miracle of healing*. Berkeley, CA: North Atlantic Books.

Lyubomirsky, S. (2008). *The how of happiness: A scientific approach to getting the life you want*. New York, NY: Penguin Press.

Martinez, G., Abma, J. C., Copen, C. E., & National Center for Health Statistics (U.S.). (2010). *Educating teenagers about sex in the United States*. Hyattsville, MD: U.S. Department of Health and Human Services.

Mikami, A. Y., & Hinshaw, S. P. (2006). Resilient adolescent adjustment among girls: Buffers of childhood peer rejection and attention-deficit/hyperactivity disorder. *Journal of Abnormal Child Psychology, 34*(6), 825–839.

Neff, K. (2011). *Self-compassion: Stop beating yourself up and leave insecurity behind*. New York, NY: Harper Collins.

Nolen-Hoeksema, S., & Girgus, J. S. (1994). The emergence of gender differences in depression during adolescence. *Psychological Bulletin, 115*(3), 424–443.

O'Sullivan, L. F. (2005). The social and relationship contexts and cognitions associated with romantic and sexual experiences of early adolescent girls. *Sexuality Research & Social Policy, 2*(3), 13–24. doi:10.1525/srsp.2005.2.3.13.

Orenstein, P., & American Association of University Women. (1994). *Schoolgirls: Young women, self-esteem, and the confidence gap*. New York, NY: Doubleday.

Orpinas, P., & Horne, A. (2006). *Bullying prevention: Creating a positive school climate and developing social competence*. Washington, DC: American Psychological Association.

O'Sullivan, L. F., Meyer-Bahlburg, H. F. L., & McKeague, I. W. (2006). The development of the sexual self-concept inventory for early adolescent girls. *Psychology of Women Quarterly, 30*(2), 139–149. doi:10.1111/j.1471 6402.2006.00277.x.

Pearson, M. R., Kholodkov, T., Henson, J. M., & Impett, E. A. (2012). Pathways to early coital debut for adolescent girls: A recursive partitioning analysis. *Journal of Sex Research, 49*(1), 13–26. doi:10.1080/00224499.2011.565428.

Petrovic, J. E., & Ballard, R. M. (2005). Unstraightening the ideal girl: Lesbians, high school, and spaces to be. In P. Bettis & N. Adams (Eds.), *Geographies of girlhood: Identities in between* (pp. 195–209). Mahwah, NJ: Lawrence Erlbaum Associates Publishers.

Pinto, K. C. (2004). Intersections of gender and age in health care: Adapting autonomy and confidentiality for the adolescent girl. *Qualitative Health Research, 14*(1), 78–99.

Pipher, M. B. (1995). *Reviving Ophelia: Saving the selves of adolescent girls*. New York, NY: Ballantine Books.

Prettyman, S. S. (2005). "We ain't no dogs": Teenage mothers (re)define themselves. In P. Bettis & N. Adams (Eds.), *Geographies of girlhood: Identities in between* (pp. 155–176). Mahwah, NJ: Lawrence Erlbaum Associates Publishers.

Resnick, M. D., Bearman, P. S., Blum, R. W., Bauman, K. E., Harris, K. M., Jones, J., Udry, J.R. (1997). Protecting adolescents from harm. Findings from the National Longitudinal Study on Adolescent Health. *JAMA: The Journal of the American Medical Association, 278*(10), 823–832.

Ricciardelli, L. A., McCabe, M. P., Holt, K. E., & Finemore, J. (2003). A biopsychosocial model for understanding body image and body change strategies among children. *Journal of Applied Developmental Psychology, 24*(4), 475–495.

Rosenthal, D. A., & Feldman, S. S. (1999). The importance of importance: Adolescents' perceptions of parental communication about sexuality. *Journal of Adolescence, 22*(6), 835–851.

Savin-Williams, R. C. (2007). Girl on girl sexuality. In B. Leadbeater & N. Way (Eds.), *Urban girls revisited: Building strengths* (pp. 301–318). New York, NY: New York University Press.

Schoenberg, J., Salmond, K., & Fleshman, P. (2008). *Change it up! What girls say about redefining leadership*. New York, NY: Girl Scouts of the USA.

Seligman, M. E. P. (1991). *Learned optimism*. New York, NY: A.A. Knopf.

Sexuality Information and Education Council of the United States, Hafner, D. (Ed.) (1995). *Facing the Facts: Sexual Health for America's Adolescents*. National Commission on Adolescent Sexual Health,. Retrieved from http://eric.ed.gov/?id=ED391779

Siegel, D. J. (2007). *The mindful brain: Reflections and attunement in the cultivation of well-being*. New York, NY: W.W. Norton & Co.

Simanski, J. W. (1998). The birds and the bees: An analysis of advice given to parents through the popular press. *Adolescence, 33*(129), 33–45.

Simmons, R. (2009). *The curse of the good girl: Raising authentic girls with courage and confidence*. New York, NY: Penguin.

Slater, A., & Tiggemann, M. (2002). A test of objectification theory in adolescent girls. *Sex Roles, 46*(9–10), 343–349.

Smith, P. H., White, J. W., & Holland, L. J. (2003). A longitudinal perspective on dating violence among adolescent and college-age women. *American Journal of Public Health, 93*(7), 1104–1109.

Stein, N. (1995). Sexual harassment in school: The public performance of gendered violence. *Harvard Educational Review, 65*(2), 145–163.

Stein, N. D. (1997). *Bullying and sexual harassment in elementary schools: It isn't just kids kissing kids*. Washington, DC: Center for Research on Women.

Steiner-Adair, C., & Barker, T. H. (2013). *The big disconnect: Protecting childhood and family relationships in the digital age*. New York, NY: Harper Collins.

Steiner-Adair, C., & Sjostrom, L. (2006). *Full of ourselves: A wellness program to advance girl power, health, and leadership*. New York, NY: Teachers College Press.

Steingard, R. J. (2013). Mood disorders and teenage girls. *Child Mind Institute*, Retrieved from http://www.childmind.org/en/posts/articles/2013-1-22-mood-disorders-teenage-girlsanxietydepression

Stokes, C. E. (2007). Representin' in cyberspace: Sexual scripts, self-definition, and hip-hop culture in black American adolescent girls' home pages. *Culture, Health & Sexuality, 9*(2), 169–184. doi:10.1080/13691050601017512.

Strahan, E. J., Lafrance, A., Wilson, A. E., Ethier, N., Spencer, S. J., & Zanna, M. P. (2008). Victoria's dirty secret: How sociocultural norms influence adolescent girls and women. *Personality and Social Psychology Bulletin, 34*(2), 288–301. doi:10.1177/0146167207310457.

Sutton, M. J., Brown, J. D., Wilson, K. M., & Klein, J. D. (2002). Shaking the tree of knowledge for forbidden fruit: Where adolescents learn about sexuality and contraception. In J. D. Brown, J. R. Steele, & K. Walsh-Childers (Eds.), *Sexual teens, sexual media: Investigating media's influence on adolescent sexuality* (pp. 22–58). Mahwah, NJ: Lawrence Erlbaum.

Taylor, B. G., Stein, N. D., Mumford, E. A., & Woods, D. (2013) Shifting Boundaries: an experimental evaluation of a dating violence prevention program in middle schools. *Prevention science: the official journal of the Society for Prevention Research, 14*(1):64–76. doi: 10.1007/s11121-012-0293-2

Taylor, J. M. L., Gilligan, C., & Sullivan, A. M. (1995). *Between voice and silence: Women and girls, race and relationship*. Cambridge, MA: Harvard University Press.

Tiggemann, M., & Lynch, J. E. (2001). Body image across the life span in adult women: The role of self-objectification. *Developmental Psychology, 37*(2), 243.

Tolman, D. L. (2002). *Dilemmas of desire: Teenage girls talk about sexuality*. Cambridge, MA: Harvard University Press.

Tolman, D. L., Spencer, R., Rosen-Reynoso, M., & Porche, M. V. (2003). Sowing the seeds of violence in heterosexual relationships: Early adolescents narrate compulsory heterosexuality. *Journal of Social Issues, 59*(1), 159–178.

Tolman, D., Striepe, M., & Harmon, T. (2003). Gender matters: Constructing a model of adolescent sexual health. *Journal of Sex Research, 40*(1), 4–12.

Underwood, M. (2003). *Social aggression among girls*. New York, NY: Guilford Press.

Vichnin, M., Freeman, E. W., Lin, H., Hillman, J., & Bui, S. (2006). Premenstrual syndrome (PMS) in adolescents: Severity and impairment. *Journal of Pediatric and Adolescent Gynecology, 19*(6), 397–402.

Ward, J. V. (2002). *The skin we're in: Teaching our children to be emotionally strong, socially smart, spiritually connected*. New York, NY: Simon & Schuster.

Ward, L. M., Day, K. M., & Epstein, M. (2006). Uncommonly good: Exploring how mass media may be a positive influence on young women's sexual health and development. In L. M. Diamond (Ed.), *Rethinking positive adolescent female sexual development* (pp. 57–70). San Francisco: Jossey-Bass.

Worell, J., & Goodheart, C. D. (2006). *Handbook of girls' and women's psychological health*. New York, NY: Oxford University Press.

World Health Organization. (1975). *Education and treatment in human sexuality: The training of health professionals*. Geneva: World Health Organization.

Zaslow, E. (2009). *Feminism, Inc: Coming of age in girl power media culture*. New York, NY: Palgrave Macmillan.

Menstruation and Premenstrual Dysphoric Disorder: Its Impact on Mood

C. Neill Epperson and Liisa Hantsoo

Introduction

In the premenstruum, many women experience symptoms such as fatigue, irritability, bloating, or breast tenderness (Angst, Sellaro, Merikangas, & Endicott, 2001; Borenstein, Chiou, Dean, Wong, & Wade, 2005; Borenstein et al., 2003). Approximately 3–8 % of women have a constellation of symptoms that are severe enough to result in decreased function in daily routine, work, or leisure activities, classified as Premenstrual Dysphoric Disorder (PMDD) (Epperson et al., 2012; Halbreich, Borenstein, Pearlstein, & Kahn, 2003; Wittchen, Becker, Lieb, & Krause, 2002; Yang et al., 2008); however, relatively little is known about biopsychological contributors to premenstrual symptoms. Recent literature has examined the potential roles of factors, such as stress or hormonal changes in the etiology or exacerbation of premenstrual symptoms. The relationships among stress, physiological factors, and psychological factors are complex, and further research is needed to unravel the biological underpinnings of premenstrual disorders (PMDs). This chapter provides an overview of the menstrual cycle, describes premenstrual disorders and their clinical presentation and impact, outlines potential biological underpinnings of these disorders, and discusses these disorders in the context of the female life span.

C.N. Epperson, M.D. (✉) • L. Hantsoo, Ph.D.
Penn Center for Women's Behavioral Wellness, Perelman School of Medicine,
University of Pennsylvania, Philadelphia, PA, USA
e-mail: cepp@mail.med.upenn.edu; LiisaHantsoo@gmail.com

The Menstrual Cycle

The human menstrual cycle is roughly 28 days and includes the follicular phase, ovulation, and luteal phase. The cycle begins with the first day of menstruation, commonly considered the onset of the follicular phase as ovarian follicles mature, producing a dominant follicle to be released at ovulation, approximately day 14. As ovarian follicles mature, they produce estrogen and the uterine lining thickens. Of the three estrogens produced by the ovary (17β-estradiol, estrone and estriol), 17β-estradiol is the most potent and well-studied estrogen with respect to mood and cognition (Amin, Canli, & Epperson, 2005). Around day 14 of the cycle, follicle stimulating hormone (FSH) and lutenizing hormone (LH) levels spike, triggering the dominant follicle to release its ovum. Following ovulation, the dominant follicle atrophies; it is then referred to as the corpus luteum, and produces progesterone. During the luteal phase, days 15–28, progesterone readies the uterine lining for implantation of a fertilized egg. If implantation has not occurred, the corpus luteum disintegrates, resulting in a large decrease in progesterone and estrogen. With these rapid decreases in estrogen and progesterone, the uterine lining is no longer supported, and menstruation begins again, allowing shedding of the uterine lining. In a typical menstrual cycle, progesterone (and thus its metabolite, allopregnanolone, ALLO) levels are low during the follicular phase. Progesterone rises through the luteal phase and then drops rapidly prior to menstruation. Estrogen rises through the follicular phase, peaks just prior to ovulation, drops, and then has a smaller rise in the luteal phase.

Many women experience physical or mood symptoms premenstrually. The most common physical symptoms are breast tenderness and bloating (Hartlage, Freels, Gotman, & Yonkers, 2012). The premenstrual phase may also exacerbate preexisting physical conditions such as epilepsy, migraines, or asthma, to name a few (Bazán, Montenegro, Cendes, Min, & Guerreiro, 2005; Haggerty, Ness, Kelsey, & Waterer, 2003; Sacco, Ricci, Degan, & Carolei, 2012). For instance, some women with migraines experience headaches only in the perimenstrual period while others may have a clustering of symptoms during this time. When these physical symptoms are accompanied by mood or behavioral changes, and are severe enough to interfere with daily functioning, it may be indicative of a more severe syndrome referred to as PMDD.

The Premenstrual Disorders

The PMDs include PMDD, premenstrual syndrome (PMS), and premenstrual exacerbation (PME) of ongoing psychiatric disorders, such as dysthymia and major depressive disorder (O'Brien et al., 2011). PMDs are characterized by physical and mood symptoms that initiate during the luteal phase, resolve during menses, and are absent in the postmenstrual week (Epperson et al., 2012; Halbreich, 2004).

Symptoms are both physical and cognitive-emotional. These disorders occur on a continuum of severity. PMDD, the more severe of the PMDs, is characterized by perimenstrual pattern of at least five physical, emotional, and/or behavioral symptoms. PMS is characterized by at least one mood or physical symptom but less than five overall symptoms. Both PMDs may have significant impact on daily function. In a study of over 4,000 women from 19 different countries, those with moderate to severe premenstrual symptoms showed increased absenteeism and decreased productivity at work (Heinemann, Minh, Heinemann, Lindemann, & Filonenko, 2012). While these disorders have long been recognized colloquially (Lurie & Borenstein, 1990), it was not until recently that formal diagnostic criteria were proposed.

The American Psychiatric Association (APA) first recognized PMDs as late luteal phase dysphoric disorder, LLPDD, and published as a set of criteria in the *Diagnostic and Statistical Manual of Mental Disorders, 3rd Edition* (*DSM-III*) appendix for diagnoses requiring further research (APA, 2000). The syndrome was renamed premenstrual dysphoric disorder in the *DSM-IV* (APA, 1994) but continued to be relegated to the appendices. In 2012, a committee of international experts on the pathophysiology and treatment of PMDD submitted to the APA DSM-5 Executive Committee a review of the state of the science regarding PMDD and with their recommendation for its inclusion in the DSM-5 as a full diagnostic category. Various bodies including the American College of Obstetricians and Gynecologists and the World Health Organization (ACOG, 2001; WHO, 2004) have also published descriptions of PMDs. Recently, attempts have been made to distinguish between typical mild premenstrual symptoms versus more severe symptoms present in PMDs (Epperson et al., 2012; O'Brien et al., 2011). Here, we will describe diagnostic criteria for both PMDD and PMS, including differential diagnosis.

Premenstrual Dysphoric Disorder

PMDD is characterized by mood and physical symptoms that are present in the luteal phase of the menstrual cycle, abate within a few days of onset of menstruation, and are absent in the postmenstrual week (Epperson et al., 2012). These symptoms must include at least one mood symptom, such as mood lability, irritability, anxiety/tension, or low mood. Other symptoms include decreased interest in usual activities, difficulty concentrating, low energy, appetite changes or food cravings, insomnia or hypersomnia, sense of overwhelm, and physical symptoms, such as breast tenderness, headaches, muscle or joint pain, or bloating. Per DSM-IV-TR guidelines, the symptoms must impair function (e.g., in social or occupational settings) and cannot merely be an exacerbation of another disorder. The DSM-5 criteria also allows for distress to be considered in addition to impairment in function, as many women report functioning at a relatively high level despite severe and distressing symptoms. Finally, symptoms must be confirmed via prospective daily ratings during at least two menstrual cycles (DSM-IV-TR & DSM-5) and be present for most menstrual cycles in the previous year.

In addition to the symptoms above, the woman should be assessed for other disorders that may better explain her symptoms, such as major depressive disorder, bipolar affective disorder, or dysthymia. In fact, PMDD is distinct from major depressive disorder and dysthymia as PMDD tends to be characterized by mood lability, irritability, anger, and/or anxiety as opposed to low mood (Angst et al., 2001; Epperson et al., 2012; Freeman et al., 2011; Landén & Eriksson, 2003). PMDD-associated symptoms are entrained to the menstrual cycle, distinguishing PMDD from bipolar and seasonal affective disorders. The clinician should also rule out medical causes, such as chronic fatigue syndrome, fibromyalgia, anemia, and migraine disorder. Although a presumptive diagnosis of PMDD can be made based upon history alone, prospective daily ratings can be invaluable in ruling out other psychiatric disorders, which may worsen premenstrually but be present to some extent throughout the menstrual cycle. The Daily Record of Severity of Problems (Endicott, Nee, & Harrison, 2006) the Calendar of Premenstrual Experiences (Feuerstein & Shaw, 2002) and the Premenstrual Assessment Form (Allen, McBride, & Pirie, 1991) are commonly used self-report questionnaires for the confirmation of PMDD diagnosis.

Premenstrual Syndrome

While PMDD represents severe symptomatology, premenstrual syndrome (PMS) represents a milder form of premenstrual symptomatology. Lay understanding of PMS may confuse normal menstrual cycle symptoms with clinically diagnosable PMS. Per American College of Obstetrics and Gynecology (ACOG) criteria, PMS diagnosis requires one physical or psychological symptom in the 5 days prior to menses (ACOG, 2001). Physical symptoms may include breast tenderness, abdominal bloating, headache, or swelling, and psychological symptoms may include depressed mood, angry outbursts, irritability, anxiety, confusion, or social withdrawal. The symptoms must occur in three consecutive menstrual cycles and must subside within 4 days of menses onset. As in PMDD, the symptom(s) must cause significant impairment, and must be verified by prospective rating for diagnosis.

Premenstrual Exacerbation

Among women with affective disorders, some experience worsening of their affective symptoms in the premenstruum. Analysis of data from the NIMH Sequenced Treatment Alternatives to Relieve Depression (STAR*D) study has provided important information on this phenomenon. In a subsample of premenopausal women with major depressive disorder (MDD) from this study, around 65 % reported premenstrual exacerbation of their depressive symptoms (Haley et al., 2013; Kornstein et al., 2005). This is also reflected in community samples, in which nearly 60 % of women in a major depressive episode experienced worsening of at least one affective symptom premenstrually (Hartlage, Brandenburg, & Kravitz, 2004).

There is also some evidence of premenstrual exacerbation of anxiety disorders, such as panic disorder, generalized anxiety disorder, and social anxiety (Hsiao, Hsiao, & Liu, 2004; van Veen, Jonker, van Vliet, & Zitman, 2009), but further research is needed (Nillni, Toufexis, & Rohan, 2011). Some have proposed that PMDs are more similar to anxiety disorders than to depressive disorders, based on their clinical features and biological profiles (Landén & Eriksson, 2003; Yonkers, 1997).

Etiology

While the etiology of the PMDs is still under investigation, it is apparent that these disorders are biologically driven and are not simply psychological or cultural phenomena. PMDD is found in women worldwide (Dambhare, Wagh, & Dudhe, 2012; Hamaideh, Al-Ashram, & Al-Modallal, 2013; Heinemann et al., 2012; Hong et al., n.d.; Schatz, Hsiao, & Liu, 2012; Takeda, Tasaka, Sakata, & Murata, 2006; Wittchen et al., 2002), indicating a biological basis. It is likely that a combination of biological factors, such as hormonal or genetic factors, as well as environmental factors, such as stress, contribute to the mood changes observed in the premenstruum. The timing of symptom onset and offset in PMDD suggests that hormonal fluctuation plays a key role in PMDD's pathogenesis. Evidence suggests that women with PMDs have altered central nervous system (CNS) sensitivity to normal hormonal fluctuations, particularly estrogen and progesterone (Cunningham, Yonkers, O'Brien, & Eriksson, 2009a; Schmidt, Nieman, Danaceau, Adams, & Rubinow, 1998). Here, we discuss several possible mechanisms for the altering of mood in the premenstruum.

CNS Sensitivity to Hormonal Fluctuations

Progesterone, Allopregnanolone

Progesterone, along with its main metabolite, allopregnanolone (ALLO), levels are low during menses and the remainder of the follicular phase. Following ovulation, progesterone and ALLO rise through the luteal phase, then drop rapidly prior to menstruation. In general, studies examining levels of ovarian steroid hormones and ALLO have not observed a significant difference between women with or without PMDD or PMS providing further evidence for the "hormonal sensitivity" theory for the etiology of PMDs (Hsiao, Liu, & Hsiao, 2004; Reame, Marshall, & Kelch, 1992; Rubinow et al., 1988; Thys-Jacobs, McMahon, & Bilezikian, 2008; Wang, Seippel, Purdy, & Bäckström, 1996). Chronic exposure followed by rapid withdrawal from ovarian hormones may be a key factor in the etiology of PMDD. In an animal model of PMDD based on progesterone withdrawal, rats in withdrawal from physiological doses of progesterone exhibited social withdrawal and anhedonia, symptoms characteristic of PMDD (Li, Pehrson, Budac, Sánchez, & Gulinello, 2012). Indeed, preclinical research demonstrates that chronic progesterone exposure followed by rapid withdrawal is associated with increased anxiety behavior and alterations in GABA-A receptor function (Gallo & Smith, 1993; Li et al., 2012; Schneider & Popik, 2009; Smith, Poschman, Cavaleri, Howell, & Yonkers, 2006) (Gulinello, Gong, & Smith, 2002; Gulinello, Orman, & Smith, 2003). This may be mediated by progesterone's main metabolite, ALLO.

ALLO, similar to alcohol or benzodiazepines, is a positive allosteric modulator of the $GABA_A$ receptor (Majewska, Harrison, Schwartz, Barker, & Paul, 1986), meaning that is has anxiolytic, anesthetic, and sedative properties (Sundström & Bäckström, 1998a; Timby et al., 2006). Accordingly, higher ALLO levels in the luteal phase are associated with lower arousal scores on the Profile of Mood States (POMS) (de Wit & Rukstalis, 1997). The short-acting benzodiazepine triazolam produced increased arousal among women with the highest luteal ALLO levels, suggesting tolerance to GABAergic neuromodulators (de Wit & Rukstalis, 1997). Whether this arousal effect holds for other short-acting benzodiazepines, such as alprazolam or oxazepam, is unknown. Women with PMS had reduced sedation response to the short-acting midazolam in the luteal phase (Sundström, Nyberg, & Bäckström, 1997), and PMD treatment studies with the short-acting alprazolam failed to show strong results (Evans, Haney, Levin, Foltin, & Fischman, 1998; Freeman, 2004). Women with PMS do show insensitivity to benzodiazepines (Sundström, Ashbrook, & Bäckström, 1997) suggesting that cross-tolerance may have developed between benzodiazepine and ALLO, both of which act via GABA receptors. Proton magnetic resonance spectroscopy (^{1}H-MRS) research indicates altered GABAergic response across the menstrual cycle in women with PMDD versus healthy controls (Epperson et al., 2002). A transcranial magnetic stimulation (TMS) study suggested that women with PMDD had reduced inhibition in the luteal phase compared to healthy controls (Smith, Adams, Schmidt, Rubinow, & Wassermann, 2003). Saccadic eye velocity (SEV), which is reduced by $GABA_A$ receptor agonists such as benzodiazepines, is reduced to a greater degree in healthy controls during the luteal phase (high ALLO levels) than in the luteal phase of women with PMDD (Sundström & Bäckström, 1998a). This reduced inhibition is suggestive of reduced GABAergic function. SSRI treatment reversed the purported sub-sensitivity to ALLO in women with PMDD, as SEV increased after treatment (Sundström & Bäckström, 1998b). These data provide further evidence of suboptimal luteal phase $GABA_A$ receptor sensitivity to neurosteroid modulation in women with PMDD.

Estrogens

Estrogens may also play a role, particularly in their role as mediators of serotonergic (5-HT) function (Watson, Alyea, Cunningham, & Jeng, 2010). During the luteal phase, women with PMDD exhibit low mood, craving and ingestion of specific foods, and impaired cognitive performance, all cognitive-affective features that may be influenced by serotonin (5-HT) (Reed, Levin, & Evans, 2008). Broadly, estrogen acts as a 5-HT agonist (Lokuge, Frey, Foster, Soares, & Steiner, 2010; Sherwin & Suranyi-Cadotte, 1990). Animal research indicates that ovarian steroid administration alters expression of the 5-HT$_{2A}$ receptor and serotonin transporter (SERT) genes (Fink, Sumner, McQueen, Wilson, & Rosie, 1998; McQueen, Wilson, & Fink, 1997), and the vesicular monoamine transporter (Rehavi, Goldin, Roz, & Weizman, 1998). Estrogen administration increased serotonin transporter mRNA in rodents within 16 h, with a 50 % increase in SERT sites in brain areas involved with emotion and behavior (McQueen et al., 1997). Conversely, low estrogen states were associated with decreased SERT gene expression (Bertrand et al., 2005; Maswood, Truitt, Hotema, Caldarola-Pastuszka, & Uphouse, 1999).

Given the CNS sensitivity model of PMDs (Schmidt et al., 1998), and estrogens' effects on the 5-HT system, it is feasible that women with PMDs are more sensitive to the effects of estrogens on 5-HT. Among healthy women, the number of 5-HT transporter platelet binding sites were lowest during the midluteal phase, and binding to platelet 5-HT transporter was significantly higher in the late follicular phase (Wihlbäck et al., 2004). Women with PMDs exhibit specific 5-HT abnormalities that are particularly apparent in the luteal phase, when estrogen is low. Clinical studies have found that women with PMS have a deficiency in whole blood 5-HT during the luteal phase, compared to non-PMS controls (Rapkin et al., 1987). Women with PMS showed blunted 5-HT production in response to L-tryptophan challenge during the luteal phase, but not during the follicular phase (Rasgon, McGuire, Tanavoli, Fairbanks, & Rapkin, 2000). Tryptophan depletion, which affects 5-HT synthesis, resulted in aggravation of premenstrual symptoms (Menkes, Coates, & Fawcett, 1994).

Genetics

There is evidence of heritability of premenstrual symptoms not accounted for by family environment (Jahanfar, Lye, & Krishnarajah, 2011; Kendler, Karkowski, Corey, & Neale, 1998; Treloar, Heath, & Martin, 2002; van den Akker, Stein, Neale, & Murray, 1987), suggesting a genetic component to PMDD; however, which genes are involved is a broader question that is still being investigated. Research to date has implicated some estrogen and 5-HT related genes. Polymorphisms in genes coding for sex steroid hormone receptors, such as estrogen receptor alpha (ESR1), may confer differential sensitivity or response to hormones. Single nucleotide polymorphisms in the ESR1 gene are associated with PMDD in preliminary research (Huo et al., 2007). A polymorphism of the *5HT$_{1A}$* gene has been associated with reduced 5-HT neurotransmission and major depression, and has recently been found to be associated with PMDD (Dhingra et al., 2007). The serotonin transporter gene length polymorphism (*5-HTTLPR*) *s* allele has been associated with reduced transcriptional efficiency of SERT, and has been associated with certain psychological features in women with PMDD (Gingnell, Comasco, Oreland, Fredrikson, & Sundström-Poromaa, 2010), but has not been associated with PMDD itself (Magnay, El-Shourbagy, Fryer, O'Brien, & Ismail, 2010; Magnay et al., 2006).

Stress

While there is likely a genetic component to PMDs, the environment must also be considered. Genetics do not operate in a vacuum, and environmental effects such as stress, hormonal fluctuation, and epigenetics likely play a role as well. History of traumatic stress has been associated with PMDD (Girdler et al., 2007; Koci & Strickland, 2007; Perkonigg, Yonkers, Pfister, Lieb, & Wittchen, 2004; Pilver, Levy, Libby, & Desai, 2011; Wittchen et al., 2002). A cross-sectional study of nearly 4,000 women found that trauma history, independent of post-traumatic stress disorder (PTSD), was associated with PMDD, although PMDD diagnosis was based on retrospective self-report (Pilver et al., 2011). Smaller studies among women seeking treatment for PMS indicated a high frequency of sexual abuse (Golding, Taylor, Menard, & King, 2000; Paddison et al., 1990). Women with a history of sexual abuse report more severe premenstrual symptomatology than those without a history of abuse (Koci & Strickland, 2007). However, other research did not find that women with PMDD had experienced greater rates of physical, emotional, or sexual abuse than the healthy controls (Segebladh et al., 2011).

In addition to past stress, current stress may also play a role. Women with PMS or PMDD were more likely to report a stressful event in the past year than women without a PMD (Potter, Bouyer, Trussell, & Moreau, 2009). Among healthy young women, those with more premenstrual symptoms reported more perceived stress (Kuczmierczyk, Labrum, & Johnson, 1992; Lustyk, Widman, & Becker Lde, 2007), and stress predicted premenstrual symptoms (Yamamoto, Okazaki, Sakamoto, & Funatsu, 2009). Women in a convenience sample with more frequent and intense premenstrual symptomatology reported greater perceived stress in the premenstruum than in the postmenstrual phase; women with lower levels of premenstrual symptomatology did not show this increase in perceived stress during the premenstrual phase (Brown & Lewis, 1993). Women with a PMD, compared to controls, perceived daily life events as more stressful during the luteal phase versus the follicular phase (Schmidt, Grover, Hoban, & Rubinow, 1990). The directionality of this relationship—whether stress promotes increased PMD symptoms, or whether increased PMD symptoms promote greater sensitivity to our perception of stress—is unclear.

Evidence suggests that early-life adversity may influence current perceived stress or stress response, perhaps via over-sensitization of the limbic-HPA axis (Girdler et al., 2007). College-aged women with an abuse history reported increased perceived stress and increased premenstrual symptoms compared to those without abuse, but perceived stress did not mediate the relationship between abuse history and premenstrual symptom severity (Lustyk et al., 2007). It is plausible that as opposed to objectively experiencing more stressors during the premenstruum, women with PMDs are more sensitive to stressors during the premenstruum. Their perception of and reaction to stress may be influenced by their affective state. Further research is needed on both affective and physiological response to stress during the premenstruum in women with PMDs.

One well-validated measure of stress response is acoustic startle. The acoustic startle response is preserved across species and provides a measure of arousal, indexed by eyeblink reflex. During the follicular phase, PMDD women did not differ from healthy controls in startle response, but in the luteal phase, PMDD women showed increased baseline startle (Epperson et al., 2007). In a similar study, PMDD women had greater arousal across the menstrual cycle compared to controls which was particularly accentuated in the luteal phase (Kask, Gulinello, Bäckström, Geyer, & Sundström-Poromaa, 2008). This suggests that women with PMDD have greater physiologic arousal during the premenstruum. Whether this increased arousal primes them for increased stress reactivity to environmental cues in the premenstruum has not yet been determined.

Cortisol response is a crucial aspect of stress response. Among healthy women, there is mixed data on variation in physiological stress response across the menstrual cycle. In studies examining cortisol response to the Trier Social Stress Test (TSST), cortisol response did not vary by menstrual cycle phase (Childs, Dlugos, & De Wit, 2010; Pico-Alfonso et al., 2007), although some studies found greater cortisol response during the luteal phase (Kirschbaum, Kudielka, Gaab, Schommer, & Hellhammer, 1999; Rohleder, Wolf, Piel, & Kirschbaum, 2003). A small number of studies have examined physiological stress variability across the menstrual cycle in PMDD women, finding lower cortisol levels during mental stress in PMDD women compared to controls (Girdler et al., 1998; Girdler, Straneva, Light, Pedersen, & Morrow, 2001), and higher baseline cortisol levels during the luteal phase (Rasgon et al., 2000). It may be that women with PMS have dysregulated cortisol response to corticotropin releasing hormone (CRH) (Facchinetti et al., 1994; Rabin et al., 1990), or altered cortisol function modulated by progesterone (Lee et al., 2012).

Brain Imaging

Imaging studies suggest differences in brain function between healthy female subjects and women with PMDD. Structurally, PMDD women had greater grey matter volume in the posterior cerebellum (Berman, London, Morgan, & Rapkin, 2013), greater grey matter density in the hippocampal cortex, and lower grey matter density in the parahippocampal cortex compared to healthy controls (Jeong, Ham, Yeo, Jung, & Joe, 2012). Not only did PMDD patients show greater prefrontal activation than healthy controls, but this correlated with degree of disability, age of onset, duration of PMDD, and differences in premenstrual and postmenstrual PMDD symptoms (Baller et al., 2013). Unlike healthy controls, women with PMDD also showed increased cerebellar activity from the follicular phase to the late luteal phase, which was correlated with worsening of mood (Rapkin et al., 2011). Women with PMDD also showed increased amygdala response to negative stimuli compared to healthy controls (Protopopescu et al., 2008). A proton magnetic resonance spectroscopy (^{1}H-MRS) study found that women with PMDD showed an increase in cortical GABA from the follicular to the luteal phases, while control women showed a decrease in cortical GABA from follicular to luteal, suggesting altered GABAergic function in PMDD (Epperson et al., 2002).

Immune Function

Depression is strongly associated with dysregulated immune function (Raison, Capuron, & Miller, 2006; Wium-Andersen, Ørsted, Nielsen, & Nordestgaard, 2013). However, there is scant research on immune function among women with PMDD and other PMDs. The luteal phase is associated with increased production of proinflammatory sIL-6R and TNF-alpha compared to the early follicular phase (O'Brien et al., 2007), and IL-6 gene expression was upregulated in the luteal phase compared to the follicular phase (Northoff et al., 2008). CRP levels vary across the menstrual cycle, and a tenfold increase in progesterone has been associated with an increase in CRP of 20–23 % (Gaskins et al., 2012; Wander, Brindle, & O'Connor, 2008). Among healthy women, serum hs-CRP was positively associated with elevated menstrual symptom scores, including mood, behavior, and physical symptoms, independent of weight and changes in circulating gonadal steroids (Puder et al., 2006). Levels of IL-6 in gingival fluid doubled from ovulation to progesterone peak (Markou, Boura, Tsalikis, Deligianidis, & Konstantinidis, 2011). In fact, some studies reveal worsening of inflammatory diseases during the premenstruum, including IBS and gingivitis (Jane, Chang, Lin, Liu, & Chen, 2011; Kane, Sable, & Hanauer, 1998; Shourie et al., 2012). Given the relationship between depression and inflammation, increased inflammatory activity in the luteal phase, and onset of PMD symptoms in the luteal phase, further study is warranted.

PMDs and the Life Span

PMDs often initiate in a woman's 20s and worsen through the mid-30s. Whether PMD symptoms worsen or improve in the menopause transition is debatable, but symptoms naturally disappear in postmenopause when hormonal fluctuations have ceased. Likewise, the lack of hormonal cyclicity during pregnancy is thought to contribute to the resolution of affective symptoms when women with PMS or PMDD become pregnant. An older cross-sectional study that focused on women with LLPDD found that premenstrual symptoms improved with age, with women ages 36–44 being less symptomatic than those 20–35 years old (Freeman, Rickels, Schweizer, & Ting, 1995). Other research indicates that premenstrual symptoms are less prevalent among women ages 45 years and older, when compared to younger women (Strine, Chapman, & Ahluwalia, 2005). However, other self-report cross-sectional research found that women aged 35–44 had more severe PMS symptoms (Tschudin, Bertea, & Zemp, 2010). It is possible that only some symptoms worsen with age, including depressed mood, feeling overwhelmed, and somatic symptoms (Sylvén, Ekselius, Sundström-Poromaa, & Skalkidou, 2013), but future longitudinal studies are needed to address this question regarding the course of PMDs with aging.

Clinical lore proposes that premenstrual mood symptoms worsen after pregnancy, and that premenstrual mood symptoms may raise the risk of postpartum depression; however, neither has been confirmed. Some premenstrual symptoms, such as irritability, decreased interest, appetite changes, and hypersomnia may increase with increasing parity (Sylvén et al., 2013), but not other symptoms. There are surprisingly few longitudinal studies on the relationship between PMS/PMDD and postpartum depression; however, a population based study found a significant concordance between retrospective self-reported premenstrual symptoms and postpartum depression (Sylvén et al., 2013). This was influenced by parity, such that multiparous women with a history of PMS or PMDD were more likely to experience postpartum depressive symptoms. Similarly, retrospective self-report of premenstrual symptoms, based on a single question, were associated with antepartum and postpartum depressive symptoms (Sugawara et al., 1997). Other research based on retrospective self-report has found similar relationships (Bloch, Rotenberg, Koren, & Klein, 2006). Both the premenstruum and postpartum are characterized by neurosteroid withdrawal, and future research may focus on determining whether this biological commonality increases risk for these disorders.

Current research has confirmed that women with premenstrual mood symptoms are more likely to have perimenopausal mood changes (Freeman, Sammel, Rinaudo, & Sheng, 2004). A longitudinal study of perimenopausal women found that premenstrual symptoms decreased with age, but that women with PMS were more likely to report perimenopausal hot flashes, depressed mood, poor sleep, and low libido than women without PMS. Estradiol fluctuation was associated with hot flashes, depressed mood, and poor sleep (Freeman et al., 2004). Retrospective self-report indicated that history of premenstrual negative affect was associated with menopausal symptoms, including vasomotor, psychological, and sexual complaints (Stone, Mazmanian, Oinonen, & Sharma, 2013). A longitudinal study of premenstrual complaints found that greater complaints were associated with a more symptomatic perimenopause symptoms, and that more symptomatic women reported more interpersonal stress, hassles, smoking, and less exercise (Morse, Dudley, Guthrie, & Dennerstein, 1998). Premenstrual complaints predicted negative mood during the menopausal transition, as did negative attitudes toward aging, menopause, and parity of one (Dennerstein, Lehert, Burger, & Dudley, 1999).

Psychosocial Factors

PMDs have been associated with a number of psychosocial features. A large sample ($n=11,648$) of cross-sectional self-report data indicates that women who reported impairing premenstrual symptoms were also more likely to report anxiety, depression, insomnia, sleepiness, pain, and were more likely to be divorced, have less education, work outside the home, smoke cigarettes, drink heavily, and be overweight or obese (Strine et al., 2005). Similar results have been found in other populations (Chuong & Burgos, 1995; Tschudin et al., 2010). PMDD has been associated with less education, history of major depressive episodes, and cigarette smoking (Cohen et al., 2002). Little research has been done on possible mechanisms among these associations, although stress is one possible causal mechanism.

PMD Treatment

Antidepressants

Pharmacotherapy is the recommended first-line treatment for PMDD, while PMS may benefit from nonmedical approaches (see below), according to the American College of Obstetricians and Gynecologists (ACOG, 2001). The selective serotonin reuptake inhibitors (SSRIs) are the gold-standard treatment for PMDD and severe mood-related PMS. Large meta-analyses of randomized clinical trials (RCTs) using continuous and luteal phase SSRI treatment reveal a sizeable effect size for continuous (standard mean difference=0.72; OR=0.28) and luteal phase (standard mean difference=0.35; OR 0.55) treatment (Brown, O' Brien, Marjoribanks, & Wyatt, 2009; Shah et al., 2008). However, some meta-analytic reviews have found small to medium effect sizes for SSRIs (Kleinstäuber, Witthöft, & Hiller, 2012), with response rates ranging from roughly 12 to 50 % (Halbreich, 2008). The clinician should consider that there are a number of side effects that may occur with SSRI use, including nausea, insomnia, and headaches, although these are typically time-limited (Brown et al., 2009).

Intermittent or Luteal Dosing

In contrast to other mood disorders, SSRIs have been shown to have a short onset of action in PMDs, taking effect within a few days or during the first cycle of treatment in most cases (Landén & Thase, 2006; Steinberg, Cardoso, Martinez, Rubinow, & Schmidt, 2012). SSRIs affect not only serotonin but also progesterone conversion to ALLO, which may explain SSRIs' rapid onset of action in PMDs. Specifically, SSRIs increase conversion of 5α-dihydroprogesterone (5α-DHP) to ALLO within minutes of exposure (Griffin & Mellon, 1999). Given this short onset of action, intermittent dosing is possible. Intermittent dosing in PMDs refers to administering the medication only during the luteal phase. In an intermittent dosing regime, a woman would take the SSRI from the time of ovulation until menstruation begins. Some studies have found intermittent dosing to be as efficacious as continuous dosing (Freeman, 2004; Kornstein, Pearlstein, Fayyad, Farfel, & Gillespie, 2006; Landén et al., 2007), although a meta-analysis found intermittent dosing was less effective than continuous dosing (Shah et al., 2008). Intermittent treatment may be particularly useful for irritability, affect lability, and mood swings, while having a weaker effect on depressed mood and somatic symptoms (Landén et al., 2007). Depressed mood and somatic symptoms may require a longer duration of SSRI treatment to show improvement.

Symptom Onset Therapy

Like intermittent dosing, symptom onset therapy involves SSRI administration only during part of the menstrual cycle. In symptom onset therapy, women take an SSRI as soon as PMD symptoms initiate and stop with menses onset. This dosing method has been examined in citalopram (Ravindran, Woods, Steiner, & Ravindran, 2007), paroxetine (Yonkers, Holthausen, Poschman, & Howell, 2006), and the serotonin/norepinephrine reuptake inhibitor (SNRI) escitalopram (Freeman, Sondheimer, Sammel, Ferdousi, & Lin, 2005). One study compared continuous, intermittent and symptom onset dosing in women with moderate to severe PMS and found that all three strategies were efficacious in reducing PMS symptoms (Kornstein et al., 2006). Further, relatively low doses (25–50 mg sertraline) were found to reduce symptoms (Kornstein et al., 2006).

Hormonal Treatment

There is minimal research evidence for the efficacy of hormonal treatment for PMDs (Cunningham et al., 2009b). Results for combined oral contraceptives have generally been negative (Bancroft & Rennie, 1993; Graham & Sherwin, 1992). A meta-analysis of studies on combined oral contraceptives containing the synthetic progestin drospirenone found that drospirenone (3 mg) plus ethinyl estradiol (20 μg) showed some benefit in reducing severe PMDD symptoms, but there was also a large placebo effect (Lopez, Kaptein, & Helmerhorst, 2012). Another set of studies on continuous dosing of levonorgestrel (90 mcg) and ethinyl estradiol (20 mcg) showed some improvement of premenstrual symptoms, but also a high placebo response rate (Freeman et al., 2012). Hormone monotherapy may be less effective than combined hormones. Meta-analyses of progesterone for PMS did not find strong evidence for progesterone use alone (Ford, Lethaby, Roberts, & Mol, 2012; Wyatt, Dimmock, Jones, Obhrai, & O'Brien, 2001), and oral micronized progesterone alone was no more effective than a placebo in treating PMS symptoms (Freeman, Rickels, Sondheimer, & Polansky, 1995). Other hormone-based interventions include gonadotropin releasing hormone (GnRH) agonists and inhibitors, which lead to postmenopausal levels of estradiol, progesterone, and ALLO. This strategy is often recommended when women continue to have troublesome symptoms or side effects with SSRI treatment. In addition, this "chemical oophorectomy" serves as a test for how a woman's PMDD symptoms would respond to a surgical menopause (Wyatt, Dimmock, Ismail, Jones, & O'Brien, 2004).

Psychotherapy

Cognitive-behavioral interventions have also been found to be helpful in reducing psychological and behavioral symptoms of PMS and PMDD. Cognitive-behavioral interventions might include modifying negative cognitions or improving coping strategies. A systematic review indicated that while SSRI was more beneficial in treating anxiety symptoms of PMDD, cognitive-behavioral therapy (CBT) was associated with increased use of cognitive-behavioral coping strategies and a shift in attribution of premenstrual symptoms (Kleinstäuber et al., 2012). CBT showed better maintenance of treatment effect at follow-up, compared to the SSRI fluoxetine (Kleinstäuber et al., 2012). Similar to SSRIs, CBT interventions produce small to medium effect sizes (Busse, Montori, Krasnik, Patelis-Siotis, & Guyatt, 2009; Kleinstäuber et al., 2012), and are superior to control conditions (Lustyk, Gerrish, Shaver, & Keys, 2009). However, it should be noted that the meta-analyses included studies in which women did not always meet *DSM* criteria for PMDD, comorbid disorders were not always excluded, and not all studies included prospective rating of premenstrual symptoms. While both pharmacologic and CBT treatment of PMDs show efficacy in symptom reduction, there appears to be no added benefit from combined treatment, based on meta-analysis (Kleinstäuber et al., 2012). For less severe PMS, ACOG recommendations include supportive therapy for PMS, although ACOG notes that supportive therapy has not been rigorously studied (ACOG, 2001). ACOG states that reassurance and informational counseling may relieve anxiety associated with milder PMS (ACOG, 2001).

Other Treatments

Less severe PMS may be managed by nonmedical treatments including relaxation training, aerobic exercise, or dietary supplementation, per ACOG guidelines (ACOG, 2001).

Future Directions

As the PMDs are unique from the major depressive disorders and may have more anxiety-like features, future research should focus on delineating the unique biological aspects of PMDs. Research might focus on the serotonergic system

(Menkes et al., 1994; Rasgon et al., 2000), neurosteroids, and the GABA system (Li et al., 2012; Turkmen, Backstrom, Wahlstrom, Andreen, & Johansson, 2011), stress response including cortisol response and acoustic startle response (Bannbers, Kask, Wikström, Risbrough, & Poromaa, 2011; Epperson et al., 2007; Kask et al., 2008; Segebladh et al., 2013), as well as immune function. Additional treatment research is also needed. As GABA may be involved in PMD pathophysiology, research on medications that impact GABA function may be beneficial. Given the PMDs' clinical features (Landén & Eriksson, 2003; Yonkers, 1997), research on cognitive-behavioral or mindfulness-based therapies focusing on irritability, anxiety, or physical symptoms in addition to low mood may be beneficial.

References

ACOG. (2001). ACOG Practice bulletin: Premenstrual syndrome. Clinical management guidelines for obstetrician-gynecologists. *International Journal of Gynecology & Obstetrics, 73*, 183–191.
Allen, S. S., McBride, C. M., & Pirie, P. L. (1991). The shortened premenstrual assessment form. *The Journal of Reproductive Medicine, 36*(11), 769–772.
Amin, Z., Canli, T., & Epperson, C. N. (2005). Effect of estrogen-serotonin interactions on mood and cognition. *Behavioral and Cognitive Neuroscience Reviews, 4*(1), 43–58. doi:10.1177/1534582305277152.
Angst, J., Sellaro, R., Merikangas, K. R., & Endicott, J. (2001). The epidemiology of perimenstrual psychological symptoms. *Acta Psychiatrica Scandinavica, 104*(2), 110–116.
APA. (1994). *Diagnostic and statistical manual of mental disorders* (4th ed.). Washington, DC: APA.
APA (2000). *Diagnostic and statistical manual of mental disorders* (4th ed., text rev.). Washington, DC: APA
Baller, E. B., Wei, S. M., Kohn, P. D., Rubinow, D. R., Alarcón, G., Schmidt, P. J., & Berman, K. F. (2013). Abnormalities of dorsolateral prefrontal function in women with premenstrual dysphoric disorder: A multimodal neuroimaging study. *The American Journal of Psychiatry, 170*(3), 305–314. doi:10.1176/appi.ajp.2012.12030385
Bancroft, J., & Rennie, D. (1993). The impact of oral contraceptives on the experience of perimenstrual mood, clumsiness, food craving and other symptoms. *Journal of Psychosomatic Research, 37*(2), 195–202.
Bannbers, E., Kask, K., Wikström, J., Risbrough, V., & Poromaa, I. S. (2011). Patients with premenstrual dysphoric disorder have increased startle modulation during anticipation in the late luteal phase period in comparison to control subjects. *Psychoneuroendocrinology, 36*(8), 1184–1192. doi:10.1016/j.psyneuen.2011.02.011.
Bazán, A. C. B., Montenegro, M. A., Cendes, F., Min, L. L., & Guerreiro, C. A. M. (2005). Menstrual cycle worsening of epileptic seizures in women with symptomatic focal epilepsy. *Arquivos de Neuro-Psiquiatria, 63*(3), 751–756. http://dx.doi.org/10.1590/S0004-282X2005000500006.
Berman, S. M., London, E. D., Morgan, M., & Rapkin, A. J. (2013). Elevated gray matter volume of the emotional cerebellum in women with premenstrual dysphoric disorder. *Journal of Affective Disorders, 146*(2), 266–271. doi:10.1016/j.jad.2012.06.038.
Bertrand, P. P., Paranavitane, U. T., Chavez, C., Gogos, A., Jones, M., & van den Buuse, M. (2005). The effect of low estrogen state on serotonin transporter function in mouse hippocampus: A behavioral and electrochemical study. *Brain Research, 1064*(1–2), 10–20. doi:10.1016/j.brainres.2005.10.018.
Bloch, M., Rotenberg, N., Koren, D., & Klein, E. (2006). Risk factors for early postpartum depressive symptoms. *General Hospital Psychiatry, 28*(1), 3–8. doi:10.1016/j.genhosppsych.2005.08.006.

Borenstein, J., Chiou, C. F., Dean, B., Wong, J., & Wade, S. (2005). Estimating direct and indirect costs of premenstrual syndrome. *Journal of Occupational and Environmental Medicine, 47*(1), 26–33.

Borenstein, J. E., Dean, B. B., Endicott, J., Wong, J., Brown, C., Dickerson, V., & Yonkers, K. A. (2003). Health and economic impact of the premenstrual syndrome. *The Journal of Reproductive Medicine, 48*(7), 515–524.

Brown, M. A., & Lewis, L. L. (1993). Cycle-phase changes in perceived stress in women with varying levels of premenstrual symptomatology. *Research in Nursing & Health, 16*(6), 423–429.

Brown, J., O' Brien, P. M. S., Marjoribanks, J., & Wyatt, K. (2009). Selective serotonin reuptake inhibitors for premenstrual syndrome. *Cochrane Database of Systematic Reviews (Online)*, (2), CD001396. doi:10.1002/14651858.CD001396.pub2

Busse, J. W., Montori, V. M., Krasnik, C., Patelis-Siotis, I., & Guyatt, G. H. (2009). Psychological intervention for premenstrual syndrome: A meta-analysis of randomized controlled trials. *Psychotherapy and Psychosomatics, 78*(1), 6–15. doi:10.1159/000162296.

Childs, E., Dlugos, A., & De Wit, H. (2010). Cardiovascular, hormonal, and emotional responses to the TSST in relation to sex and menstrual cycle phase. *Psychophysiology, 47*(3), 550–559. doi:10.1111/j.1469-8986.2009.00961.x.

Chuong, C. J., & Burgos, D. M. (1995). Medical history in women with premenstrual syndrome. *Journal of Psychosomatic Obstetrics and Gynaecology, 16*(1), 21–27.

Cohen, L. S., Soares, C. N., Otto, M. W., Sweeney, B. H., Liberman, R. F., & Harlow, B. L. (2002). Prevalence and predictors of premenstrual dysphoric disorder (PMDD) in older premenopausal women. The Harvard Study of Moods and Cycles. *Journal of Affective Disorders, 70*(2), 125–132.

Cunningham, J., Yonkers, K. A., O'Brien, S., & Eriksson, E. (2009). Update on research and treatment of premenstrual dysphoric disorder. *Harvard Review of Psychiatry, 17*(2), 120–137. doi:10.1080/10673220902891836.

Dambhare, D. G., Wagh, S. V., & Dudhe, J. Y. (2012). Age at menarche and menstrual cycle pattern among school adolescent girls in Central India. *Global Journal of Health Science, 4*(1), 105–111.

de Wit, H., & Rukstalis, M. (1997). Acute effects of triazolam in women: Relationships with progesterone, estradiol, and allopregnanolone. *Psychopharmacology, 130*(1), 69–78.

Dennerstein, L., Lehert, P., Burger, H., & Dudley, E. (1999). Mood and the menopausal transition. *The Journal of Nervous and Mental Disease, 187*(11), 685–691.

Dhingra, V., Magnay, J. L., O'Brien, P. M. S., Chapman, G., Fryer, A. A., & Ismail, K. M. K. (2007). Serotonin receptor 1A C(-1019)G polymorphism associated with premenstrual dysphoric disorder. *Obstetrics and Gynecology, 110*(4), 788–792. doi:10.1097/01.AOG.0000284448.73490.ac.

Endicott, J., Nee, J., & Harrison, W. (2006). Daily record of severity of problems (DRSP): Reliability and validity. *Archives of Women's Mental Health, 9*(1), 41–49. doi:10.1007/s00737-005-0103-y.

Epperson, C. N., Haga, K., Mason, G. F., Sellers, E., Gueorguieva, R., Zhang, W., ... Krystal, J. H. (2002). Cortical gamma-aminobutyric acid levels across the menstrual cycle in healthy women and those with premenstrual dysphoric disorder: A proton magnetic resonance spectroscopy study. *Archives of General Psychiatry, 59*(9), 851–858.

Epperson, C., Pittman, B., Czarkowski, K. A., Stiklus, S., Krystal, J. H., & Grillon, C. (2007). Luteal-phase accentuation of acoustic startle response in women with premenstrual dysphoric disorder. *Neuropsychopharmacology, 32*(10), 2190–2198. doi:10.1038/sj.npp.1301351.

Epperson, C., Steiner, M., Hartlage, S. A., Eriksson, E., Schmidt, P. J., Jones, I., & Yonkers, K. A. (2012). Premenstrual dysphoric disorder: Evidence for a new category for DSM-5. *The American Journal of Psychiatry, 169*(5), 465–475.

Evans, S. M., Haney, M., Levin, F. R., Foltin, R. W., & Fischman, M. W. (1998). Mood and performance changes in women with premenstrual dysphoric disorder: Acute effects of alprazolam. *Neuropsychopharmacology, 19*(6), 499–516. doi:10.1016/S0893-133X(98)00064-5.

Facchinetti, F., Fioroni, L., Martignoni, E., Sances, G., Costa, A., & Genazzani, A. R. (1994). Changes of opioid modulation of the hypothalamo-pituitary-adrenal axis in patients with severe premenstrual syndrome. *Psychosomatic Medicine, 56*(5), 418–422.

Feuerstein, M., & Shaw, W. S. (2002). Measurement properties of the calendar of premenstrual experience in patients with premenstrual syndrome. *The Journal of Reproductive Medicine, 47*(4), 279–289.

Fink, G., Sumner, B. E., McQueen, J. K., Wilson, H., & Rosie, R. (1998). Sex steroid control of mood, mental state and memory. *Clinical and Experimental Pharmacology & Physiology, 25*(10), 764–775.

Ford, O., Lethaby, A., Roberts, H., & Mol, B. W. J. (2012). Progesterone for premenstrual syndrome. *Cochrane Database of Systematic Reviews (Online), 3*, CD003415. doi:10.1002/14651858.CD003415.pub4.

Freeman, E. W. (2004). Luteal phase administration of agents for the treatment of premenstrual dysphoric disorder. *CNS Drugs, 18*(7), 453–468.

Freeman, E. W., Halberstadt, S. M., Rickels, K., Legler, J. M., Lin, H., & Sammel, M. D. (2011). Core symptoms that discriminate premenstrual syndrome. *Journal of Women's Health (2002), 20*(1), 29–35. doi:10.1089/jwh.2010.2161.

Freeman, E. W, Halbreich, U., Grubb, G. S., Rapkin, A. J., Skouby, S. O., Smith, L., ... Constantine, G. D. (2012). An overview of four studies of a continuous oral contraceptive (levonorgestrel 90 mcg/ethinyl estradiol 20 mcg) on premenstrual dysphoric disorder and premenstrual syndrome. *Contraception, 85*(5), 437–445. doi:10.1016/j.contraception.2011.09.010

Freeman, E. W., Rickels, K., Schweizer, E., & Ting, T. (1995). Relationships between age and symptom severity among women seeking medical treatment for premenstrual symptoms. *Psychological Medicine, 25*(2), 309–315.

Freeman, E. W., Rickels, K., Sondheimer, S. J., & Polansky, M. (1995). A double-blind trial of oral progesterone, alprazolam, and placebo in treatment of severe premenstrual syndrome. *JAMA: The Journal of the American Medical Association, 274*(1), 51–57.

Freeman, E. W., Sammel, M. D., Liu, L., Gracia, C. R., Nelson, D. B., & Hollander, L. (2004). Hormones and menopausal status as predictors of depression in women in transition to menopause. *Archives of General Psychiatry, 61*(1), 62–70. doi:10.1001/archpsyc.61.1.62.

Freeman, E. W., Sammel, M. D., Rinaudo, P. J., & Sheng, L. (2004). Premenstrual syndrome as a predictor of menopausal symptoms. *Obstetrics and Gynecology, 103*(5 Pt 1), 960–966. doi:10.1097/01.AOG.0000124804.81095.7f.

Freeman, E. W., Sondheimer, S. J., Sammel, M. D., Ferdousi, T., & Lin, H. (2005). A preliminary study of luteal phase versus symptom-onset dosing with escitalopram for premenstrual dysphoric disorder. *The Journal of Clinical Psychiatry, 66*(6), 769–773.

Gallo, M. A., & Smith, S. S. (1993). Progesterone withdrawal decreases latency to and increases duration of electrified prod burial: A possible rat model of PMS anxiety. *Pharmacology, Biochemistry, and Behavior, 46*(4), 897–904.

Gaskins, A. J., Wilchesky, M., Mumford, S. L., Whitcomb, B. W., Browne, R. W., Wactawski-Wende, J., ... Schisterman, E. F. (2012). Endogenous reproductive hormones and C-reactive protein across the menstrual cycle: The BioCycle Study. *American Journal of Epidemiology, 175*(5), 423–431. doi:10.1093/aje/kwr343

Gingnell, M., Comasco, E., Oreland, L., Fredrikson, M., & Sundström-Poromaa, I. (2010). Neuroticism-related personality traits are related to symptom severity in patients with premenstrual dysphoric disorder and to the serotonin transporter gene-linked polymorphism 5-HTTPLPR. *Archives of Women's Mental Health, 13*(5), 417–423. doi:10.1007/s00737-010-0164-4.

Girdler, S. S., Leserman, J., Bunevicius, R., Klatzkin, R., Pedersen, C. A., & Light, K. C. (2007). Persistent alterations in biological profiles in women with abuse histories: Influence of premenstrual dysphoric disorder. *Health Psychology, 26*(2), 201–213. doi:10.1037/0278-6133.26.2.201.

Girdler, S. S., Pedersen, C. A., Straneva, P. A., Leserman, J., Stanwyck, C. L., Benjamin, S., & Light, K. C. (1998). Dysregulation of cardiovascular and neuroendocrine responses to stress in premenstrual dysphoric disorder. *Psychiatry Research, 81*(2), 163–178. doi:10.1016/S0165-1781(98)00074-2

Girdler, S. S., Straneva, P. A., Light, K. C., Pedersen, C. A., & Morrow, A. L. (2001). Allopregnanolone levels and reactivity to mental stress in premenstrual dysphoric disorder. *Biological Psychiatry, 49*(9), 788–797.

Golding, J. M., Taylor, D. L., Menard, L., & King, M. J. (2000). Prevalence of sexual abuse history in a sample of women seeking treatment for premenstrual syndrome. *Journal of Psychosomatic Obstetrics and Gynaecology, 21*(2), 69–80.

Graham, C. A., & Sherwin, B. B. (1992). A prospective treatment study of premenstrual symptoms using a triphasic oral contraceptive. *Journal of Psychosomatic Research, 36*(3), 257–266.

Griffin, L. D., & Mellon, S. H. (1999). Selective serotonin reuptake inhibitors directly alter activity of neurosteroidogenic enzymes. *Proceedings of the National Academy of Sciences of the United States of America, 96*(23), 13512–13517.

Gulinello, M., Gong, Q. H., & Smith, S. S. (2002). Progesterone withdrawal increases the alpha4 subunit of the GABA(A) receptor in male rats in association with anxiety and altered pharmacology—a comparison with female rats. *Neuropharmacology, 43*(4), 701–714.

Gulinello, M., Orman, R., & Smith, S. S. (2003). Sex differences in anxiety, sensorimotor gating and expression of the alpha4 subunit of the GABAA receptor in the amygdala after progesterone withdrawal. *The European Journal of Neuroscience, 17*(3), 641–648.

Haggerty, C. L., Ness, R. B., Kelsey, S., & Waterer, G. W. (2003). The impact of estrogen and progesterone on asthma. *Annals of Allergy, Asthma & Immunology, 90*(3), 284–291; quiz 291–293, 347. doi:10.1016/S1081-1206(10)61794-2

Halbreich, U. (2004). The diagnosis of premenstrual syndromes and premenstrual dysphoric disorder—clinical procedures and research perspectives. *Gynecological Endocrinology, 19*(6), 320–334.

Halbreich, U. (2008). Selective serotonin reuptake inhibitors and initial oral contraceptives for the treatment of PMDD: Effective but not enough. *CNS Spectrums, 13*(7), 566–572.

Halbreich, U., Borenstein, J., Pearlstein, T., & Kahn, L. S. (2003). The prevalence, impairment, impact, and burden of premenstrual dysphoric disorder (PMS/PMDD). *Psychoneuroendocrinology, 28*(Suppl 3), 1–23.

Haley, C. L., Sung, S. C., Rush, A. J., Trivedi, M. H., Wisniewski, S. R., Luther, J. F., & Kornstein, S. G. (2013). The clinical relevance of self-reported premenstrual worsening of depressive symptoms in the management of depressed outpatients: a STAR*D report. *Journal of Women's Health (2002), 22*(3), 219–229. doi:10.1089/jwh.2011.3186

Hamaideh, S. H., Al-Ashram, S. A., & Al-Modallal, H. (2013). Premenstrual syndrome and premenstrual dysphoric disorder among Jordanian women. *Journal of Psychiatric and Mental Health Nursing.* doi:10.1111/jpm.12047.

Hartlage, S. A., Brandenburg, D. L., & Kravitz, H. M. (2004). Premenstrual exacerbation of depressive disorders in a community-based sample in the United States. *Psychosomatic Medicine, 66*(5), 698–706. doi:10.1097/01.psy.0000138131.92408.b9.

Hartlage, S. A., Freels, S., Gotman, N., & Yonkers, K. (2012). Criteria for premenstrual dysphoric disorder: Secondary analyses of relevant data sets. *Archives of General Psychiatry, 69*(3), 300–305. doi:10.1001/archgenpsychiatry.2011.1368.

Heinemann, L. A. J., Minh, T. D., Heinemann, K., Lindemann, M., & Filonenko, A. (2012). Intercountry assessment of the impact of severe premenstrual disorders on work and daily activities. *Health Care for Women International, 33*(2), 109–124. doi:10.1080/07399332.2011.610530.

Hong, J., Park, S., Wang, H.-R., Chang, S., Sohn, J., Jeon, H., … Cho, M. (n.d.). Prevalence, correlates, comorbidities, and suicidal tendencies of premenstrual dysphoric disorder in a nationwide sample of Korean women. *Social Psychiatry and Psychiatric Epidemiology,* 1–9. doi:10.1007/s00127-012-0509-6

Hsiao, M.-C., Hsiao, C.-C., & Liu, C.-Y. (2004). Premenstrual symptoms and premenstrual exacerbation in patients with psychiatric disorders. *Psychiatry and Clinical Neurosciences, 58*(2), 186–190.

Hsiao, C.-C., Liu, C.-Y., & Hsiao, M.-C. (2004). No correlation of depression and anxiety to plasma estrogen and progesterone levels in patients with premenstrual dysphoric disorder. *Psychiatry and Clinical Neurosciences, 58*(6), 593–599. doi:10.1111/j.1440-1819.2004.01308.x.

Huo, L., Straub, R. E., Roca, C., Schmidt, P. J., Shi, K., Vakkalanka, R., ... Rubinow, D. R. (2007). Risk for premenstrual dysphoric disorder is associated with genetic variation in ESR1, the estrogen receptor alpha gene. *Biological Psychiatry, 62*(8), 925–933. doi:10.1016/j.biopsych.2006.12.019

Jahanfar, S., Lye, M.-S., & Krishnarajah, I. S. (2011). The heritability of premenstrual syndrome. *Twin Research and Human Genetics, 14*(5), 433–436. doi:10.1375/twin.14.5.433.

Jane, Z.-Y., Chang, C.-C., Lin, H.-K., Liu, Y.-C., & Chen, W.-L. (2011). The association between the exacerbation of irritable bowel syndrome and menstrual symptoms in young Taiwanese women. *Gastroenterology Nursing, 34*(4), 277–286. doi:10.1097/SGA.0b013e3182248708.

Jeong, H.-G., Ham, B.-J., Yeo, H. B., Jung, I.-K., & Joe, S.-H. (2012). Gray matter abnormalities in patients with premenstrual dysphoric disorder: An optimized voxel-based morphometry. *Journal of Affective Disorders, 140*(3), 260–267. doi:10.1016/j.jad.2012.02.010.

Kane, S. V., Sable, K., & Hanauer, S. B. (1998). The menstrual cycle and its effect on inflammatory bowel disease and irritable bowel syndrome: A prevalence study. *The American Journal of Gastroenterology, 93*(10), 1867–1872. doi:10.1111/j.1572-0241.1998.540_i.x.

Kask, K., Gulinello, M., Bäckström, T., Geyer, M. A., & Sundström-Poromaa, I. (2008). Patients with premenstrual dysphoric disorder have increased startle response across both cycle phases and lower levels of prepulse inhibition during the late luteal phase of the menstrual cycle. *Neuropsychopharmacology, 33*(9), 2283–2290. doi:10.1038/sj.npp.1301599.

Kendler, K. S., Karkowski, L. M., Corey, L. A., & Neale, M. C. (1998). Longitudinal population-based twin study of retrospectively reported premenstrual symptoms and lifetime major depression. *The American Journal of Psychiatry, 155*(9), 1234–1240.

Kirschbaum, C., Kudielka, B. M., Gaab, J., Schommer, N. C., & Hellhammer, D. H. (1999). Impact of gender, menstrual cycle phase, and oral contraceptives on the activity of the hypothalamus-pituitary-adrenal axis. *Psychosomatic Medicine, 61*(2), 154–162.

Kleinstäuber, M., Witthöft, M., & Hiller, W. (2012). Cognitive-behavioral and pharmacological interventions for premenstrual syndrome or premenstrual dysphoric disorder: A meta-analysis. *Journal of Clinical Psychology in Medical Settings, 19*(3), 308–319. doi:10.1007/s10880-012-9299-y.

Koci, A., & Strickland, O. (2007). Relationship of adolescent physical and sexual abuse to perimenstrual symptoms (PMS) in adulthood. *Issues in Mental Health Nursing, 28*(1), 75–87. doi:10.1080/01612840600996281.

Kornstein, S. G., Harvey, A. T., Rush, A. J., Wisniewski, S. R., Trivedi, M. H., Svikis, D. S., ... Harley, R. (2005). Self-reported premenstrual exacerbation of depressive symptoms in patients seeking treatment for major depression. *Psychological Medicine, 35*(5), 683–692.

Kornstein, S. G., Pearlstein, T. B., Fayyad, R., Farfel, G. M., & Gillespie, J. A. (2006). Low-dose sertraline in the treatment of moderate-to-severe premenstrual syndrome: Efficacy of 3 dosing strategies. *The Journal of Clinical Psychiatry, 67*(10), 1624–1632.

Kuczmierczyk, A. R., Labrum, A. H., & Johnson, C. C. (1992). Perception of family and work environments in women with premenstrual syndrome. *Journal of Psychosomatic Research, 36*(8), 787–795.

Landén, M., & Eriksson, E. (2003). How does premenstrual dysphoric disorder relate to depression and anxiety disorders? *Depression and Anxiety, 17*(3), 122–129. doi:10.1002/da.10089.

Landén, M., Nissbrandt, H., Allgulander, C., Sörvik, K., Ysander, C., & Eriksson, E. (2007). Placebo-controlled trial comparing intermittent and continuous paroxetine in premenstrual dysphoric disorder. *Neuropsychopharmacology, 32*(1), 153–161. doi:10.1038/sj.npp.1301216.

Landén, M., & Thase, M. E. (2006). A model to explain the therapeutic effects of serotonin reuptake inhibitors: The role of 5-HT2 receptors. *Psychopharmacology Bulletin, 39*(1), 147–166.

Lee, E. E., Nieman, L. K., Martinez, P. E., Harsh, V. L., Rubinow, D. R., & Schmidt, P. J. (2012). ACTH and cortisol response to Dex/CRH testing in women with and without premenstrual dysphoria during GnRH agonist-induced hypogonadism and ovarian steroid replacement. *The Journal of Clinical Endocrinology and Metabolism, 97*(6), 1887–1896. doi:10.1210/jc.2011-3451.

Li, Y., Pehrson, A. L., Budac, D. P., Sánchez, C., & Gulinello, M. (2012). A rodent model of premenstrual dysphoria: Progesterone withdrawal induces depression-like behavior that is differentially sensitive to classes of antidepressants. *Behavioural Brain Research, 234*(2), 238–247. doi:10.1016/j.bbr.2012.06.034.

Lokuge, S., Frey, B. N., Foster, J. A., Soares, C. N., & Steiner, M. (2010). The rapid effects of estrogen: A mini-review. *Behavioural Pharmacology, 21*(5–6), 465–472. doi:10.1097/FBP.0b013e32833da5c3.

Lopez, L. M., Kaptein, A. A., & Helmerhorst, F. M. (2012). Oral contraceptives containing drospirenone for premenstrual syndrome. *Cochrane Database of Systematic Reviews (Online), 2*, CD006586. doi:10.1002/14651858.CD006586.pub4.

Lurie, S., & Borenstein, R. (1990). The premenstrual syndrome. *Obstetrical & Gynecological Survey, 45*(4), 220–228.

Lustyk, M. K. B., Gerrish, W. G., Shaver, S., & Keys, S. L. (2009). Cognitive-behavioral therapy for premenstrual syndrome and premenstrual dysphoric disorder: A systematic review. *Archives of Women's Mental Health, 12*(2), 85–96. doi:10.1007/s00737-009-0052-y.

Lustyk, M. K. B., Widman, L., & Becker Lde, L. (2007). Abuse history and premenstrual symptomatology: Assessing the mediating role of perceived stress. *Women & Health, 46*(4), 61–80.

Magnay, J. L., El-Shourbagy, M., Fryer, A. A., O'Brien, S., & Ismail, K. M. K. (2010). Analysis of the serotonin transporter promoter rs25531 polymorphism in premenstrual dysphoric disorder. *American Journal of Obstetrics and Gynecology, 203*(2), 181.e1–5. doi:10.1016/j.ajog.2010.02.043

Magnay, J. L., Ismail, K. M. K., Chapman, G., Cioni, L., Jones, P. W., & O'Brien, S. (2006). Serotonin transporter, tryptophan hydroxylase, and monoamine oxidase A gene polymorphisms in premenstrual dysphoric disorder. *American Journal of Obstetrics and Gynecology, 195*(5), 1254–1259. doi:10.1016/j.ajog.2006.06.087.

Majewska, M. D., Harrison, N. L., Schwartz, R. D., Barker, J. L., & Paul, S. M. (1986). Steroid hormone metabolites are barbiturate-like modulators of the GABA receptor. *Science (New York, N.Y.), 232*(4753), 1004–1007.

Markou, E., Boura, E., Tsalikis, L., Deligianidis, A., & Konstantinidis, A. (2011). The influence of sex hormones on proinflammatory cytokines in gingiva of periodontally healthy premenopausal women. *Journal of Periodontal Research, 46*(5), 528–532. doi:10.1111/j.1600-0765.2011.01369.x.

Maswood, S., Truitt, W., Hotema, M., Caldarola-Pastuszka, M., & Uphouse, L. (1999). Estrous cycle modulation of extracellular serotonin in mediobasal hypothalamus: Role of the serotonin transporter and terminal autoreceptors. *Brain Research, 831*(1–2), 146–154.

McQueen, J. K., Wilson, H., & Fink, G. (1997). Estradiol-17 beta increases serotonin transporter (SERT) mRNA levels and the density of SERT-binding sites in female rat brain. *Brain Research. Molecular Brain Research, 45*(1), 13–23.

Menkes, D. B., Coates, D. C., & Fawcett, J. P. (1994). Acute tryptophan depletion aggravates premenstrual syndrome. *Journal of Affective Disorders, 32*(1), 37–44.

Morse, C. A., Dudley, E., Guthrie, J., & Dennerstein, L. (1998). Relationships between premenstrual complaints and perimenopausal experiences. *Journal of Psychosomatic Obstetrics and Gynaecology, 19*(4), 182–191.

Nillni, Y. I., Toufexis, D. J., & Rohan, K. J. (2011). Anxiety sensitivity, the menstrual cycle, and panic disorder: A putative neuroendocrine and psychological interaction. *Clinical Psychology Review, 31*(7), 1183–1191. doi:10.1016/j.cpr.2011.07.006.

Northoff, H., Symons, S., Zieker, D., Schaible, E. V., Schäfer, K., Thoma, S., ... Fehrenbach, E. (2008). Gender- and menstrual phase dependent regulation of inflammatory gene expression in response to aerobic exercise. *Exercise Immunology Review, 14*, 86–103.

O'Brien, P. M. S., Bäckström, T., Brown, C., Dennerstein, L., Endicott, J., Epperson, C. N., ... Yonkers, K. (2011). Towards a consensus on diagnostic criteria, measurement and trial design of the premenstrual disorders: The ISPMD Montreal consensus. *Archives of Women's Mental Health, 14*(1), 13–21. doi:10.1007/s00737-010-0201-3

O'Brien, S. M., Fitzgerald, P., Scully, P., Landers, A., Scott, L. V., & Dinan, T. G. (2007). Impact of gender and menstrual cycle phase on plasma cytokine concentrations. *Neuroimmunomodulation, 14*(2), 84–90. doi:10.1159/000107423.

Paddison, P. L., Gise, L. H., Lebovits, A., Strain, J. J., Cirasole, D. M., & Levine, J. P. (1990). Sexual abuse and premenstrual syndrome: Comparison between a lower and higher socioeconomic group. *Psychosomatics, 31*(3), 265–272. doi:10.1016/S0033-3182(90)72162-7.

Perkonigg, A., Yonkers, K. A., Pfister, H., Lieb, R., & Wittchen, H.-U. (2004). Risk factors for premenstrual dysphoric disorder in a community sample of young women: The role of traumatic events and posttraumatic stress disorder. *The Journal of Clinical Psychiatry, 65*(10), 1314–1322.

Pico-Alfonso, M. A., Mastorci, F., Ceresini, G., Ceda, G. P., Manghi, M., Pino, O., ... Sgoifo, A. (2007). Acute psychosocial challenge and cardiac autonomic response in women: The role of estrogens, corticosteroids, and behavioral coping styles. *Psychoneuroendocrinology, 32*(5), 451–463. doi:10.1016/j.psyneuen.2007.02.009

Pilver, C. E., Levy, B. R., Libby, D. J., & Desai, R. A. (2011). Posttraumatic stress disorder and trauma characteristics are correlates of premenstrual dysphoric disorder. *Archives of Women's Mental Health, 14*(5), 383–393. doi:10.1007/s00737-011-0232-4.

Potter, J., Bouyer, J., Trussell, J., & Moreau, C. (2009). Premenstrual syndrome prevalence and fluctuation over time: Results from a French population-based survey. *Journal of Women's Health (2002), 18*(1), 31–39. doi:10.1089/jwh.2008.0932.

Protopopescu, X., Tuescher, O., Pan, H., Epstein, J., Root, J., Chang, L., ... Silbersweig, D. (2008). Toward a functional neuroanatomy of premenstrual dysphoric disorder. *Journal of Affective Disorders, 108*(1–2), 87–94. doi:10.1016/j.jad.2007.09.015

Puder, J. J., Blum, C. A., Mueller, B., De Geyter, C., Dye, L., & Keller, U. (2006). Menstrual cycle symptoms are associated with changes in low-grade inflammation. *European Journal of Clinical Investigation, 36*(1), 58–64. doi:10.1111/j.1365-2362.2006.01591.x.

Rabin, D. S., Schmidt, P. J., Campbell, G., Gold, P. W., Jensvold, M., Rubinow, D. R., & Chrousos, G. P. (1990). Hypothalamic-pituitary-adrenal function in patients with the premenstrual syndrome. *Journal of Clinical Endocrinology and Metabolism, 71*(5), 1158–1162.

Raison, C. L., Capuron, L., & Miller, A. H. (2006). Cytokines sing the blues: Inflammation and the pathogenesis of depression. *Trends in Immunology, 27*(1), 24–31. doi:10.1016/j.it.2005.11.006.

Rapkin, A. J., Berman, S. M., Mandelkern, M. A., Silverman, D. H. S., Morgan, M., & London, E. D. (2011). Neuroimaging evidence of cerebellar involvement in premenstrual dysphoric disorder. *Biological Psychiatry, 69*(4), 374–380. doi:10.1016/j.biopsych.2010.09.029.

Rapkin, A. J., Edelmuth, E., Chang, L. C., Reading, A. E., McGuire, M. T., & Su, T. P. (1987). Whole-blood serotonin in premenstrual syndrome. *Obstetrics and Gynecology, 70*(4), 533–537.

Rasgon, N., McGuire, M., Tanavoli, S., Fairbanks, L., & Rapkin, A. (2000). Neuroendocrine response to an intravenous L-tryptophan challenge in women with premenstrual syndrome. *Fertility and Sterility, 73*(1), 144–149.

Ravindran, L. N., Woods, S.-A., Steiner, M., & Ravindran, A. V. (2007). Symptom-onset dosing with citalopram in the treatment of premenstrual dysphoric disorder (PMDD): A case series. *Archives of Women's Mental Health, 10*(3), 125–127. doi:10.1007/s00737-007-0181-0.

Reame, N. E., Marshall, J. C., & Kelch, R. P. (1992). Pulsatile LH secretion in women with premenstrual syndrome (PMS): Evidence for normal neuroregulation of the menstrual cycle. *Psychoneuroendocrinology, 17*(2–3), 205–213.

Reed, S. C., Levin, F. R., & Evans, S. M. (2008). Changes in mood, cognitive performance, and appetite in the late luteal and follicular phases of the menstrual cycle in women with and without PMDD (premenstrual dysphoric disorder). *Hormones and Behavior, 54*(1), 185–193. doi:10.1016/j.yhbeh.2008.02.018.

Rehavi, M., Goldin, M., Roz, N., & Weizman, A. (1998). Regulation of rat brain vesicular monoamine transporter by chronic treatment with ovarian hormones. *Brain Research. Molecular Brain Research, 57*(1), 31–37.

Rohleder, N., Wolf, J. M., Piel, M., & Kirschbaum, C. (2003). Impact of oral contraceptive use on glucocorticoid sensitivity of pro-inflammatory cytokine production after psychosocial stress. *Psychoneuroendocrinology, 28*(3), 261–273. doi:10.1016/S0306-4530(02)00019-7.

Rubinow, D. R., Hoban, M. C., Grover, G. N., Galloway, D. S., Roy-Byrne, P., Andersen, R., & Merriam, G. R. (1988). Changes in plasma hormones across the menstrual cycle in patients with menstrually related mood disorder and in control subjects. *American Journal of Obstetrics and Gynecology, 158*(1), 5–11.

Sacco, S., Ricci, S., Degan, D., & Carolei, A. (2012). Migraine in women: The role of hormones and their impact on vascular diseases. *The Journal of Headache and Pain, 13*(3), 177–189. doi:10.1007/s10194-012-0424-y.

Schatz, D. B., Hsiao, M.-C., & Liu, C.-Y. (2012). Premenstrual dysphoric disorder in East Asia: A review of the literature. *International Journal of Psychiatry in Medicine, 43*(4), 365–380.

Schmidt, P. J., Grover, G. N., Hoban, M. C., & Rubinow, D. R. (1990). State-dependent alterations in the perception of life events in menstrual-related mood disorders. *The American Journal of Psychiatry, 147*(2), 230–234.

Schmidt, P. J., Nieman, L. K., Danaceau, M. A., Adams, L. F., & Rubinow, D. R. (1998). Differential behavioral effects of gonadal steroids in women with and in those without premenstrual syndrome. *The New England Journal of Medicine, 338*(4), 209–216. doi:10.1056/NEJM199801223380401.

Schneider, T., & Popik, P. (2009). An animal model of premenstrual dysphoric disorder sensitive to antidepressants. *Current Protocols in Neuroscience/Editorial Board, Jacqueline N. Crawley ... [et al.], Chapter 9*, Unit 9.31. doi:10.1002/0471142301.ns0931s46

Segebladh, B., Bannbers, E., Kask, K., Nyberg, S., Bixo, M., Heimer, G., & Sundström-Poromaa, I. (2011). Prevalence of violence exposure in women with premenstrual dysphoric disorder in comparison with other gynecological patients and asymptomatic controls. *Acta Obstetricia et Gynecologica Scandinavica, 90*(7), 746–752. doi:10.1111/j.1600-0412.2011.01151.x

Segebladh, B., Bannbers, E., Moby, L., Nyberg, S., Bixo, M., Bäckström, T., & Sundström Poromaa, I. (2013). Allopregnanolone serum concentrations and diurnal cortisol secretion in women with premenstrual dysphoric disorder. *Archives of Women's Mental Health*. doi:10.1007/s00737-013-0327-1

Shah, N. R., Jones, J. B., Aperi, J., Shemtov, R., Karne, A., & Borenstein, J. (2008). Selective serotonin reuptake inhibitors for premenstrual syndrome and premenstrual dysphoric disorder: A meta-analysis. *Obstetrics and Gynecology, 111*(5), 1175–1182. doi:10.1097/AOG.0b013e31816fd73b.

Sherwin, B. B., & Suranyi-Cadotte, B. E. (1990). Up-regulatory effect of estrogen on platelet 3H-imipramine binding sites in surgically menopausal women. *Biological Psychiatry, 28*(4), 339–348.

Shourie, V., Dwarakanath, C. D., Prashanth, G. V., Alampalli, R. V., Padmanabhan, S., & Bali, S. (2012). The effect of menstrual cycle on periodontal health—a clinical and microbiological study. *Oral Health & Preventive Dentistry, 10*(2), 185–192.

Smith, Adams, Schmidt, Rubinow, & Wassermann (2003). Abnormal luteal phase excitability of the motor cortex in women with premenstrual syndrome. Biol Psychiatry. *54*(7):757–62.

Smith, M., Poschman, K., Cavaleri, M., Howell, H., & Yonkers, K. (2006). Symptoms of posttraumatic stress disorder in a community sample of low-income pregnant women. *American Journal of Psychiatry, 163*(5), 881–884.

Steinberg, E. M., Cardoso, G. M. P., Martinez, P. E., Rubinow, D. R., & Schmidt, P. J. (2012). Rapid response to fluoxetine in women with premenstrual dysphoric disorder. *Depression and Anxiety, 29*(6), 531–540. doi:10.1002/da.21959.

Stone, S. E., Mazmanian, D., Oinonen, K. A., & Sharma, V. (2013). Past reproductive events as predictors of physical symptom severity during the menopausal transition. *Menopause (New York, N.Y.)*. doi:10.1097/GME.0b013e31827e18b8.

Strine, T. W., Chapman, D. P., & Ahluwalia, I. B. (2005). Menstrual-related problems and psychological distress among women in the United States. *Journal of Women's Health (2002), 14*(4), 316–323. doi:10.1089/jwh.2005.14.316.

Sugawara, M., Toda, M. A., Shima, S., Mukai, T., Sakakura, K., & Kitamura, T. (1997). Premenstrual mood changes and maternal mental health in pregnancy and the postpartum period. *Journal of Clinical Psychology, 53*(3), 225–232.

Sundström, I., Ashbrook, D., & Bäckström, T. (1997). Reduced benzodiazepine sensitivity in patients with premenstrual syndrome: A pilot study. *Psychoneuroendocrinology, 22*(1), 25–38.

Sundström, I., & Bäckström, T. (1998a). Patients with premenstrual syndrome have decreased saccadic eye velocity compared to control subjects. *Biological Psychiatry, 44*(8), 755–764.

Sundström, I., & Bäckström, T. (1998b). Citalopram increases pregnanolone sensitivity in patients with premenstrual syndrome: An open trial. *Psychoneuroendocrinology, 23*(1), 73–88.

Sundström, I., Nyberg, S., & Bäckström, T. (1997). Patients with premenstrual syndrome have reduced sensitivity to midazolam compared to control subjects. *Neuropsychopharmacology, 17*(6), 370–381. doi:10.1016/S0893-133X(97)00086-9.

Sylvén, S. M., Ekselius, L., Sundström-Poromaa, I., & Skalkidou, A. (2013). Premenstrual syndrome and dysphoric disorder as risk factors for postpartum depression. *Acta Obstetricia et Gynecologica Scandinavica, 92*(2), 178–184. doi:10.1111/aogs.12041.

Takeda, T., Tasaka, K., Sakata, M., & Murata, Y. (2006). Prevalence of premenstrual syndrome and premenstrual dysphoric disorder in Japanese women. *Archives of Women's Mental Health, 9*(4), 209–212. doi:10.1007/s00737-006-0137-9.

Thys-Jacobs, S., McMahon, D., & Bilezikian, J. P. (2008). Differences in free estradiol and sex hormone-binding globulin in women with and without premenstrual dysphoric disorder. *The Journal of Clinical Endocrinology and Metabolism, 93*(1), 96–102. doi:10.1210/jc.2007-1726.

Timby, E., Balgård, M., Nyberg, S., Spigset, O., Andersson, A., Porankiewicz-Asplund, J., … Poromaa, I. S. (2006). Pharmacokinetic and behavioral effects of allopregnanolone in healthy women. *Psychopharmacology, 186*(3), 414–424. doi:10.1007/s00213-005-0148-7

Treloar, S. A., Heath, A. C., & Martin, N. G. (2002). Genetic and environmental influences on premenstrual symptoms in an Australian twin sample. *Psychological Medicine, 32*(1), 25–38.

Tschudin, S., Bertea, P. C., & Zemp, E. (2010). Prevalence and predictors of premenstrual syndrome and premenstrual dysphoric disorder in a population-based sample. *Archives of Women's Mental Health, 13*(6), 485–494. doi:10.1007/s00737-010-0165-3.

Turkmen, S., Backstrom, T., Wahlstrom, G., Andreen, L., & Johansson, I.-M. (2011). Tolerance to allopregnanolone with focus on the GABA-A receptor. *British Journal of Pharmacology, 162*(2), 311–327. doi:10.1111/j.1476-5381.2010.01059.x.

van den Akker, O. B., Stein, G. S., Neale, M. C., & Murray, R. M. (1987). Genetic and environmental variation in menstrual cycle: Histories of two British twin samples. *Acta Geneticae Medicae et Gemellologiae, 36*(4), 541–548.

van Veen, J. F., Jonker, B. W., van Vliet, I. M., & Zitman, F. G. (2009). The effects of female reproductive hormones in generalized social anxiety disorder. *International Journal of Psychiatry in Medicine, 39*(3), 283–295.

Wander, K., Brindle, E., & O'Connor, K. A. (2008). C-reactive protein across the menstrual cycle. *American Journal of Physical Anthropology, 136*(2), 138–146. doi:10.1002/ajpa.20785.

Wang, M., Seippel, L., Purdy, R. H., & Bäckström, T. (1996). Relationship between symptom severity and steroid variation in women with premenstrual syndrome: Study on serum pregnenolone, pregnenolone sulfate, 5 alpha-pregnane-3,20-dione and 3 alpha-hydroxy-5 alpha-pregnan-20-one. *The Journal of Clinical Endocrinology and Metabolism, 81*(3), 1076–1082.

Watson, C. S., Alyea, R. A., Cunningham, K. A., & Jeng, Y.-J. (2010). Estrogens of multiple classes and their role in mental health disease mechanisms. *International Journal of Women's Health, 2*, 153–166.

WHO, W. H. O. (2004). *The ICD-1 classification of mental, behavioral and developmental disorders* (2nd ed., 10th revision). Geneva, Switzerland.

Wihlbäck, A.-C., Sundström Poromaa, I., Bixo, M., Allard, P., Mjörndal, T., & Spigset, O. (2004). Influence of menstrual cycle on platelet serotonin uptake site and serotonin2A receptor binding. *Psychoneuroendocrinology, 29*(6), 757–766. doi:10.1016/S0306-4530(03)00120-3.

Wittchen, H. U., Becker, E., Lieb, R., & Krause, P. (2002). Prevalence, incidence and stability of premenstrual dysphoric disorder in the community. *Psychological Medicine, 32*(1), 119–132.

Wium-Andersen, M. K., Ørsted, D. D., Nielsen, S. F., & Nordestgaard, B. G. (2013). Elevated C-reactive protein levels, psychological distress, and depression in 73, 131 individuals. *JAMA Psychiatry, 70*(2), 176–184. doi:10.1001/2013.jamapsychiatry.102.

Wyatt, K. M., Dimmock, P. W., Ismail, K. M. K., Jones, P. W., & O'Brien, P. M. S. (2004). The effectiveness of GnRHa with and without "add-back" therapy in treating premenstrual syndrome: A meta analysis. *BJOG, 111*(6), 585–593. doi:10.1111/j.1471-0528.2004.00135.x.

Wyatt, K., Dimmock, P., Jones, P., Obhrai, M., & O'Brien, S. (2001). Efficacy of progesterone and progestogens in management of premenstrual syndrome: Systematic review. *BMJ (Clinical Research ed.), 323*(7316), 776–780.

Yamamoto, K., Okazaki, A., Sakamoto, Y., & Funatsu, M. (2009). The relationship between premenstrual symptoms, menstrual pain, irregular menstrual cycles, and psychosocial stress among Japanese college students. *Journal of Physiological Anthropology, 28*(3), 129–136.

Yang, M., Wallenstein, G., Hagan, M., Guo, A., Chang, J., & Kornstein, S. (2008). Burden of premenstrual dysphoric disorder on health-related quality of life. *Journal of Women's Health (2002), 17*(1), 113–121. doi:10.1089/jwh.2007.0417.

Yonkers, K. A. (1997). Anxiety symptoms and anxiety disorders: How are they related to premenstrual disorders? *Journal of Clinical Psychiatry, 58*(Suppl. 3), 62–67; discussion 68–69.

Yonkers, K. A., Holthausen, G. A., Poschman, K., & Howell, H. B. (2006). Symptom-onset treatment for women with premenstrual dysphoric disorder. *Journal of Clinical Psychopharmacology, 26*(2), 198–202. doi:10.1097/01.jcp.0000203197.03829.ae.

Part II
The Reproductive Years

The Psychological Gestation of Motherhood

Diana Lynn Barnes

Introduction

Pregnancy and childbirth are a time of heightened emotional sensitivity for most women (Gavin et al., 2005). A number of studies show more psychiatric admissions around the childbearing years than at any other time in the female life cycle (Munk-Olsen, Laursen, Pedersen, Mors, & Mortensen, 2006; O'Hara & Stuart, 1999). Along with the physiological changes that occur during pregnancy, there also comes a period of psychological gestation as women begin to embrace the idea that their lives will be forever changed by the physically and emotionally demanding role requirements of motherhood.

This transition to motherhood has been described as a crisis by some authors (Bibring, 1959; Blum, 1980; Hollway, 2010; Leiffer, 1977; Villanci & Ryan, 1997). Some commentary contends that the use of the word crisis as part of the psychosocial discourse of motherhood has led to faulty assumptions that pivotal life transitions invariably produce illness; ultimately this thinking becomes embedded in the cultural expose about the mothering experience (Monk, 2013). Perhaps it is not the transition itself, or even the use of the word crisis, that creates vulnerability to psychiatric illness around the perinatal period, but rather our cultural insistence to remain hushed about the truth of women's experiences around their entrée into mothering.

Although becoming a mother is generally filled with joy and fulfillment, it is also a time of tremendous biological, social, and psychological vulnerability that represents a dramatic turning point in a woman's life. No two pregnancies are alike, and a woman's reactions to impending motherhood are most often affected by her individual circumstances, her relationship with her partner and her family, her feelings about herself, and her desire to become a mother in addition to what she believes

D.L. Barnes, Psy.D. (✉)
The Center for Postpartum Health, 13743 Riverside Drive, Sherman Oaks, CA 91423, USA
e-mail: dlbarnes@postpartumhealth.com

society expects of her in this new role. The growing realization that she will be forever transformed by the birth of her child is quite often psychologically destabilizing (Raphael-Leff, 1991).

Many women find their adaptation to motherhood disruptive and overwhelming (Barnes & Balber, 2007; Nicholson, 1999; Oakley, 1979); they feel largely unprepared to cope with the dynamic shifts created by this life-altering transition to motherhood (Nelson, 2003). One study by researcher Amy Rossiter (1988) that looked at this transition concluded there were several psychological dimensions to new motherhood and they included shock, panic, anxiety, feeling unprepared, unknowledgeable, and out of control. The initial shock ignited by the birth of a baby often results in a longing, frequently unexpressed, for the life that existed before. Consequently, the new mother, overwhelmed because she is experiencing the unexpected loss of her remembered life, finds herself wedged between two worlds and sworn to her own private world of secrecy for fear of being judged, not only by other mothers but by society in general. These identified losses that stir emotions such as anxiety, sadness, anger, and guilt often leave new mothers vulnerable to psychological distress (Taubman-Ben-Ari et al., 2009; Tedeshi & Calhoun, 2004). Only recently has the notion that motherhood and anguish could be emotional partners even been challenged (Held & Rutherford, 2012).

While this psychological gestation creates enormous upheaval and social disruption for many women, pregnancy is also recognized as a time that provides the opportunity for positive change and the potential for personal growth (Nelson, 2003; Parens, 1975; Taubman-Ben-Ari et al., 2009). A study by Bailey (1999) identified a connection between a woman's recognition of her pregnancy and an increasing level of self-awareness not previously available to many of the women in this study. Her research found that the physical markers of pregnancy afford women the opportunity to rewrite their life narratives and introduce preferred story lines; motherhood seems to "excuse" women from the need to stay entrenched in old ideas about self and self in relation to others (Bailey, p. 348). Raphael-Leff describes a psychoanalytic process of rebirth that facilitates a reorganization of self as women reintegrate both past and present into a different formulation of self (Raphael-Leff, 1991).

Becoming a mother is both a conscious and an unconscious process that often begins months and even years before the actual birth of a child (Darvill, Skirton, & Farrand, 2010; Maushart, 2000). A mother's identity emerges within the context of a developmental progression as she strives to make psychological sense of her altered body and her changing perspective of herself in the world. How she makes sense of the profound experience of sharing her physical space as well as her emotional space with this baby she has yet to know, predicts the psychological dimensions of her pregnancy (Raphael-Leff, 1991).

The dynamic process of becoming a mother is not an event that happens at the moment of birth; instead, it takes place gradually over time and is an outcome of the growing confidence in maternal abilities that emerges through accumulated experience, observation, and the shared wisdom of those who entered the world of motherhood before us (Maushart, 2000). The following discussion addresses the psychological and emotional experience of new mothers as they make their way through pregnancy. It examines the impact of social and cultural belief systems on women's meanings of motherhood and "the good mother," and also considers the significance of women's earliest attachment experiences on the construction of individual meaning. This chapter also looks at the developmental progression that takes place as women adapt to their new role as mother.

Historical Perspectives on Motherhood

Beliefs about the role of mothers and the meanings attached to motherhood are born out of the sociopolitical and cultural tenor of any particular historical period. In the eighteenth century, women in Britain and France not only had charge for the well-being of their own families but were portrayed as the backbone of the political structure and essential to the vigor of the nation (Yeo, 1999).

Other meanings associated with motherhood find their origins in writings as early as the Bible when Eve was told, "In sorrow will you bear children" (Genesis 3:16). Over time, this foreboding message about what awaits women during childbirth evolved into a more expansive historical and cultural perspective about motherhood as synonymous with suffering. Centuries later, threads of this belief continue to permeate ideologies about motherhood. In her classic feminist treatise on motherhood, *Of Woman Born: Motherhood as Experience and Institution*, Adrienne Rich maintains that the strength of this primary identification of mother as sufferer was "so necessary to the emotional grounding of human society that the mitigation, or removal, of that suffering, that identification, must be fought at every level, including the level of refusing to question it at all" (Rich, 1976, p. 30). Her comments suggest that the societal need to idealize mothers and motherhood is a defensive reaction to the darker sides of this life-altering experience that somewhere along the way we have found too unbearable to tolerate.

Some of the early ideologies stand in stark contrast with our more modern ideas about mothers. Hagar (2011) identifies a change in perspective between pre-nineteenth century and post nineteenth century thinking about mothers. According to Hagar, until the nineteenth century in Western Europe, a woman fulfilled her maternal role simply by giving birth. Infants were taken from their mothers and left in the care of women of lower social standing who nursed them and "mothered them." It was only after a period of at least 2 years, and sometimes even as long as 5 years, that these children were returned to their families. Hager argues that while this practice may seem abhorrent, and even abusive, in light of modern ideas about the relentlessly available mother who believes that any indication of her physical or emotional absence will be injurious to her child's development; however, mothers of the seventeenth and eighteenth century behaved according to the prevailing beliefs of their time as to how children should be raised. The milk of the peasant woman was considered substantially more nutritious than that of the aristocratic mother and the country environment was seen to be preferable and much healthier than the polluted city, believed to be plagued by disease (Hager, 2011). Until the nineteenth century in Western Europe, the idea that women were expected to love their children and take care of them was not part of the cultural repertoire of maternal behavior.

The striving to be a "good mother," advanced a dramatic shift in mid-nineteenth century thinking inculcating the idea that only trained medical and scientific professionals understood the complicated requirements of children. In order to excel at mothering, mothers must look to the conclusions drawn from scientific observation and data (Apple, 2006; Noon, 2004; Miller, 2005; Villanci & Ryan, 1997). Any ideas about women as the foremost experts on their own children vanished from view. As mothers turned increasingly more often to books on childcare, their anxiety about doing the right thing for their children increased as well (Stearns, 2002).

Motherhood as a Social Construction

A woman's experience of motherhood is shaped by the social and cultural context within which she lives. Some writings contend that the advent of motherhood is a necessary step in female development and the proclamation of her adult status (Redshaw & Martin, 2001; Woolett & Phoenix, 1991). Among feminist authors, there are those who argue that the desire to join the ranks of "mother" is socially constructed and not biologically driven (Chodorow, 1978, Glenn, Chang, & Forcey, 1994; Rich, 1976). Along with this social construction exists a cultural assumption that all women want to be mothers; therefore, to remain childless is considered unnatural, "so deeply inscribed and culturally scripted are essentialist ideas about womanhood" (Miller, 2005, p. 58). The word "Mother" is imbued with such powerful and almost mystical meaning that whether a woman chooses that path or not, "motherhood is central to the ways in which they are defined by others and to their perceptions of themselves" (Phoenix, Woolett, & Lloyd, 1991, p. 13).

What the good mother looks like and how she should behave is continually redefined as each era or society sees her differently (Douglas & Michaels, 2004; Redshaw & Martin, 2001; Thurer, 1994). By the early twentieth century, the idea that motherhood was evidence of womanliness was a fundamental tenet of psychoanalytic theory (Glenn et al., 1994). It was a view that remained popular for decades. The mother of the 1950s epitomized femininity and perfection (Villanci & Ryan, 1997). Maternal icons like June Cleaver, Harriet Nelson, and Donna Reed stayed at home, were never frazzled or exhausted, they wore dresses and makeup with their hair always neatly coifed. Motherhood was touted as a woman's destiny and the only source of her identity. Child-care guru Dr. Benjamin Spock reinforced the societal standard because he believed that women belonged at home, especially during the early years of a child's life. Not only the traditional mother of this time denied her needs in the service of her children, her husband, and her family, but any bid for self-fulfillment was seen as selfish and contradictory to good mothering. Mothering became an altruistic pursuit (Villanci & Ryan, 1997). In the 1960s, as the women's movement for freedom and choice opened the door to the 1970s archetype of the supermom; women were told they could have everything they wanted and achieve anything they desired (Villanci & Ryan, 1997). The 1970s mothers were expected to multitask with finesse and make "doing it all" and "having it all" seem easy.

In the following decade, becoming a mother was perceived as the path to self-fulfillment and mothers had a crucial role in the social and psychological development of their children. By the 1990s, most mothers were also working outside of the home which created a cultural contradiction that promoted another myth—mothers who work do not love their children as much as those mothers who devote themselves to full-time mothering. Social researcher Sharon Hays coined the term "intensive mothering" (Hays, 1996) to describe the mothering ideology of the time. Intensive mothering regards mothers as the ideal caregivers; it is a process that is "child centered, expert guided, emotionally absorbing, labor intensive, and financially expensive" (Hays, 1996, p. 8). It implies, however, that the mothering of children is a commitment to a life of self-sacrifice, limited to those women who have enough time, stamina, and money to stay at home (Medina & Magnuson, 2009). A study that looked at this issue actually found that mothers do value work and motherhood simultaneously and that the importance of each is positively correlated (McQuillan, Greil, Shreffler, & Tichenor, 2008).

Because the meanings attached to motherhood are socially prescribed, they establish an ideal for "normal mothering" that almost never accounts for the realities of women's individual and unique experiences (Phoenix, Woolett, & Lloyd, 1991). Heisler and Ellis (2008) write about the constructed faces of motherhood, faces that are intended to shield women from their fears of judgment or rejection by others. Mommy faces are tantamount to a facade that keeps women's private vulnerabilities hidden from public view. Their research concludes that women work with the messages they receive about motherhood and create faces in order to ensure acceptance from others about their mothering capabilities. Reluctant to reveal their actual feelings, many mothers struggle to maintain an image that often leaves them feeling as though they are actors in their own lives (Heisler & Ellis, 2008).

Maushart (2000) also suggests that in order to maintain the socially constructed expectations about good mothers, women ultimately mask the emotional truth about their experience. "The mask of motherhood is an assemblage of fronts—mostly brave, serene, and all knowing that we use to disguise the chaos and complexity of our lived experience" (p. 2). According to Maushart, it is this composition of false selves that keeps women silent about what they really feel. Inevitably, their silence breeds shame.

Social attitudes about motherhood evolve into a social conviction about the right way to mother. The social edict creates a mythical ideology about mothers and mothering which inevitably becomes internalized (Villanci & Ryan, 1997). As these cultural beliefs are solidified, they continue to reinforce societal norms so that they remain unopposed. Myths about good and bad mothers become synonymous with ideas about good and bad women (Choi, Henshaw, Baker, & Tree, 2005). The myths about motherhood invariably create expectations in the minds of most women that are impossible to fulfill. These cultural ideals become a yardstick by which women measure their sense of competence and confidence in their maternal role. The "Motherhood Crisis" (Villanci & Ryan, 1997) evolves from an assortment of myths about perfection that inevitably result in a mother's sense of failure at her inability to achieve the impossible (p. 4).

There is the idea that mothering is instinctive and that good mothers just know what to do and how to respond to their infant. There is a pervasive belief that capable mothers are always attuned; they possess an inherent and exquisite sensibility so they never feel out of step with their baby. Cultural ideas about good babies that rarely cry become inextricably linked with self-worth when the mother who has tried for hours to calm a fussing baby is unable to do so. Consequently, the new mother's good feelings about herself are contingent on her perceived capacity to mother; perceptions that have been shaped by social attitudes (Letherby, 1994).

The societal myth that mothering comes naturally promotes an auxiliary belief that it is unnatural for mothers to feel stress or anger, frustration or boredom; consequently, when the ordinary and expected relational disruptions occur between a mother and her infant, women are likely to feel inadequate. It is this profound fear of failure that leaves new mothers believing they must try even harder and this idea ultimately maintains the societal idealization of motherhood even more (Choi et al., 2005).

Not only does this social construction of motherhood interfere with women's understanding of the true day-to-day realities of mothering, but it also fails to acknowledge the expected and normal occurring period of adaptation to this extraordinary life cycle event. A study by Rogan, Shmied, Barclay, Everitt, and Wylie (1997) analyzed the experiences of 55 first-time mothers in Australia and identified six elements that embody the acute process of change experienced by most women. There was the initial realization as to how much their lives had changed and a corollary feeling that they were unready to take on these enormous changes dictated by the birth of their infants. Because they were overwhelmed by change, they began to feel drained which then elicited feelings of isolation and loss; experiencing the loss of the lives they once knew made women feel even more alone and more drained. Through this emotional progression, however, women eventually confronted the challenges of motherhood and started "working it out" (p. 877); all of these dimensions are interwoven throughout the psychological adjustment to motherhood (Rogan et al., 1997).

Because the myths about motherhood do not paint an honest and balanced portrait of women's experiences, they have a powerful impact on women's lives. As new mothers come face to face with the discrepancies between prevailing myth, expectations that originate from those myths, and the actual realities of motherhood, they frequently lose their balance in a whirlwind of anxiety, guilt, and even despair, which subsequently taints their overall experience of new motherhood (Birns & Hay, 1988). This psychological maelstrom is often the precursor for a downward spiral into depression. It is this mismatch between expectations about motherhood and the actual experience that often results in a crisis of identity (Barnes, 2012; Maushart, 2000; Smith, 1999).

Developing a Motherhood Identity

A woman's identity as a mother is ultimately influenced not only by social messages but also by life experiences and her interactions with others. Pregnancy, particularly in the last trimester, is often seen as a time of reflection (Bailey, 1999; Barnes, 2012). The physical changes of pregnancy give rise to the psychological processes inherent in this life-altering transition. For some women, pregnancy and entry into motherhood confirms their female identity (Van Busell, Spit, & Demyttenaere, 2009). Others consider, often with concern, whether motherhood will change their view of themselves in the world and alter their feelings about themselves in relation to important others in their lives. Bailey (1999) maintains that pregnancy opens the door to a newly found awareness about different aspects of self and speaks of this naturally occurring developmental process as a "refraction of self." She identifies six elements of change: mothering identity, bodily change, the working woman, practices of the self, the relational self, and altered experience of space and time. These dimensions of experience bring different facets of personality into view and deepen an understanding of self that was previously out of a woman's awareness (Bailey, 1999).

Another earlier study by Smith (1999) found that the development of a mothering identity paralleled the three trimesters of pregnancy. In data collected from four case studies of British women moving through pregnancy toward motherhood, the first trimester was found to be a time of adjustment and uncertainty. During middle pregnancy, expectant mothers begin to immerse themselves in a process of psychological preparation and a changing perception of self while in the third trimester the experience seems less about their inner world and more intensely about the upcoming birth, often with ambivalent feelings that swing between excitement and apprehension about the forthcoming changes they are about to confront (Smith, 1999). The growing insights about impending motherhood has also been described as an unfolding three-stage process of realization that accompanies the bodily changes of pregnancy; from initial recognition that there is a pregnancy to an awareness of the fetus and finally the reality of the baby (Raphael-Leff, 1991). Postpartum, the introspections of pregnancy tend to result in a transformation of the new mother's priorities and options. Other studies echo this transformation of self (Nelson, 2003; Sethi, 1995; Taubman-Ben-Ari et al., 2009).

Alterations in self-perception are not the exclusive domain of the pregnant woman; even those mothers-to-be, through surrogacy, adoption, and step parenting who do not experience the physical dimensions of pregnancy find themselves moving through the same developmental process (Heisler & Ellis, 2008). Their research on the construction of a "mommy identity" recognized four themes that emerge from women's remembered messages about motherhood. These themes converge to formulate a global picture of the good mother. The overarching themes establish motherhood as a priority over any other life pursuits, with certain behaviors and characteristics that exemplify what the good mother looks like. Motherhood is seen as one-dimensional and does not allow for the expression of any other parts of self. Finally, motherhood involves an ongoing discourse about self-worth. In many ways, a mother's interactions with her children and how she is perceived as a good mother by others becomes the barometer that assesses the degree of her good feelings about herself (Heisler & Ellis, 2008).

Who Is the Good Mother, Really?

The discourse around motherhood ideology invariably includes a discussion about what constitutes a good mother. For the traditional mother of the last century, her understanding about what embodies a good mother was clearly defined and extremely restrictive; she stayed at home full-time and felt entirely fulfilled in her maternal and domestic role; demographically, she was white and middle class (Johnston & Swanson, 2006). The diverse mothering experiences of women living in poverty, single mothers, women of color, or the lesbian mother were not even a consideration.

Adrienne Rich (1976) also writes about this view of the traditional mother whose only identity is a maternal one. She has attuned herself so exquisitely to the needs of others that she has become virtually invisible. In her book, *The Cultural Contradictions of Motherhood*, Sharon Hays (1996) echoes this theme of self-sacrifice that seems to pervade much of the literature on motherhood. The cultural sanctioning of good mothers exists within Hay's construct of "intensive mothering," in which children's needs take precedence over the individual needs of their mothers (p. 46). The idea that mothers exist only for their children (Elvin-Nowak & Thomsson, 2001) is closely linked with another concept about good mothers as always and ever available.

Held and Rutherford (2012) argue that in an attempt to explain the developmental needs of children and the ideal conditions under which children thrive, psychoanalytic literature has also promoted child-centered mothering and omnipresent availability as critical for normal psychological growth. According to this theoretical perspective, a child's healthy ego development rests on the consistent availability and reliable responsiveness of the adequately attuned mother (Ainsworth, Blehar, Waters, & Wall, 1978; Bowlby, 1969; Winnicott, 1987). John Bowlby, the grandfather of Attachment Theory posited that any prolonged separations between a mother and her child in the first years of life had potentially life-long negative repercussions for a child's social and emotional development (Bowlby, 1969). British pediatrician D. W. Winnicott (1987) spoke of a phenomenon that he termed, "primary maternal pre-occupation." According to Winnicott, it is a period of intense focus when mothers screen out the world so they may attune themselves to the needs of their infants. Similarly, the research of Mary Ainsworth, a protégé of Bowlby, addresses the issue of maternal sensitivity and responsiveness (Ainsworth et al., 1978). Contemporary researchers also emphasize the critical significance of a mother's ability to read her baby and respond appropriately, authentically, and reliably (Main, 2000; Sroufe, 2000; Stern, 1994).

While the consensus of the research community rightfully confirms the importance of maternal–infant attachment and understands that creating less than optimal conditions for this delicate emotional connection between mother and child has developmental implications, it also has fed some of the motherhood myths, particularly the myth that "good mothers" always understand their babies' cues and are never at a loss as to how to respond. Although Bowlby spoke about the detriment in lengthy separations, many mothers feel guilt-ridden at the thought of being away from their babies for even an hour. A mother's self-care, that is absolutely critical in order to remain attuned and emotionally present, takes a back seat to the entrenched idea of ever present and always available. Held and Rutherford contend that the ideologies of the psychoanalytic community have been influential in establishing a "clear good mother versus bad mother dynamic that defined how the normal mother should feel and act" (Held & Rutherford, 2012, p. 111).

Contemporary mothers, however, find themselves in the midst of a "socially constructed paradox" between the traditional image of the self-sacrificing mother and the modern career woman with needs of her own and a desire for an identity that exists apart from her children (Ex & Janssens, 2000, p. 884). Elvin-Nowak and Thomsson (2001) identified three distinct perspectives reflecting contemporary mothering beliefs about the good mother among employed mothers in Sweden. One group of mothers held a conviction that a mother's accessibility to her children is critical to their healthy psychological development. A second group took the stance that motherhood involves personal fulfillment beyond the needs of the child. Another group of women offered an additional perspective focusing on women's adult roles such that motherhood and work are valued as individual spheres for identity fulfillment. A study by Johnston and Swanson (2006) had findings that were notably consistent with those in the Swedish study. The results also seem to suggest that mothers construct their ideas about good mothers on the basis of their employment status; the stay-at-home mothers' definition of good mothering as "always being there," automatically disqualifies full-time working mothers from the ranks of good mothers. The construction of the happy mother with happy children by part-time and full-time employed mothers eliminates the mother at home from the category of "happy," because she has failed to develop her identity apart from her children. The researchers concluded that these narrowly defined constructions of good and bad mothers have limited women's freedom of choice.

The Birth of a Mother

There is an ongoing conversation in the psychological literature about the psychodynamic process that unfolds as women move through their pregnancies towards motherhood. For some women, this delicately unfolding psychological process that accompanies her emerging identity as a mother began many years before conception. For others, it begins to materialize more distinctly during pregnancy and continues many months beyond birth as she assumes the responsibilities of caring for her infant and steps officially into this new role called mother. Raphael-Leff (1980) speaks about a deepening sense of relationship that embodies the transition to motherhood, beginning with a connection to the physical pregnancy, followed by a growing connection to the fetus and finally the baby.

The journey towards motherhood entails a developmental process in which there is no return to one's former sense of self; many women talk about feeling "lost." It has been described as a psychological metamorphosis (Block, 1991) that leaves women uncertain about their capacities to handle the future that lies ahead of them. One study that sought to examine the experiences of first time mothers (Sethi, 1995) identified a four-stage psychosocial process involving a reconfiguration of self that emerges as women make the transition to becoming a mother. The dialectic begins with a "giving of self," as new mothers turn themselves over to the needs of their infants. It is through their care giving that they go on to redefine self, redefine other relationships, and redefine their own professional goals (Sethi, 1995).

Within these broader categories of change lie the emotional nuances that are an integral part of women's developing ideas about themselves as mothers. They may initially feel overwhelmed by an encroaching sense of loneliness and confinement because the "spur of the moment" moments have seemingly vanished. While it may feel as though they are teetering between two worlds with no way to turn back, new mothers may also be swept away by the amazement of it all and the joy and love inherent in welcoming a baby into their lives. The experiences of new mothers often reflect a range of contradictory feelings, whether excitement or uncertainty, fear or confidence, frustration or flexibility, that many find confusing and then voice as evidence of some failure on their parts.

Each mother's reactions and anxieties may differ; these emotional disparities vary from woman to woman and often reflect their psychological management of previous times of change and transition. At the same time that major life transitions awaken strong emotions like sadness, anxiety, and a longing for the life that came before, the need to adapt to the highly stressful circumstances surrounding motherhood frequently generates positive change and personal growth (Tedeshi & Calhoun, 2004). Raphael-Leff's model of adjustment suggests two different maternal orientations that frame a woman's psychological experience of pregnancy (1980)—the Facilitator who surrenders to the emotional challenges of pregnancy, greeting the changes with openness and hopefulness about the future. In contrast, there is the Regulator whose pregnancy leaves her so apprehensive about the future that she is thrown into a state of emotional upheaval, fervently resisting any notion that her pregnancy could provide an opportunity for positive change.

A seminal study by Regina Lederman in which she looked at the psychosocial adaptation to pregnancy (1996) concluded that a positive identification with mothering involves a conscious process of visualization in which the expectant mother is able to see herself in the motherhood role. Lederman's research also suggests that a positive adjustment to motherhood requires that women are able to think about the qualities they believe are essential for a mother to have and be able to look ahead to the many ways in which their lives will be forever different following the birth of their infant.

Daniel Stern, who has written extensively about adaptation to motherhood, describes the psychological preparation that fully emerges with the birth of a child as a compilation of dialogues that he termed the "motherhood constellation" (Stern, 1995). According to Stern, the motherhood constellation consists of four related themes and a "motherhood trilogy" which he refers to as the internal and external discourse that enters the minds of most expectant and new mothers. This discourse includes a mother's dialogue with her own mother, focusing mostly on their relationship when the new mother was a child; in addition, there is her conversation with herself as a new mother and her discourse with her own infant as she takes on the maternal role.

The four themes that materialize during this psychologically delicate period are the life growth theme, the primary relatedness theme, the supporting matrix theme, and the identity reorganization theme. The life growth theme involves the new mother's concerns as to whether she is sufficiently capable of protecting her infant and keeping him alive; a mother's inner dialogue as to whether she feels nurturing enough to foster her infant's healthy psychological development is the focus of the primary relatedness theme. The supporting matrix theme refers to her capacity to create the necessary social supports to bolster a smoother transition to motherhood. A woman's growing recognition that motherhood involves a reorganization of self in relation to others is the fourth fundamental theme in this constellation.

Attachment History and Its Role in the Psychological Construction of Mothers

The attachment relationship between a mother and her child begins to take shape during pregnancy. An infant's birth acts as a catalyst for a new mother's remembrances about herself as a child. Consequently, the transition to motherhood requires a deepening understanding regarding the expectant mother's memories of her emotional attachment with her own mother as she moves from daughter to mother, partner to mother, and often, from career woman to mother (Stern, 1995). Stern's emphasis on the new mother's earliest attachment relationship is supported by other researchers who also conclude that the examination of a mother's own childhood attachments is an integral part of her growing psychological comfort with her maternal role (Lederman, 1996; Shereshefsky & Yarrow, 1973; Siegel, 2003). Because the birth of a child brings most mothers to a level of heightened sensitivity, unresolved issues between the expectant mother and her own mother play a significant role in the quality of the adjustment period postpartum (Barnes, 2000). When a woman becomes pregnant, it is as though she steps into the shoes of her mother and joins the club.

A study by Shereshefsky and Yarrow (1973) acknowledged that the details of a woman's early relationship experience with her own mother provided insight into the ease with which she adapted to motherhood. They evaluated the mother–daughter relationship by rating items based on the expectant mother's feelings about their early relationship, which they termed the "perception of experience in being mothered" scale. They looked at her appraisal of her mother's empathy and closeness to her, how her mother felt about her own mothering, and the extent to which the mother-to-be felt that her mother met her emotional needs up to age 12 and then again from age 12 until she became pregnant. The researchers concluded there was a definite connection between a woman's positive experience of being mothered and her confidence in assuming the maternal role. Furthermore, a positive relationship enhanced her ability to manage, with minimal anxiety, any of her fears that surfaced during the pregnancy. In contrast, an emotionally unsatisfying and difficult relationship with her own mother often leaves the new mother feeling isolated and believing that she lacks the necessary coping skills to nurture her newborn, leaving her more vulnerable to the onset of child-bearing related mood disorders (Barnes, 2000).

A woman's subjective experience of her own attachment history influences her perceptions about the future relationship between herself and her infant (Siegel, 2012; Sroufe, 2000). Those expectant mothers who are not able to see any relevance between their history and their experience of pregnancy and motherhood are very likely to dismiss their own history and how they were mothered. As a result, they tend to distance themselves from their feelings in order to cope. Other women become so enmeshed in their experience of motherhood that they lose perspective. This emotional fusion between a mother and her baby is often reflected in her recollections about her relationship with her mother. They are more likely not only to remain enmeshed with their mothers but also to mirror that enmeshment with their children when they become mothers. Those new mothers who are securely attached are able to evaluate their feelings and experiences in what has been referred to as a "cohesive narrative" of their attachment history (Main, 2000; Siegel, 2012).

Because attachment styles are generationally transmitted, new mothers who express security in their attachments are more likely to experience their own competence in the maternal role while managing the normal and expected stress that accompanies mothering (Behringer, Reiner, & Spangler, 2011; Taubman-Ben-Ari et al., 2009). Those mothers, who are insecurely attached, however, tend to experience increasingly more anxiety with more difficulty managing their emotional distress when faced with stressful circumstances (Mikulincer & Florian, 1999). During pregnancy, securely attached mothers are more likely to establish a positive relationship with their fetus and are better able to create support systems, which also act as a buffer against stressful feelings (Taubman-Ben-Ari et al., 2009).

Maternal Ambivalence

> My children cause me the most exquisite suffering of which I have any experience. It is the suffering of ambivalence: the murderous alternation between bitter resentment and raw-edged nerves, and blissful gratification and tenderness. (Adrienne Rich, 1976, 1986, p. 21)

The societal push to idealize mothers has promulgated a belief that any ambivalence a mother might feel as she approaches motherhood is worrisome and indicative of an underlying pathological process at work. However, it is a belief that silences any normally occurring contradictory feelings that may exist in the minds of women as they step into the unfamiliar world of motherhood. The idea that excitement and fear, love and hate can coexist stands in stark contrast with the cultural need to put a positive spin on the challenges inherent in mothering work and to deny any negative associations. Maternal ambivalence, however, is a normal phenomenon, and given the pressures and performance expectations hurled upon mothers by cultural dictates, ambivalence is quite understandable and predictable.

There is no single emotion that mothers feel towards their children (Arendell, 2000). Despite cultural folklore that the devoted mother feels only love, being a mother is emotionally unpredictable and feelings can vary even within the course of a day and certainly over the course of the relationship between a mother and her children. The emotional life of a mother is vulnerable to shifts that are contingent on circumstance, supports, and children's behaviors. One study found greater expressions of anger in mothers as compared with childless women (Galambos & Krahn, 2008).

Even within the supposedly blissful state that mothers are expected to experience in the days and weeks following childbirth, many mothers talk about feeling trapped with no apparent way to extricate themselves from the reality, for some quite terrifying, that they are now responsible for the physical and emotional survival of another human being. It is akin to feeling "emotionally and physically disabled," writes Susan Maushart (2000, p. 114). And yet, new mothers, especially those in treatment with child-bearing related mood disorders, feel shame, anxiety, and guilt about the whirlwind of conflicted feelings, and unless asked, will rarely disclose those thoughts and feelings they believe are reflective of poor character. Roszika Parker, who has written extensively about maternal ambivalence, finds the roots of ambivalence in the differing needs between mother and child. Giving women permission to voice the contest of needs engenders a thought process which Parker maintains actually leads to more attuned mothering (Parker, 1995).

Conclusion

Because cultural belief seems to set the gold standard for how all good mothers should behave, mothers are generally identified "not by how they feel, but by what they try to do" (Ruddick, 1994, p. 34). However, the true voice of motherhood lies within each woman's individual experience. Becoming a mother and being a mother are emotionally intense experiences that do not begin with pregnancy nor end with childbirth. The motherhood mandate which insists that women slip into the world of mothering in a state of exultation more often throws them into a world of uncertainty, leaving them more vulnerable to the onset of illness postpartum. The foremost comment from women who have come to treatment postpartum is, "no one ever told me it would be like this!"

The 9 months of pregnancy offers a clearly defined period during which mothers and fathers can prepare for change. Some research indicates that pregnancy allows for an adaptive process in which individuals actively seek information so as to construct their experience and make sense of the anticipated changes (Deutsch, Ruble, Fleming, Brooks-Gunn, & Stangor, 1987). Understanding the psychological story underlying each woman's pregnancy is critical to helping her make a more comfortable transition to the all-encompassing world of motherhood.

References

Ainsworth, M. D. S., Blehar, M. C., Waters, E., & Wall, S. (1978). *Patterns of attachment: A psychological study of the strange situation.* Hillsdale, NJ: Lawrence Erlbaum Associates.
Apple, R. (2006). *Perfect motherhood: Science and childrearing in America.* New Brunswick, NJ: Rutgers University Press.
Arendell, T. (2000). Conceiving and investigating motherhood: The decade's scholarship. *Journal of Marriage and the Family, 62,* 1192–1207.
Bailey, L. (1999). Refracted selves? A study of changes in self-identity in the transition to motherhood. *Sociology, 33*(2), 335–352.
Barnes, D. L. (2000). *Ambivalence as a risk factor in postpartum depression.* Poster presentation, Marce' Society, International Conference, London, UK.
Barnes, D. L. (2012). Women's reproductive mental health: The myth of maternal bliss. *Family Therapy, 11*(3), 17–19.
Barnes, D. L., & Balber, L. G. (2007). *The journey to parenthood: Myths, reality, and what really matters.* Oxford: Radcliffe Publishing.
Behringer, J., Reiner, I., & Spangler, G. (2011). Maternal representations of past and current attachment relationships and emotional experiences across the transition to motherhood: A longitudinal study. *Journal of Family Psychology, 25*(2), 210–219.
Bibring, G. (1959). Some considerations of the psychological process in pregnancy. *The Psychoanalytic Study of the Child, 14,* 113–121.
Birns, E., & Hay, D. F. (1988). *The different faces of motherhood.* New York, NY: Plenum Press.
Block, J. (1991). *Motherhood as metamorphosis: Change and continuity in the life of a new mother.* New York, NY: Penguin.
Blum, B. L. (Ed.). (1980). *Psychological aspects of pregnancy, birthing, and bonding.* New York, NY: Human Sciences Press.
Bowlby, J. (1969). *Beginning of attachment behavior: Attachment and loss: Vol. 1: Attachment* (pp. 265–330). New York, NY: Basic Books.
Chodorow, N. (1978). *The reproduction of mothering.* Berkeley, CA: University of California Press.
Choi, P., Henshaw, C., Baker, S., & Tree, J. (2005). Supermum, superwife, supereverything: Performing femininity in the transition to motherhood. *Journal of Reproductive and Infant Psychology, 23*(2), 167–180.
Darvill, R., Skirton, H., & Farrand, P. (2010). Psychological factors that impact on women's experiences of first-time motherhood: A qualitative study of the transition. *Midwifery, 26,* 357–366.
Deutsch, F. M., Ruble, D. N., Fleming, A., Brooks-Gunn, J., & Stangor, C. (1987). Information-seeking and maternal self-definition during the transition to motherhood. *Journal of Personality and Social Psychology, 55*(3), 420–431.
Douglas, S. J., & Michaels, M. W. (2004). *The mommy myth: The idealization of motherhood and how it has undermined women.* New York, NY: Free Press.
Elvin-Nowak, Y., & Thomsson, H. (2001). Motherhood as idea and practice: A discursive understanding of employed mothers in Sweden. *Gender & Society, 15,* 407–428.
Ex, C. T. G. M., & Janssens, J. M. A. M. (2000). Young females' images of motherhood. *Sex Roles, 43*(11/12), 865–890.

Galambos, N. L., & Krahn, H. J. (2008). Depression and anger trajectories during the transition to adulthood. *Journal of Marriage and Family, 70*(1), 15–27.

Gavin, N., Gaynes, N. B., Lohr, K., Meltzer-Brody, S., Gartlehner, G., & Swinson, T. (2005). Perinatal depression: A systematic review of prevalence and incidence. *Obstetrics and Gynecology, 106*(5), 1071–1083.

Glenn, N. E., Chang, G., & Forcey, L. R. (Eds.). (1994). *Mothering, ideology, experience, and agency.* New York, NY: Routledge.

Hager, T. (2011). Making sense of an untold story: A personal deconstruction of the myth of motherhood. *Qualitative Inquiry, 17*(1), 35–44.

Hays, S. (1996). *The cultural contradictions of motherhood.* New Haven, CT: Yale University Press.

Heisler, J. M., & Ellis, J. B. (2008). Motherhood and the construction of "mommy identity": Messages about motherhood and face negotiation. *Communication Quarterly, 56*(4), 445–467.

Held, L., & Rutherford, A. (2012). Can't a mother sing the blues? Postpartum depression and the construction of motherhood in late 20th century America. *History of Psychology, 15*(2), 107–123.

Hollway, W. (2010). Conflict in the transitions to becoming a mother: A psychosocial approach. *Psychoanalysis, Culture, and Society, 15*(2), 136–155.

Johnston, D. D., & Swanson, D. H. (2006). Constructing the "good mother": The experience of mothering ideologies by work status. *Sex Roles, 54,* 509–519.

Lederman, R. P. (1996). *Psychosocial adaptation in pregnancy: Assessment of seven dimensions of maternal development* (2nd ed.). New York, NY: Springer.

Leiffer, M. (1977). Psychological changes accompanying pregnancy and motherhood. *Genetic Psychology Monographs, 95,* 55–96.

Letherby, G. (1994). Mother or not, mother or what? Problems of definition and identity. *Women's Studies International Forum, 17*(5), 525–532.

Main, M. (2000). The adult attachment interview: Fear, attention, safety and discourse processes. *Journal of the American Psychoanalytic Association, 48*(4), 1055–1096.

Maushart, S. (2000). *The mask of motherhood: How becoming a mother changes our lives and why we never talk about it.* New York, NY: Penguin.

McQuillan, J., Greil, A. L., Shreffler, K. M., & Tichenor, V. (2008). The importance of motherhood among women in the contemporary United States. *Gender & Society, 22*(4), 477–496.

Medina, S., & Magnuson, S. (2009). Motherhood in the 21st century: Implications for counselors. *Journal of Counseling & Development, 87,* 90–96.

Mikulincer, M., & Florian, V. (1999). Appraisal and coping with a real life stressful situation: The contribution of attachment styles. *Personality and Social Psychology Bulletin, 2,* 408–416.

Miller, T. (2005). *Making sense of motherhood: A narrative approach.* Cambridge: Cambridge University Press.

Monk, H. (2013). Marketing mothering as 'crisis': Professions saving us from the 'danger' of becoming mothers. *Journal of Prenatal and Perinatal Psychology and Health, 27*(3), 180–192.

Munk-Olsen, T., Laursen, T. M., Pedersen, C. B., Mors, O., & Mortensen, P. B. (2006). New parents and mental disorders: A population-based register study. *Journal of the American Medical Association, 296*(21), 2582–2589.

Nelson, A. M. (2003). Transition to motherhood. *Journal of Obstetric, Gynecologic, and Neonatal Nursing, 32*(4), 465–477.

Nicholson, P. (1999). Loss happiness and postpartum depression: The ultimate paradox. *Canadian Psychology, 40,* 162–178.

Noon, D. H. (2004). Situating gender and professional identity in American child study, 1880–1910. *History of Psychology, 7*(2), 107–129.

O'Hara, M. W., & Stuart, S. (1999). Pregnancy and postpartum. In R. G. Robinson & W. R. Yates (Eds.), *Psychiatric treatment of the medically ill* (pp. 253–277). New York, NY: Marcel Dekker.

Oakley, A. (1979). *Becoming a mother.* Oxford: Martin Robertson.

Parens, H. (1975). Parenthood as a developmental phase. *Journal of the American Psychoanalytic Association, 23,* 154–165.

Parker, R. (1995). *Mother love/mother hate: The power of maternal ambivalence*. New York, NY: Basic Books.
Phoenix, A., Woolett, A. & Lloyd, E. (eds). (1991). *Motherhood: Meaning, practices & ideologies*. London: Sage Publications.
Raphael-Leff, J. (1991). *Psychological processes of childbearing*. New York, NY: Chapman & Hall.
Redshaw, M., & Martin, C. (2001). Motherhood: A natural progression and a major transition. *Journal of Reproductive and Infant Psychology, 29*(4), 305–307.
Rich, A. (1976). *Of woman born: Motherhood as experience and institution*. New York, NY: Norton.
Rogan, F., Shmied, V., Barclay, L., Everitt, L., & Wylie, A. (1997). 'Becoming a mother'—developing a new theory of early motherhood. *Journal of Advanced Nursing, 25*, 877–885.
Rossiter, A. (1988). *From private to public: A feminist exploration of early mothering*. Toronto, ON: The Women's Press.
Ruddick, S. (1994). Thinking mothers/conceiving birth. In D. Bassin, M. Honey, & M. M. Kaplan (Eds.), *Representations of motherhood* (pp. 29–46). New Haven, CT: Yale University Press.
Sethi, S. (1995). The dialectic in becoming a mother: Experiencing a postpartum phenomenon. *The Scandinavian Journal of Caring Sciences, 9*(4), 235–244.
Shereshefsky, P. M., & Yarrow, I. J. (Eds.). (1973). *Psychological aspects of a first pregnancy and early postnatal adaptation*. New York, NY: Raven.
Siegel, D. J. (2003). An interpersonal neurobiology of psychotherapy. In M. F. Solomon & D. J. Siegel (Eds.), *Healing trauma: Attachment, mind, body, and brain*. New York, NY: W.W. Norton & Company.
Siegel, D. J. (2012). *Pocket guide to interpersonal neurobiology to interpersonal neurobiology: An integrative handbook of the mind*. New York, NY: W.W. Norton & Company.
Smith, J. A. (1999). Identity development during the transition to motherhood: An interpretative phenomenological analysis. *Journal of Reproductive and Infant Psychology, 17*(3), 281–299.
Stearns, P. N. (2002). *Anxious parents: A history of modern childrearing in America*. New York, NY: New York University Press.
Stern, D. N. (1994). One way to build a clinically relevant baby. *Infant Mental Health Journal, 15*(1), 9–25.
Stern, D. N. (1995). *The motherhood constellation: A unified view of parent-infant psychotherapy*. New York, NY: Basic Books.
Sroufe, A. L. (2000). Early relationships and the development of children. *Infant Mental Health Journal, 21*(1–2), 67–74.
Taubman-Ben-Ari, O., Shlomo, S. B., Sivan, S., & Dolizki, M. (2009). The transition to motherhood—a time for growth. *Journal of Social and Clinical Psychology, 28*(8), 943–970.
Tedeshi, R. G., & Calhoun, L. G. (2004). Posttraumatic growth: Conceptual foundations and empirical evidence. *Psychological Inquiry, 15*(1), 1–18.
Thurer, S. L. (1994). *Myths of motherhood: How culture reinvents the good mother*. Boston, MA: Houghton-Miflin.
Van Busell, J. C. H., Spit, B., & Demyttenaere, K. (2009). Anxiety in pregnant and postpartum women: An exploratory study of the role of maternal orientations. *Journal of Affective Disorders, 114*, 232–242.
Villanci, S. L., & Ryan, J. E. (1997). *Motherhood at the crossroads: Meeting the challenge of changing roles*. New York, NY: Insight Books.
Winnicott, D. W. (1987). *Babies and their mothers*. New York, NY: Addison-Wesley.
Woolett, A., & Phoenix, A. (1991). Psychological view of mothering. In A. Phoenix & A. Woolett (Eds.), *Motherhood: Meanings, practices and ideologies*. Sage Publications: London.
Yeo, E. J. (1999). The creation of 'motherhood' and women's responses in Britain and France 1750–1914. *Women's History Review, 8*(2), 201–217.

Screening and Risk Assessment for Perinatal Mood Disorders

Carol Henshaw

Introduction

Postpartum depression, PPD, is the most common medical complication of childbirth with a mean prevalence of 13 % (O'Hara & Swain, 1996). Rates are higher in populations with extreme social adversity and some migrant groups. The postpartum period is also a high-risk time for recurrence of severe mood disorders. As many as 67 % of women with bipolar disorder experience a recurrence after delivery with an increased risk of requiring psychiatric admission (Freeman et al., 2002; Munk-Olsen et al., 2009). Ninety percent of all postpartum bipolar relapses occur within the first 4 weeks after delivery (Harlow et al., 2007).

Less severe but more common mood disorders such as unipolar depression are associated with poor outcomes for both mother and infant: prenatal depression is associated with adverse outcomes including increased activity, delayed growth, preterm birth, and low birth weight (Field, Diego, & Hernanzez-Rief, 2006; Grote et al., 2010), and maternal depression in the first year of a child's life can result in compromised child care practices including feeding (especially breastfeeding), sleep routines, attendance at well-child visits, immunization rates, and safety practices (Field, 2010). In low-income countries, depression is associated with poor infant growth (Stewart, 2007). When mothers are depressed, the disruption in the attachment relationship increases the risk for child cognitive and behavioral problems (Grace, Evindar, & Stewart, 2003). Hence, screening and risk assessment of pregnant and postpartum women with mood disorders are imperative.

C. Henshaw, M.B., Ch.B., M.D., F.R.C.Psych. (✉)
Liverpool Womens NHS Foundation Trust & University of Liverpool, Liverpool, UK
e-mail: chenshaw@doctors.org.uk

Preconception Care

Both medication and an untreated mental disorder may pose risks to the fetus during pregnancy, breastfeeding, and early life. These risks can be reduced if women with mood disorders who are of childbearing age and those taking psychotropic medication are counselled about the risks in the event they should become pregnant and the need for contraception until they wish to embark on a pregnancy. Those planning a pregnancy should receive preconception counselling to determine any risk for a recurrence during pregnancy and the postpartum period in relation to their medication, a strategy recommended by several national guidelines (e.g., American Psychiatric Association, 2002; Royal College of Obstetricians and Gynaecologists, 2011; Scottish Intercollegiate Guidelines Network (SIGN), 2012). Some of the mood-stabilizing drugs used in bipolar disorder, e.g., valproate and carbamazepine, are teratogenic and could have an adverse effect on a fetus later in pregnancy, whereas the risk associated with lithium has been overestimated in the past. As the evidence base changes rapidly, it is important that physicians ensure that they are up to date and have read and understood the relevant studies, not merely scanned the abstract. Many women read accessed Internet headlines regarding the medication they are taking (e.g., antidepressants taken in pregnancy cause autism), and while they may be vaguely familiar with a particular study, they are unable to appreciate how robust the study is and whether all confounding variables have been controlled for.

For bipolar women, the risk of a postpartum episode increases the closer a hospitalization has been prior to pregnancy, the number of previous hospitalizations, and the duration of the most recent illness (Harlow et al., 2007). Puerperal episodes run in families. There is a 24-fold increase in the risk of a postpartum episode if a first-degree relative has bipolar disorder (Munk-Olsen, Laursen, Pederson, Mors, & Mortensen, 2007); if a sibling has suffered from PPD, this also increases the risk of depression after delivery (Murphy-Eberenz et al., 2006). Therefore, taking a family history becomes as important as taking a careful personal psychiatric history. Any risk assessment should include a look at the outcome of any previous medications that have been discontinued. If mood stabilizers are stopped, a woman is at a higher risk of a pregnancy episode. Most episodes during pregnancy are depressive or dysphoric mania. Pregnancy is not protective against relapse. A study of euthymic pregnant, bipolar women who stopped mood-stabilizing medication compared with those who continued it reported that the risk of an episode during pregnancy was 2.3 times greater if medication had been discontinued. The median time to recurrence after stopping medication was 9 weeks (Viguera et al., 2007), and those women affected spent a greater proportion of their pregnancy ill. Delaying conception and using contraception until a stable period has elapsed may reduce the risk.

This also allows other risk factors to be assessed, and interventions to reduce the risk can be implemented, for example, smoking cessation, weight reduction (if the woman is overweight or obese), or ceasing alcohol and illicit drug intake. Folic acid is often prescribed but does not eliminate the risk of neural tube defects in infants born to those women taking anticonvulsants in the first trimester of pregnancy. If drugs are going to be withdrawn, planning ahead allows this to be done slowly, which reduces the risk of recurrence compared with a rapid cessation (Viguera et al., 2007). Monotherapy, a single drug rather than multiple drugs, is preferable during pregnancy if possible, as very little is known about the risks of more than one drug either taken concomitantly or sequentially.

If a drug a woman has responded to is withdrawn prior to, or early in, pregnancy, consideration must be given to when it is to be reinstated: either later in pregnancy or in the immediate postpartum period. There should be a clear plan to augment the dose if symptoms occur. Where there is a high risk of recurrence on discontinuation and a woman stays on her mood stabilizer, changes in the monitoring regime may be required (e.g., more frequent monitoring of lithium levels and monitoring of lamotrigine levels). Women who have first-trimester exposure to lithium or anticonvulsants will require high-level ultrasound screening.

Forty-five percent of women with bipolar disorder in one US study were advised against pregnancy by a health professional, including psychiatrists, other mental health professionals, primary care physicians, or obstetricians (Viguera, Cohen, Bouffard, Whitfield, & Baldessarini, 2002). Among women who consulted with a health care provider that specialized in perinatal and reproductive care, 63 % subsequently attempted a pregnancy (Viguera et al., 2002).

Pregnancy Screening and Risk Assessment

Depression in pregnancy is as common as it is postpartum, and at least 15 % of postpartum episodes occur during pregnancy. Gavin et al. (2005) reported that the incidence of new-onset depression in pregnancy (14.5 %) was the same as the incidence in the first 3 months after delivery and Bennett, Einarson, Taddio, Koren, and Einarson (2004) observed prevalence rates of 7.4 %, 12.8 %, and 12.0 % for the first, second, and third trimesters, respectively. A large study of pregnant women in the USA found 30 % with depressive symptoms, but only 13.8 % of these were in active treatment (Marcus, Flynn, Blow, & Barry, 2003). Stowe, Hostetter, and Newport (2005) observed that although almost 90 % of the women they studied had a past history of depression and over 50 % had a history of PPD, they had not been referred for psychiatric evaluation during pregnancy.

Frequently, when there is no systematic screening protocol in place during pregnancy, women and the clinicians who treat them mistakenly attribute symptoms of depression to those of pregnancy. Even when depression has been recognized, treatment is often delayed in order to avoid fetal antidepressant exposure. Others have noted that when current depression is identified by obstetricians or midwives, it was included on the problem list for only 24 % of the depressed women (Lyell et al., 2012); however, midwives were more likely to include depression on the problem list than obstetricians.

Screening for Current Mood Disorder

In England and Wales, the National Institute for Clinical Excellence (2007) states that at a woman's first contact with services in the antenatal period, health care professionals (including midwives, obstetricians, health visitors, and GPs) should ask about:

- Past or present severe mental illness including severe depression, schizophrenia, bipolar disorder, and/or psychosis in the postnatal period
- Any previous treatment by a psychiatrist/specialist mental health team including inpatient care
- A family history of perinatal mental illness

At her initial assessment, the health care professional evaluating her should also ask the following two questions to identify possible depression:

- During the past month, have you often been bothered by feeling down, depressed, or hopeless?
- During the past month, have you often been bothered by having little interest or pleasure in doing things?

A third question should be considered if the woman answers "yes" to either of the initial questions:

- Is this something you feel you need or want help with?

The above questions aim to detect current depression. If there is a current problem or significant past history, further assessment and referral are advised with recommendations for written care plans for those with serious problems. The Scottish recommendations are very similar but do not advise on the use of any specific tool for assessing depression in pregnancy save to say that as a minimum, women should be asked about their mood when being assessed and accepted for pregnancy care (SIGN, 2012).

The Australian guidelines (Austin, Colton, Priest, Reilly, & Hadzi-Pavlovic, 2013) advise using the Edinburgh Postnatal Depression Scale (EPDS) to assess depression during pregnancy with recommendations for further evaluation and care for those scoring 13 or more. The American College of Obstetricians and Gynecologists, ACOG, states that "at this time there is insufficient evidence to support a firm recommendation for universal antepartum or postpartum screening" (ACOG, 2010).

A program in the USA, "Identify, Screen, Intervene, Support" (ISIS), is aimed to screen all pregnant women at 32 weeks of gestation with the EPDS. High scorers were assessed further, including assessment of suicidal risk, and referred on as appropriate to a brief psychosocial intervention for those with mild-to-moderate problems and to the psychiatric team if more severe or complex problems exist. The program managed to screen 75 % of patients (Thoppil, Riutcel, & Nalesnik, 2005). Altshuler et al. (2008) developed the observer-rated Pregnancy Depression Scale for use by clinicians to assess pregnant women. The scale had satisfactory validity, but this study only explored validity in 201 women who were already known to be depressed.

Antenatal Screening for the Risk of PPD

Austin and Lumley (2003) reviewed 16 studies which evaluated instruments used to screen women during pregnancy in order to identify those who are at risk of PPD. Eleven of the studies had devised instruments specifically for this purpose, in seven a study-specific instrument was combined with a standard self-report measure, three used a self-report measure alone, and three used a diagnostic interview. The conclusion was that no instrument met the criteria for routine population screening during pregnancy and postulated that this might have occurred because key risk predictors (personality traits, past history of abuse, depression, and severe blues) were not included in many of the screening instruments in question.

Subsequently, Austin and colleagues devised the Pregnancy Risk Questionnaire, PRQ, which included identified risk factors and carried out a validation study (Austin, Hadzi-Pavolvic, Saint, & Parker, 2005). They concluded that the PRQ's sensitivity and specificity are better than previous scales, but the positive predictive value remains limited. More recently, in order to develop a shorter self-report instrument, they extracted 12 items from the PRQ and validated the resulting self-report Antenatal Risk Questionnaire, ANRQ, against a diagnostic interview. They reported that the ANRQ is an acceptable tool aiding in the identification of those women at risk for PPD and is useful as part of a psychosocial screening assessment when used with the EPDS and questions on alcohol and illicit drug consumption and domestic violence (Austin, Middleton, Reilly, & Highet, 2013).

In Canada, the Antenatal Psychosocial Health Assessment, ALPHA, was developed to screen women in relation to 15 risk factors and to identify those most at risk for a poorer psychosocial outcome. When compared with usual care in a randomized controlled trial, staffs identified more psychosocial concerns by using the ALPHA, particularly those relating to family violence (Carroll et al., 2005). However, 65 % of clinicians refused to take part in the trial, which raises questions about how easy more routine or widespread use would be.

The Postpartum Depression Predictors Inventory, PDPI, based on 13 risk factors has been developed, revised the PDPI-R, and had its psychometrics properties tested (Beck, Records, & Rice, 2006; Records, Rice, & Beck, 2007). It is designed to be the basis of an interview and is not a self-report scale. The PDPI performed well in pregnancy when validated against the EPDS and a cutoff of 10.5 is recommended, but it has not been validated against a standardized interview. A Japanese translation is now available (Ikeda & Kamibeppu, 2013).

Postpartum Screening

Many national guidelines advocate screening for depression in the postpartum period, and there is evidence that when compared to routine clinical evaluation at 6 months postpartum, screening using the EPDS detected a higher incidence of depression (35.4 % vs. 6.3 %) (Evins, Theofrastous, & Galvin, 2000). While some guidelines, like those in Australia, advocate the use of a specific instrument (e.g., the EPDS), others have argued that screening in the UK primary care is not cost effective (Hewitt & Gilbody, 2009; Paulden, Palmer, Hewitt, & Gilbody, 2009). Who undertakes postpartum screening depends on the organization of services in that country and which professional is in contact with mothers. In the UK, health visitors are the appropriate professionals, whereas in the USA, where women routinely take their infants to well-baby checkups, it might be the pediatrician (see below).

Regardless of the specific guidelines of any particular health care system, it is essential that all clinicians who screen have been trained to use the instrument they have chosen and are able to carry out further clinical inquiry should a woman score above the threshold of the screen being used. Without proper resources for treatment, positive screening results have minimum value; it is critical that health care providers know their local referral pathways.

The Role of Pediatricians

Several studies have examined the role of pediatricians in screening for maternal depression. Having a preterm or a sick infant or a multiple birth increases the risk of mothers' depression, and clinicians working in neonatal intensive care have a significant role in recognizing and screening for depression in the mothers of the infants in their care (Beck, 2003). Other opportunities for screening for maternal depression exist during well-child clinic visits.

Olsen et al. (2002) surveyed pediatricians in the USA regarding their role in screening for maternal depression. Of those who responded, 57 % felt responsible for recognizing maternal depression and 45 % were confident in their ability to do this. However, only 32 % felt confident in actually diagnosing postpartum depression. Depressed mothers with higher symptom scores were younger, living alone, or were receiving public assistance. Those depressed mothers who have been seen by the clinician more often and who have an established relationship are more likely to be identified as depressed by their pediatrician (Heneghan, Johnson, Bauman, & Stein, 2000). Time constraints and lack of training were reported barriers, while a more psychosocially orientated interview style promotes mothers' disclosure of the emotional issues that may be affecting them (Wissow, Roter, & Wilson, 1994). Although many mothers welcome the opportunity to discuss their own emotional health with their child's physician, others who fear being reported to child protection services may be much less likely to disclose anything (Heneghan, Mercer, & DeLeone, 2004). Rychnovsky and Brady (2007) advised pediatricians to consider using either the EPDS or the Postpartum Depression Screening Scale (PDSS) to screen for maternal depression, and the American Academy of Pediatrics is endorsing screening at well-baby care visits.

Screening Instruments

A number of self-report instruments have been used to screen for PPD, some specifically devised for this purpose and others for depression in the general population (reviewed by Boyd, Le, & Somberg, 2005). Women scoring above threshold on these scales all require further assessment and clinical evaluation; therefore, those carrying out screening must have sufficient skills to carry this out. A high score on any screening instrument is never a substitute for skilled clinical judgment and does not equate to a diagnosis of depression.

The Edinburgh Postnatal Depression Scale

The EPDS was developed in the 1980s to overcome the limitations of other instruments not developed specifically for use in pregnancy or the postpartum period (Cox, Holden, & Sagovsky, 1987). It consists of ten items and is easily completed in a few minutes. It is free to use and, provided the validation study reference is included on the scale, can be copied without breaching copyright. Training is required in order to use it most effectively, and guidance for its use is contained in the second edition of the manual (Cox, Holden, & Henshaw 2014).

The EPDS is the most extensively researched instrument and since 1987 has been validated for use in pregnancy (Murray & Cox, 1990) as well as a variety of other populations: e.g., fathers (Ballard, Davis, Cullen, Mohan & Dean, 1994), non-postnatal women (Cox, Chapman, Murray, & Jones, 1996), following miscarriage (Lee et al., 1997), perimenopausal women (Becht et al., 2001), and mothers with intellectual disability (Gaskin & James, 2006). It has now been translated into at least 60 languages (Cox, Holden, & Henshaw, 2013).

The Postpartum Depression Screening Scale

The PDSS was developed by Beck and Gable in 2000. A Likert-type scale, it consists of 35 items and takes 5–10 min to complete. The test gives an overall severity score in one of the three ranges: normal adjustment, significant symptoms of PPD, and positive screen for PPD. It also scores seven symptom areas and has an inconsistent responding index, which serves to identify women who are just checking items at random. The first seven items have been used as a short form (Beck & Gable, 2002). Like the Edinburgh, this scale has also been translated into several languages and is distributed for a fee by Western Psychological Services.

Other Screening Instruments

The Patient Health Questionnaire, PHQ-9, a widely used screening instrument in primary care, has now been validated for use in pregnancy (Sidebottom et al., 2012). Several other instruments including the Beck Depression Inventory, BDI; Center for Epidemiologic Studies Depression Scale, CES-D; General Health Questionnaire, GHQ; Hospital Anxiety and Depression Scale, HAD; Profile of Mood States, POMS; and Zung Depression Scale, ZDS, have been used in screening for PPD and their psychometric properties (reviewed by Boyd et al., 2005).

Comparisons Between Scales

Several studies (see below) have compared the EPDS and PDSS with other measures in different populations.

BDI and EPDS

Harris, Huckle, Thomas, Johns, and Fung (1989) compared the ability of the EPDS and the BDI in identifying women with major depression in the UK. The sensitivity of the EPDS was 95 % and its specificity 93 %; the sensitivity of the BDI was 68 % and its specificity 88 %. They concluded that the performance of the BDI was markedly inferior in this application. In a Canadian study, Lussier, David, Saucier, and Borgeat (1996) reported a low concordance between the BDI and the EPDS and distinct response patterns belonging to divergent subgroups, suggesting that the two instruments were differently attuned to aspects of the presentation of PPD. More recently Lam et al. (2009) compared the two scales in pregnant women in Peru concluding that both had good internal consistency and an acceptable Pearson correlation. Su et al. (2007) found 13/14 to be the optimal cutoff for the EPDS in pregnant Taiwanese women in the second trimester and 12/13 in the third trimester with no variation by trimester with the BDI. In a study of African-American low-income postpartum women, Tandon, Cluxton-Keller, Leis, Lee, and Perry (2012) concluded that the EPDS and BDI-II performed equally well.

HAD and EPDS

A UK study (Thompson, Harris, Lazarus, & Richards, 1998) reported that the EPDS was superior to the HAD in identifying depression and similar to the observer-rated Hamilton Rating Scale for Depression, HRSD, which it matched for sensitivity to change in mood over time. An Australian group (Condon & Corkindale, 1997) found little agreement between the EPDS, the depression subscale of the HAD, the ZDS, and the depression subscale of the POMS and concluded that this might reflect the different emphasis in the item content of the questionnaires.

GHQ, CES-D, and EPDS

In France, Guedeney, Fermanian, Guelfi, and Kumar (2000) compared the EPDS with the GHQ-28 and the CES-D. The EPDS appeared better at identifying depression in postnatal women with anhedonic and anxious symptomatology but less satisfactory for those with psychomotor retardation. Navarro et al. (2007) concluded that both the EPDS and GHQ were valid instruments to detect PPD, anxiety, and adjustment disorders in their study of women at 6 weeks postpartum, whereas Logsdon and Myers (2010) reported the EPDS to perform better in adolescent mothers. When studied in women who had miscarried, Lee et al. (1997) observed that both scales had good sensitivity and specificity, concurrent validity, and internal consistency, but the EPDS only detected major depression while the GHQ detected both depression and anxiety disorders.

Kessler 10 Scale of Psychological Distress and EPDS

When the K-10 scale was compared with the EPDS against a DSM-IV diagnosis when screening pregnant women in rural India, both scales performed equally well (Fernandes et al., 2011).

ZDS, Symptom Checklist Revised (SCL-90-R), and EPDS

Despite Condon and Corkindale (1997) reporting little agreement between the EPDS and ZDS, others have found that they performed equally (Muzik et al., 2000) in an Austrian population.

Self-Reporting Questionnaire and EPDS

A study in rural Ethiopia reported that the EPDS performed less well than the Self-Reporting Questionnaire (SRQ) (Hanlon et al., 2008), but in a later study in Addis Ababa (an urban setting), the EPDS performed better (Tesfaye, Hanlon, Wondimagegn, & Alem, 2010). Pollock, Manaseki, and Patel (2006) observed a better performance by the SRQ in a literate urban population in Mongolia.

When used with nonliterate and impoverished women in Pakistan, both instruments were effective but the health workers administering them preferred to use the SRQ because of its simpler format (Rahman, Iqbal, Lovel, & Shah, 2005). Both instruments were equally valid when used in a Brazilian sample 3 months after delivery (Santos et al., 2007).

PHQ-9 and EPDS

Flynn, Sexton, Ratliff, Porter, and Zivin (2011) found few differences between the scales' performance when assessing major depression in pregnant and postpartum women in a US psychiatric outpatient setting. However, another study found that 17 % of scores were discordant. This was predicted by being younger than 30 and having a lower educational level (Yawn et al., 2009). Hanusa, Scholle, Haskett, Spadaro, and Wisner (2008) found the EPDS and short form of the Postpartum Depression Screening Scale (PDSS-SF) to be more accurate than the PHQ-9. A community-based study of postpartum women (most of whom were not literate) in Ghana reported that while internal consistency was equivalent, the PHQ-9 had better test–retest reliability and criterion validity when compared with the EPDS (Weobong et al., 2009).

PDSS, EPDS, BDI, and PHQ-9

Beck and Gable (2001) compared these three scales PDSS, EPDS and BDI, reporting that the PDSS yielded the highest combination of sensitivity of 91 % and specificity of 72 %. Also in the USA, Hanusa et al. (2008) compared the seven-item PDSS, EPDS and BDI. They concluded that the EPDS was the most accurate scale and that the EPDS and PDSS were more accurate than the PHQ-9. Chaudron et al. (2010) screened young black women in an urban setting with the EPDS, BDI, and PDSS. While all three scales performed equally well as continuous measures, the optimal cutoff for detecting major depressive disorder with the EPDS was ≤ 9 and for major and minor depression, ≤ 7.

Visual Analogue Scales and EPDS

A small study of 34 women compared scores on visual analogue scales (VAS), a continuous line between two end points; the respondent makes a mark at a point corresponding with how much agreement there is with the endpoint items at 15–21 days after delivery and the EPDS at 4 weeks postpartum. Responses on all six VAS items were significantly correlated with EPDS scores, and regression analysis showed that

61 % of the variability of EPDS scores was explained by the VAS questions (McCoy et al., 2005). It is likely that some of the differences in performance between studies and scales reflect differences in the population investigated. Clinicians should check whether the scale they plan to use has been validated in the population they are planning to screen and, if several have, which performs best.

Readability

It is important to consider the reading level of any self-rated instrument used in screening. Logsdon and Hutti (2006) assessed the EPDS, PDSS, CES-D, and BDI and reported that all were below the US 6th grade (equivalent to age 11 or 12), which is recommended for public documents. This is similar to the assessment of the ZDS (Shumway, Sentell, Unick, & Bamberg, 2004) who also reported the PHQ-9 as having a readability score at 7th grade.

Telephone and Internet Screening

Telephone screening is an option for women who find it difficult to access settings where screening is taking place face to face, i.e., those in rural areas or those reliant on public transport. The PDSS (Mitchell, Mittelstaedt, & Schott-Baer, 2006) has been shown to have good reliability when used over the telephone. An electronic version of the EPDS was first produced and validated by Glaze and Cox (1991). They reported that women were happy to complete the scale in this way. There is now an Internet version, which has been validated (Spek, Nikliček, Cuijpers, & Pop, 2008). A small mixed-methods study has explored the use of an online version of the EPDS: after receiving an e-mail prompt, the woman completes it and then receives the score and referral information (Drake, Howard, & Kinsey, 2013). The authors suggest that this may reduce the stigma associated with depression as it can be done privately in the woman's own time and also improves access for rural and disadvantaged women. Internet use of the PDSS has also been explored and found to have satisfactory validity (Le, Perry, & Sheng, 2009). In this small US study, it was noted that a higher proportion of Hispanic and Asian women participated in the Internet arm compared to the arm of the study where women completed a pen-and-paper PDSS.

Adolescent Mothers

Adolescent mothers may be more vulnerable to PPD. Research on adolescent mothers shows increasing rates of depressive symptoms in the postnatal period, particularly for those with more family conflict, fewer social supports, and low self-esteem at a time when they are negotiating the challenges of adolescence (Reid & Meadows-Oliver, 2007). DeRosa and Logsdon (2006) reviewed several screening instruments for use with adolescent mothers concluding that no scale was perfect, but using the CES-D and the EPDS together might be the best option until further data in this population is available.

Mothers Who Do Not Speak English

Migrant along with some minority groups have higher rates of depression, are often disadvantaged, and may have both practical and culturally determined barriers in accessing care (O'Mahoney & Donnelly, 2010). The EPDS and PDSS are available in several languages but have not been validated in all, so they may not be accurate or culturally appropriate. In the UK, the booklets, *How are you feeling?*, were developed initially for pregnant or postpartum women whose first language was not English, but now they are used with those who are not literate or who have an intellectual disability (Community Practitioners' and Health Visitor's Association, 2004). In addition to text, they are pictorial, and each one was designed to be culturally appropriate for speakers of that language (Arabic, Bengali, Chinese, English, Somali, and Urdu). Like rating scales, they do not replace clinical judgement and their successful use requires the time to talk, with an interpreter if needed. Clinicians need good interview skills, an understanding of the woman's cultural and personal circumstances, and the same knowledge of mood disorders and care pathways as anyone screening with a rating scale.

Women's Experiences with Screening

Several studies have explored women's views of being screened for PPD. The UK qualitative studies report that 54 % found screening with the EPDS unacceptable (Shakespeare, Blake & Garcia, 2003). Women with negative views preferred an opportunity to talk; some felt unprepared, and others were anxious about the consequences of being screened, including being thought of as a bad mother or being offered unacceptable treatment such as antidepressants (Chew-Graham, Sharp, Chamberlain, Folkes, & Turner, 2009). Consequently, they were reluctant to answer questions honestly. Most preferred screening at home rather than in the baby clinic that they felt lacked privacy. Some resented the intrusion into their personal lives, and some did not want to admit to PPD, which they felt was stigmatized.

The relationship with the person carrying out the screening is especially important; women reported that it was difficult if they had not met that person before or felt that they could not trust them (Poole, Mason, & Osborn, 2006). Two much larger Australian quantitative studies of the acceptability of screening with the EPDS have reported that the majority of women felt comfortable with the EPDS and had no difficulties in completing it. Those with high scores were more likely to report discomfort with screening (Buist et al., 2006; Gemmill, Leigh, Ericksen et al., 2006).

Risk Assessment

Suicide is the leading cause of maternal death in industrialized countries, and any pregnant or postpartum woman with a mood disorder must be evaluated regarding suicidal ideation risks to herself as well as risks to others, including her infant and any older children she might have. Out of 4,150 women completing the EPDS, 9 % reported some suicidal ideation, and 4 % reported that this was occurring "sometimes" or "quite often" (Howard, Flach, Mehay, Sharp, & Tylee, 2011). Suicidal ideation was associated with being younger, having a higher parity, and having higher levels of depressive symptoms. Postpartum women who commit suicide use violent methods such as self-immolation, hanging, or jumping from a height (Oates & Cantwell, 2011), unlike women in the general population who are more likely to use nonviolent methods such as a drug overdose. Much less is known about nonfatal deliberate self-harm in pregnant and postpartum women. One recent small study found that pregnant women who self-harmed during a previous episode of PPD are six times more likely to do so in the next postpartum period (Healey et al., 2013).

Conclusions

Given the problems associated with untreated maternal depression during pregnancy and the postpartum outlined above and the risks associated with childbearing for women with bipolar disorder, it is essential that sufferers are identified and treated. Studies have shown that screening detects more cases than are identified during routine clinical care. There are now validated instruments which can be used to facilitate this either face to face or via electronic means. Providing those carrying out the screening have been trained appropriately, a difference can be made in the lives of women with mood disorders.

References

Altshuler L. L., Cohen L. S., Vitonis A. F., Faraone, S.V., Harlow, B.L., Suri, R., … Stowe, Z.N. (2008). The pregnancy depression scale: A screening tool for depression in pregnancy. *Archives Women's Mental Health, 11*(4), 277–285.

American College of Obstetricians and Gynecologists. (2010). Screening for depression during and after pregnancy. *Committee Opinion No. 453. Obstetrics & Gynecology, 115*, 394–395.

American Psychiatric Association. (2002). Practice guideline for the treatment of patients with bipolar disorder. Second Edition. Available via Psychiatry online: http://psychiatryonline.org/content.aspx?bookid=28&sectionid=1669577. Accessed May 9 2013.

Austin, M. P., Colton, J., Priest, S., Reilly, N., & Hadzi-Pavlovic, D. (2013). The Antenatal Risk Questionnaire (ANRQ): Acceptability and use for psychosocial risk assessment in the maternity setting. *Women and Birth, 26*(1), 17–25.

Austin, M. P., Hadzi-Pavolvic, D., Saint, K., & Parker, G. (2005). Antenatal screening for the prediction of postnatal depression: Validation of psychosocial pregnancy risk questionnaire. *Acta Psychiatrica Scandinavica, 112*(4), 310–317.

Austin, M. P., & Lumley, J. (2003). Antenatal screening for postnatal depression: A systematic review. *Acta Psychiatrica Scandinavica, 107*(1), 10–17.

Austin, M. P., Middleton, M., Reilly, N. M., & Highet, N. J. (2013). Detection and management of mood disorders in the maternity setting: The Australian clinical practice guidelines. *Women and Birth, 26*(1), 2–9.

Ballard, C. G., Davis, R., Cullen, P. C., Mohan, R. N., & Dean, C. (1994). Prevalence of postnatal psychiatric morbidity in mothers and fathers. *British Journal of Psychiatry, 164*, 782–788.

Becht, M. C., Van Erp, C. F., Teeuwisse, T. M., et al. (2001). Measuring depression in women around menopausal age: towards a validation of the Edinburgh Postnatal depression scale. *Journal of Affective Disorders, 63*, 209–213.

Beck, C. T. (2003). Recognizing and screening for postpartum depression in mothers of NICU infants. *Advances in Neonatal Care, 3*(1), 37–46.

Beck, C. T., & Gable, R. K. (2000). Postpartum depression screening scale: Development and psychometric testing. *Nursing Research, 49*(5), 272–282.

Beck, C. T., & Gable, R. K. (2001). Comparative analysis of the performance of the postpartum depression screening scale with two other depression instruments. *Nursing Research, 50*(4), 242–250.

Beck, C. T., & Gable, R. K. (2002). *Postpartum depression scale screening manual*. Los Angeles: Western Psychological Services.

Beck, C. T., Records, K., & Rice, M. (2006). Further development of the postpartum depression predictors inventory-revised. *Journal of Obstetric, Gynecologic, & Neonatal Nursing, 35*(6), 735–745.

Bennett, H. A., Einarson, A., Taddio, A., Koren, G., & Einarson, T. R. (2004). Prevalence of depression during pregnancy: Systematic review. *Journal of Obstetrics & Gynecology, 103*(4), 698–709.

Boyd, R. C., Le, H. N., & Somberg, R. (2005). Review of screening instruments for postpartum depression. *Archives of Women's Mental Health, 8*(3), 141–153.

Buist, A., Condon, J., Brooks, J., Speedman, C., Milgrom, J., Hayes, B., … Bilszta, J. (2006). Acceptability of routine screening for postnatal depression: An Australia-wide study. *Journal of Affective Disorders, 93*(1), 233–237.

Carroll, J. C., Reid, A. J., Biringer, A., Midmer, D., Glazer, R. H., Wilson, L., … Stewart, D. E. (2005). Effectiveness of the Antenatal Psychosocial Health Assessment (ALPHA) form in detecting psychosocial concerns: A randomized controlled trial. *Canadian Medical Association Journal, 173*(3), 253–259.

Chaudron, L. H., Szilagyi, P. G., Tang, W., Ansone, E., Talbot, N. L., Wadkins, H. I., … Wisner, K. L. (2010). Accuracy of depression screening tools for identifying postpartum depression among urban mothers. *Pediatrics, 125*(3), e609–e617.

Chew-Graham, C. A., Sharp, D., Chamberlain, E., Folkes, L., & Turner, K. M. (2009). Disclosures of symptoms of postnatal depression, the perspectives of health professionals and women: A qualitative study. *BMC Family Practice, 10*(1), 7.

Community Practitioners' and Health Visitor's Association. (2004). *How are you feeling? Supporting the emotional and social health of minority women. A resource and training pack*. London: CPHVA.

Condon, J. T., & Corkindale, C. J. (1997). The assessment of depression in the postnatal period: A comparison of four self-report questionnaires. *Australian New Zealand Journal of Psychiatry, 31*(3), 353–359.

Cox, J. L., Chapman, G., Murray, D., & Jones, P. (1996). Validation of the Edinburgh Postnatal Depression Scale (EPDS) in non-postnatal women. *Journal of Affective Disorders, 39*(3), 185–189.

Cox, J. L., Holden, J. M., & Sagovsky, R. (1987). Detection of postnatal depression: Development of the 10-item Edinburgh postnatal depression scale. *British Journal of Psychiatry, 150*(6), 782–786.

Cox, J., Holden, J., Henshaw, C. (2014). Perinatal Mental Health: the Edinburgh Postnatal Depression Scale (EPDS) Manual. RCPsych Publications: London

DeRosa, N., & Logsdon, C. (2006). A comparison of screening instruments for depression in postpartum adolescents. *Journal of Child & Adolescent Psychiatric Nursing, 19*(1), 13–20.

Drake, E., Howard, E., & Kinsey, E. (2013). Online screening and referral for postpartum depression: An exploratory study. *Community Mental Health Journal, 50*(3), 305–311.

Evins, G. G., Theofrastous, J. F., & Galvin, S. L. (2000). Postpartum depression: A comparison of screening and routine clinical evaluation. *American Journal of Obstetrics & Gynecology, 182*(5), 1080–1082.

Fernandes, M., Srinivasan, K., Stein, S., Menezes, G., Sumithra, R. S., & Ramchandani, P. (2011). Assessing prenatal depression in the rural developing world: A comparison of two screening measures. *Archives of Women's Mental Health, 14*(3), 209–216.

Field, T. (2010). Postpartum depression effects on early interactions, parenting, and safety practices: A review. *Infant Behavior & Development, 33*(1), 1–6.

Field, T., Diego, M., & Hernanzez-Rief, M. (2006). Prenatal depression effects on the fetus and newborn: A review. *Infant Behavior & Development, 29*, 445–455.

Flynn, H. A., Sexton, M., Ratliff, S., Porter, K., & Zivin, K. (2011). Comparative performance of the Edinburgh postnatal depression scale and the patient health questionnaire-9 in pregnant and postpartum women seeking psychiatric services. *Psychiatry Research, 187*(1–2), 130–134.

Freeman, M. P., Smith, K. W., Freeman, S. A., McElroy, S. L., Kmetz, G. E., Wright, R., et al. (2002). The impact of reproductive events on the course of bipolar disorder in women. *Journal of Clinical Psychiatry, 63*(4), 284–287.

Gaskin, K., & James, H. (2006). Using the Edinburgh postnatal depression scale with learning disabled mothers. *Journal of Community Practice, 79*(12), 1462–2815.

Gavin, N., Gaynes, B., Lohr, K., Meltzer-Brody, S., Gartlehner, G., & Swinson, T. (2005). Perinatal depression: A systematic review of prevalence and incidence. *Obstetrics & Gynecology, 106*(5 Part I), 1071–1083.

Gemmill, A. W., Leigh, B., Ericksen, J., et al. (2006). A survey of the clinical acceptability of screening for postnatal depression in depressed and non-depressed women. *BMC Public Health, 6*, 211.

Glaze, R., & Cox, J. L. (1991). Validation of a computerised version of the 10-item (self-rating) Edinburgh Postnatal Depression Scale. *Journal of Affective Disorders, 22*(102), 73–77.

Grace, S. L., Evindar, A., & Stewart, D. E. (2003). The effect of postpartum depression on child cognitive development and behavior: A review and critical analysis of the literature. *Archives of Women's Mental Health, 6*(4), 263–274.

Grote, N. K., Bridge, J. A., Gavin, A. R., Melville, J. L., Iyengar, S., & Katon, W. J. (2010). A meta-analysis of depression during pregnancy and the risk of preterm birth, low birth weight, and intrauterine growth restriction. *Archives of General Psychiatry, 67*(10), 1012–1024.

Guedeney, N., Fermanian, J., Guelfi, J. D., & Kumar, R. C. (2000). The Edinburgh Postnatal Depression Scale (EPDS) and the detection of major depressive disorders in early postpartum: Some concerns about false negatives. *Journal of Affective Disorders, 61*(1), 107–112.

Hanlon, C., Medhin, G., Alem, A., Araya, M., Abdulahi, A., Hughes, M., … Prince, M. (2008). Detecting perinatal common mental disorders in Ethiopia: Validation of the self-reporting questionnaire and Edinburgh Postnatal Depression Scale. *Journal of Affective Disorders, 108*(3), 251–262.

Hanusa, B. H., Scholle, S. H., Haskett, R. F., Spadaro, K., & Wisner, K. L. (2008). Screening for depression in the postpartum period: A comparison of three instruments. *Journal of Women's Health, 17*(4), 585–596.

Harlow, B. L., Vitonis, A. F., Sparen, P., Cnattingius, S., Joffe, H., & Hultman, C. M. (2007). Incidence of hospitalization for postpartum psychotic and bipolar women with and without prior pregnancy or prenatal psychiatric hospitalisations. *Archives of General Psychiatry, 64*(1), 42–48.

Harris, B., Huckle, P., Thomas, R., Johns, S., & Fung, H. (1989). The use of rating scales to identify post-natal depression. *British Journal of Psychiatry, 154*, 813–817.

Healey, C., Morriss, R., Henshaw, C., Wadoo, O., Sajjad, A. Scholefield, H., ... Kinderman, P. (2013). Self-harm in postpartum depression: An audit of referrals to a perinatal mental health team. *Archives of Women's Mental Health, 16*(3), 237–245.

Heneghan, A. M., Johnson, E. J., Bauman, L. J., & Stein, R. E. (2000). Do pediatricians recognize mothers with depressive symptoms? *Pediatrics, 106*(6), 1367–1373.

Heneghan, A. M., Mercer, M., & DeLeone, N. L. (2004). Will mothers discuss parenting stress and depressive symptoms with their child's pediatrician? *Pediatrics, 113*(3), 460–467.

Hewitt, C. E., & Gilbody, S. M. (2009). Is it clinically and cost effective to screen for postnatal depression: A systematic review of controlled clinical trials and economic evidence. *British Journal of Obstetrics & Gynecology, 116*(8), 1019–1027.

Howard, L. M., Flach, C., Mehay, A., Sharp, D., & Tylee, A. (2011). The prevalence of suicidal ideation identified by the Edinburgh Postnatal Depression Scale in postpartum women in primary care: Findings from the RESPOND trial. *BMC Pregnancy & Childbirth, 11*(1), 57.

Ikeda, M., & Kamibeppu, K. (2013). Measuring the risk factors for postpartum depression: Development of the Japanese version of the Postpartum Depression Predictors Inventory-Revised (PDPI-R-J). *BMC Pregnancy & Childbirth, 13*(1), 112.

Lam, N., Contreras, H., Mori, E., Cuesta, F., Gutierrez, C., Neyra, M., ... Córdova, G. (2009). Comparison of two self report questionnaires for depressive symptoms detection in pregnant women. *Anales de la Facultdad Medicina, 80*, 28–32.

Le, H. N., Perry, D. F., & Sheng, X. (2009). Using the internet to screen for postpartum depression. *Maternal Child Health Journal, 13*(2), 213–221.

Lee, D. T., Wong, C. K., Ungvari, G. S., Cheung, L. P., Haines, C. J., & Chung, T. K. (1997). Screening psychiatric morbidity after miscarriage: Application of the 30-item general health questionnaire and the Edinburgh postnatal depression scale. *Psychosomatic Medicine, 59*, 207–210.

Logsdon, M. C., & Hutti, M. H. (2006). Readability: An important issue impacting healthcare for women with postpartum depression. *American Journal of Maternal Child Nursing, 31*(6), 351–355.

Logsdon, M. C., & Myers, J. A. (2010). Comparative performance of two depression screening instruments in adolescent mothers. *Journal of Women's Health, 19*(6), 1123–1128.

Lussier, V., David, H., Saucier, J. F., & Borgeat, F. (1996). Self-rating assessment of postnatal depression: A comparison of the beck depression inventory and the Edinburgh postnatal depression scale. *The Journal of Prenatal and Perinatal Psychology and Health, 11*, 81–91.

Lyell, D. J., Chambers, A. S., Steidtman, D., Tsai, E., Caughey, A. B., Wong, A., & Mauber, R. (2012). Antenatal identification of major depressive disorder: A cohort study. *American Journal of Obstetrics & Gynecology, 207*(6), 506, e1–e6.

Marcus, S. M., Flynn, H. A., Blow, F. C., & Barry, K. L. (2003). Depressive symptoms among pregnant women screened in obstetrics settings. *Journal of Women's Health, 12*(4), 373–380.

McCoy, S. J., Beal, J. M., Peyton, M. E., Stewart, A. L., DeMers, A. M., & Watson, G. H. (2005). Correlations of visual analog scales with Edinburgh postnatal depression scale. *Journal of Affective Disorders, 86*(2–3), 295–297.

Mitchell, A. M., Mittelstaedt, M. E., & Schott-Baer, D. (2006). Postpartum depression: The reliability of telephone screening. *American Journal of Maternal Child Nursing, 31*, 382–387.

Munk-Olsen, T., Laursen, T. M., Mendelson, T., Pederson, C. B., Mors, O., & Mortensen, P. B. (2009). Risks and predictors of readmission for a mental disorder during the postpartum period. *Archives of General Psychiatry, 66*(2), 189–195.

Munk-Olsen, T., Laursen, T. M., Pederson, C. B., Mors, O., & Mortensen, P. B. (2007). Family and partner psychopathology and risk of postpartum mental disorders. *Journal of Clinical Psychiatry, 68*, 1947–1953.

Murphy-Eberenz, K., Zandi, P. P., March, D., Crowe, R. R., Scheftner, W. A., Alexander, M., ... Levinson, D. F. (2006). Is perinatal depression familial? *Journal of Affective Disorders, 90*(1), 49–55.

Murray, D., & Cox, J. L. (1990). Identifying depression during pregnancy with the Edinburgh Postnatal Depression Scale (EPDS). *Journal of Reproductive Infant Psychology, 8*, 99–107.

Muzik, M., Klier, C. M., Rosenblum, K. L., Holzinger, A., Umek, W., & Katschnig, H. (2000). Are commonly used self-report inventories suitable for screening postpartum depression and anxiety disorders? *Acta Psychiatrica Scandinavica, 102*, 71–73.

National Institute for Health and Clinical Excellence. (2007). *Antenatal and postnatal mental health: Clinical management and service guidance.* London: National Institute for Health and Clinical Excellence.

Navarro, P., Ascaso, C., Garcia, E. L., Aguado, J., Torres, A., & Martin-Santos, R. (2007). Postnatal psychiatric morbidity: A validation study of the GHQ-12 and the EPDS as screening tools. *General Hospital Psychiatry, 29*(1), 1–7.

O'Hara, M. W., & Swain, A. M. (1996). Rates and risks of postpartum depression: A meta-analysis. *International Review of Psychiatry, 8*, 37–54.

O'Mahoney, J., & Donnelly, T. (2010). Immigrant and refugee women's post-partum depression help-seeking experiences and access to care: A review and analysis of the literature. *Journal of Psychiatric Mental Health Nursing, 17*(10), 917–928.

Oates, M., & Cantwell, R. (2011). Deaths from psychiatric causes. *British Journal of Obstetrics & Gynecology, 118*, 1–203.

Olsen, A. L., Kemper, K. J., Kellejer, K. J., Hammond, C. S., Zuckerman, B. S., & Dietrich, A. J. (2002). Primary care pediatricians' roles and perceived responsibilities in the identification and management of maternal depression. *Pediatrics, 110*(6), 1169–1176.

Paulden, M., Palmer, S., Hewitt, C., & Gilbody, S. (2009). Screening for postnatal depression in primary care: Cost effective analysis. *British Medical Journal, 339*, b5203.

Pollock, J. I., Manaseki, H. S., & Patel, V. (2006). Detection of depression in women of child-bearing age in non-western cultures: A comparison of the Edinburgh postnatal depression scale and the self-reporting questionnaire-20 in Mongolia. *Journal of Affective Disorders, 92*(2–3), 267–271.

Poole, H., Mason, L., & Osborn, T. (2006). Women's views of being screened for postnatal depression. *Journal of Community Practice, 79*(11), 363–367.

Rahman, A., Iqbal, Z., Lovel, H., & Shah, M. A. (2005). Screening for postnatal depression in the developing world: A comparison of the WHO self-reporting questionnaire (SRQ20) and the Edinburgh postnatal depression screen (EPDS). Journal of Pakistan Psychiatric Society, 2(2), 69.

Records, K., Rice, M., & Beck, C. T. (2007). Psychometric assessment of the postpartum depression predictors inventory–revised. *Journal of Nursing Measurement, 15*(3), 189–202.

Reid, V. & Meadows, O. M. (2007). Postpartum depression in adolescent mothers: an integrative review of the literature. *Journal of Pediatric Health Care 21*, 289–298.

Royal College of Obstetricians and Gynaecologists. (2011). *Management of women with mental health issues during pregnancy and the postnatal period, 14.* London: RCOG.

Rychnovsky, J. D., & Brady, M. A. (2007). Choosing a postpartum screening instrument for your pediatric practice. *Journal of Pediatric Health Care, 22*(1), 64–67.

Santos, I. S., Matijasevich, A., Tavares, B. F., da Cruz Lima, A. C., Rieger, R. E., & Lopes, B. C. (2007). Comparing validity of Edinburgh scale and SRQ20 in screening for post-partum depression. *Clinical Practice & Epidemiology in Mental Health, 3*, 18.

Scottish Intercollegiate Guidelines Network. (2012). *Management of perinatal mood disorders.* Edinburgh: Scottish Intercollegiate Guidelines Network.

Shakespeare, J., Blake, F., & Garcia, J. (2003). A qualitative study of the acceptability of routine screening of postnatal women using the Edinburgh postnatal depression scale. *British Journal of General Practice, 53*(493), 614–619.

Shumway, M., Sentell, T., Unick, G., & Bamberg, W. (2004). Cognitive complexity of self-administered depression measures. *Journal of Affective Disorders, 83*(2), 191–198.

Sidebottom, A. C., Harrison, P. A., Godecker, A., et al. (2012). Validation of the Patient Health Questionnaire (PHQ)-9 for prenatal depression screening. *Archives of Women's Mental Health, 15*, 1434–1816.

Spek, V., Nikliček, I., Cuijpers, P., & Pop, V. (2008). Internet administration of the Edinburgh depression scale. *Journal of Affective Disorders, 106*(3), 301–305.

Stewart, R. (2007). Maternal depression and infant growth: A review of recent evidence. *Maternal Child Nutrition, 3*(2), 94–107.

Stowe, Z. N., Hostetter, A. L., & Newport, D. J. (2005). The onset of postpartum depression: Implications for clinical screening in obstetrical and primary care. *American Journal of Obstetrics & Gynecology, 192*(2), 522–526.

Su, K. P., Chiu, T. H., Huang, C. L., Ho, M., Lee, C. C., Wu, P.L., ... Pariante, C. M. (2007). Different cutoff points for different trimesters? The use of Edinburgh Postnatal Depression Scale and Beck Depression Inventory to screen for depression in pregnant Taiwanese women. *General Hospital Psychiatry, 29*(5), 436–441.

Tandon, S. D., Cluxton-Keller, F., Leis, J., Lee, H. N., & Perry, D. F. (2012). A comparison of three screening tools to identify perinatal depression among low-income African American women. *Journal of Affective Disorders, 136*(102), 155–162.

Tesfaye, M., Hanlon, C., Wondimagegn, D., & Alem, A. (2010). Detecting postnatal common mental disorders in addis Ababa, Ethiopia: Validation of the Edinburgh postnatal depression scale and Kessler scales. *Journal of Affective Disorders, 122*(1–2), 102–108.

Thompson, W. M., Harris, B., Lazarus, J., & Richards, C. (1998). A comparison of the performance of rating scales used in the diagnosis of postnatal depression. *Acta Psychiatrica Scandinavica, 98*(3), 224–227.

Thoppil, J., Riutcel, T. L., & Nalesnik, S. W. (2005). Early intervention for perinatal depression. *American Journal of Obstetrics & Gynecology, 192*(5), 1446–1448.

Viguera, A. C., Cohen, L. S., Bouffard, S., Whitfield, T. H., & Baldessarini, R. J. (2002). Reproductive decisions by women with bipolar disorder after prepregnancy psychiatric consultation. *American Journal of Psychiatry, 159*(12), 2102–2104.

Viguera, A. C., Whitfield, T., Baldessarini, F. J., Newport, D., Stowe, Z., Reminick, A., ... Cohen, L. (2007). Risk of recurrence in women with bipolar disorder during pregnancy: Prospective study of mood stabilizer discontinuation. *American Journal of Psychiatry, 164*(12), 1817–1824.

Weobong, B., Akpalu, B., Doku, V., Owusu-Asyei, S., Hurt, L., Kirkwood, B., ... Prince, M. (2009). The comparative validity of screening scales for postnatal common mental disorder in Kintampo, Ghana. *Journal of Affective Disorders, 113*(1-2), 109–117.

Wissow, L. S., Roter, D. L., & Wilson, M. E. H. (1994). Pediatrician interview style and mothers' disclosure of psychosocial issues. *Pediatrics, 93*(2), 289–295.

Yawn, B. P., Pace, W., Wollan, P. C., Bertram, S., Kurland, M., Graham, D., et al. (2009). Concordance of Edinburgh postnatal depression scale EPDS and patient health questionnaire PHQ-9 to assess increased risk of depression among postpartum women. *Journal of the American Board of Family Medicine, 22*(5), 483–491.

Postpartum Adjustment: What Is Normal and What Is Not

Lucy J. Puryear

Introduction

Women have been becoming pregnant and delivering babies since the beginning of time. Though it happens every day, all over the world, it is a complicated process both physically and psychologically. Even when everything goes as expected, there are physical, biochemical, and hormonal adjustments the body must make after birth as well as enormous psychological transitions. A woman's body is never the same as it was before birth, and who she is as a person is changed forever. For all women the postpartum period is a time of physical recovery and psychological adjustment and can span many weeks or months with challenges along the way.

Sometimes all does not go as expected; babies come earlier than they were meant to, may need to be born via caesarean section, or may have their own physical or neurological challenges. The psychological and physical challenges all mothers face may turn into more serious difficulties, including depression and anxiety.

What is normal? The transition from pregnancy to new motherhood happens in a moment. The experiences vary from woman to woman. For some, the moment is described as euphoric and the feeling of love for their newborn is immediate and overwhelming. Many women describe this feeling as the most intense emotion they have ever experienced. For other women the exertion of labor and delivery may overshadow the joy of having a newborn baby, and the relief of having the baby delivered is accompanied by a sense of unreality that a real living baby has been put in her arms. It may take several days for the new mother to slowly warm up to the idea that this baby is hers.

L.J. Puryear, M.D. (✉)
Department of Obstetrics and Gynecology and Menninger
Department of Psychiatry Baylor College of Medicine, Medical Director Center
for Reproductive Psychiatry The Pavilion for Women, Texas Children's Hospital,
Houston, TX, USA
e-mail: ljpuryea@texaschildrens.org

Both responses are normal, and no one should be judged for how quickly or how slowly she falls in love. It is a huge adjustment to become a mother, and everyone adjusts at her own pace. Bringing a newborn home is a major shift in a woman's identity, and it can take time to become accustomed to the new paradigm. Many factors of a woman's past and current history make the experience uniquely hers.

Along with joy can come a sense of loss, ambivalence, and fear. All of these responses are part of the normal process of becoming a parent. Although some of these feelings may be seen as more negative, this does not mean that they are not normal. Having a baby may have been planned and eagerly awaited, but acknowledging that negative feelings also accompany this process is important. It is important for the mother and her support system to know the difference between normal negative feelings and those that are more serious and require intervention. A more detailed discussion of the common psychological adjustments that accompany becoming a mother is discussed in chapter "The Psychological Gestation of Motherhood."

The Baby Blues

It is estimated that 80 % of women will experience symptoms of the baby blues (Nonacs & Cohen, 1998). These statistics are similar to the percentage of women who experience the symptoms of premenstrual syndrome (Steiner, Peer, Macdougall, & Haskett, 2011). Neither of these symptom complexes qualify as a psychiatric illness; most women will experience the mild emotional ups and downs that can go along with normal hormonal changes of the menstrual cycle and delivering a baby.

The baby blues occur during the first 2 weeks after delivery, and many women describe experiencing a change in mood 24–48 h after birth. The symptoms include crying for no reason, emotions changing from happy to tearful within minutes, mild irritability and frustration, anxiety, and feelings of being overwhelmed by all of the new responsibilities that come with having a baby (Beck, 2006). The baby blues is not the same as depression. The symptoms generally subside with time as the mother becomes more comfortable with herself and her new baby and as a more regular schedule emerges. Though tearful at times, the new mother feels excited and happy about the changes in her life, even if there is some adjustment to her new role.

There is no clear scientific evidence as to why the baby blues occur, although there is speculation that it is related to the huge hormonal changes that occur within the first 3 days after delivery. During pregnancy, estrogen and progesterone levels climb higher than at any other time in a woman's life only to fall precipitously with the delivery of the placenta (Skalkidou, Hellgren, Comasco, Sylven, & Sundstrom Poromaa, 2012). It is this hormonal change that likely precipitates the tearfulness and mood lability of the baby blues, along with the psychological stressors of new parenthood and sleep deprivation. Over the first 2 weeks, as the hormonal changes become less dramatic, the symptoms of the baby blues typically resolve. By the end of the baby's first 2 weeks, both mother and baby have more of a rhythm established, breastfeeding is usually going well, and reality of being a parent is less overwhelming. Women with the baby blues do not need to seek medical attention.

Postpartum Depression

While the percentages vary depending on the study, for about 13–19 % of women, more serious mood symptoms occur that are much more debilitating than the milder tearfulness and transient symptoms of the baby blues (O'Hara et al., 2012). Postpartum depression, PPD, is a serious illness that must be recognized as such and treated. Although PPD does not have a diagnostic code in the *Diagnostic and Statistical Manual, Version 5*, DSM-5 (American Psychiatric Association & American Psychiatric Association DSM-5 Task Force, 2013), separate from major depressive disorder, mothers with PPD and those who treat them know that there are unique features of depression during the postpartum period that are especially difficult for the new mother with a new baby at home.

PPD is not prolonged baby blues. Baby blues almost always resolve within 2 weeks, and any symptoms of tearfulness or depressed mood that continue beyond that time must be investigated. The Edinburgh Postpartum Depression Scale, EPDS, is a reliable and validated screening tool used by many clinicians to screen mothers for PPD (Cox, Holden, & Sagovsky, 1987). It is a self-rating scale easily answered by a new mother and can help identify those women who may need further help. Many hospitals and health care providers are using this scale routinely to aid in the recognition of PPD, and some states require all women who deliver a baby to be screened. This recommendation is controversial given the lack of resources available for mental health treatment in many communities.

Women with PPD may have many of the same symptoms as depression experienced at other times during a woman's life: depressed mood, low energy, appetite changes, sleep difficulties, lack of interest in usual activities, guilt, feelings of worthlessness and hopelessness, feeling agitated, and thoughts of death. For this reason, and because to date there has been limited evidence (Jones, Cantwell & Nosology Working Group, Royal College of Psychiatrists Perinatal Section, 2010) indicating that this is a biologically distinct illness, PPD has been classified as a modifier under the category of major depressive disorder. However, in the context of a new baby, some of these symptoms may be especially significant and specific for PPD and have a different quality given the environment in which they occur.

Sleep disturbance may be one of the hallmark symptoms of PPD (Ross, Murray, & Steiner, 2005; Swanson, Pickett, Flynn, & Armitage, 2011). Sleep is at a premium, and most new mothers long for the chance to sleep longer than 2 or 3 h at a time. For mothers with depression, they find it difficult to sleep even when the baby is sleeping. Ruminating about the baby is common, and it is difficult to turn off those thoughts in order to fall asleep. As sleep becomes more elusive, the mother becomes more sleep deprived, which many believe may contribute to worsening her depression (Swanson et al., 2011).

For some new mothers one of the most disturbing symptoms of PPD may be their feeling of detachment or not feeling love for their newborn. She feels distant and removed, which is exactly the opposite of how she thought she would feel. Guilt accompanies this feeling of detachment along with the belief that she is a terrible mother and should never have had a baby. These thoughts are often kept hidden due to the shame a new mother experiences because of what she perceives as a lack of love for her baby. These feelings may lead the mother to believe that the baby and the rest of her family would be better off without her, and suicidal thoughts may become more prominent (Healey et al., 2013). Some mothers, however, feel very emotionally connected to their infant and describe that is the one thing that is keeping them from experiencing complete despair.

For any woman with depression it is imperative that she be asked if she is having thoughts of hurting herself or hurting her baby. Although not common, new mothers do attempt suicide and these thoughts are not likely to be volunteered. There are times when a woman may feel badly about leaving her baby without a mother and will take the baby's life prior to taking her own. Suicide is a tragic consequence of untreated depression, particularly when it is a new mother and her newborn or even other children in the family. Many of these tragic events can be prevented with the appropriate recognition and treatment (Spinelli, 2004). Most women with PPD will recover from this debilitating illness when receiving proper care.

Risk Factors

It is important that women at risk for PPD be identified prior to delivery. With identification, measures can be put into place to decrease the risk of PPD occurring or to identify those women who need special attention after delivery for quick recognition of symptoms before they get worse. Studies have shown that the following situations may make a woman at increased risk for a postpartum illness:

1. Previous episode of depression in a woman's life.
2. If there has been a previous episode of PPD, there is about a 50 % risk of another episode.
3. Severe premenstrual syndrome: It is believed that there is a subset of women who are vulnerable to mood symptoms with normal hormonal shifts. These women are also vulnerable to mood symptoms around the time of menopause.
4. Family history of bipolar disorder.
5. Poor relationship support (Beck, 2001; O'Hara & McCabe, 2013; Stowe & Nemeroff, 1995).

Some women may have none of the above risk factors, and yet PPD can still occur.

Cause

Similar to baby blues, it is believed that the rapid hormonal changes that occur in the first few days postpartum are responsible for triggering mood symptoms in susceptible women (Skalkidou et al., 2012). It is hypothesized that there is something biologically unique about women with PPD that makes them vulnerable to mood changes as a result of changes in hormones (Bloch et al., 2000). The differences may be due to genetic alterations in serotonin and/or estrogen receptors in the brain (Moses-Kolko et al., 2008). Women with PPD are also at risk for symptoms around the time of perimenopause when hormonal levels are again fluctuating (Studd & Nappi, 2012).

Newer research is attempting to locate genes that may predispose women to PPD, biochemical alterations in oxytocin or glutamate in the brain (Jonas et al., 2013), and differing functional activity of the brain in women with PPD when compared to normal controls (Engineer et al., 2013; Jonas et al., 2013; Pinheiro et al., 2013; Suda, Segi-Nishida, Newton, & Duman, 2008; Westberg & Eriksson, 2008). The goal is to find out what causes PPD, to identify those who are at risk for developing it, and to put measures in place to prevent it from occurring.

Biological mechanisms are not the only explanations for PPD; environmental factors may contribute to a genetic or a biologic risk. In many studies poor psychosocial support is confirmed as a risk factor for PPD, along with any stressor during the year (Dennis & Dowswell, 2013; Misri et al., 2012).

Treatment

Depression is a treatable illness; the sooner the symptoms are recognized the less severe they may become and the more quickly remission may be achieved. Early recognition and treatment also reduce the risk of suicide.

Restoration of quality sleep is an integral part of treatment. In some cases of mild depression, 4–5 h of uninterrupted sleep for 2 or 3 days may be enough to start the woman on the road to recovery (Khazaie, Ghadami, Knight, Emamian, & Tahmasian, 2013; Ross et al., 2005). Protecting sleep is important for any new mother; family members and other support systems are critical in supporting a mother suffering with depression and making sure that she has time to sleep.

Given the disruption in sleep that accompanies having a newborn, strategies must be put in place to ensure that when the baby is sleeping the mother can also sleep. This often means putting the baby in another room with a family member so that if the baby awakens before it is time to be fed, it can be soothed and comforted by someone else, away from the mother's hearing. At night, baby nurses or postpartum doulas can minimize the amount of time a nursing mother is awake by bringing the baby to her for feeding, then changing the baby, and putting it back to sleep afterward. These options may be expensive, but partners and other family members can function in the same way. Not being able to sleep when the baby is sleeping can be an early indication that PPD or anxiety is present and needs further investigation.

Psychotherapy is another important option for the treatment of depression. There are several types of therapy shown to be specifically effective for PPD (Nanzer et al., 2012; Nonacs & Cohen, 2002; O'Mahen, Himle, Fedock, Henshaw, & Flynn, 2013). Interpersonal psychotherapy focuses on the role transition that occurs with motherhood and helps process the losses that accompany any change in role. A new mother needs support as she moves into her new identity of motherhood (Dennis et al., 2012; Reay et al., 2012; Stuart, 2012). Even if medication is necessary, the combination of therapy and medication has been shown to be more effective than either used alone (Weissman et al., 1979). Support groups are useful; women hear from other women who are experiencing similar feelings and can interact with women who have recovered (Shaw et al., 2006). Many hospitals, clinics, and community organizations are forming support groups for new mothers, thus making these types of interventions more readily available.

For more serious depression, when the mother is not able to take care of herself or her baby, or is having frequent suicidal thoughts, medication is often necessary. The antidepressants used to treat major depression are effective for PPD as well. Research shows that many of the antidepressants, particularly the serotonin reuptake inhibitors, SRIs, are safe to take while breastfeeding (Birnbaum et al., 1999; Gentile, 2005; Worsley, Gilbert, Gavrilidis, Naughton, & Kulkarni, 2013). Given the reassuring literature, mothers may not have to choose between breastfeeding and treating their depression.

Other alternative modalities have been studied for the treatment of PPD including omega-3 fatty acids, acupuncture, massage, and light therapy (Freeman, 2009; Markhus et al., 2013). These options may be less effective for severe depression, but they can be complementary additions to medication therapy and psychotherapy.

Anxiety

One of the universal aspects of parenthood is anxiety. Many parents report that they never stop worrying, even when their children are grown and out of the house and have children of their own. For anyone who has ever brought a newborn baby home, anxiety is pervasive, particularly if it is their first child. This is reasonable given that a newborn baby is helpless, and a parent is responsible for insuring that it is fed, warm, and pain free and that nothing in the environment can cause the baby harm. It is very common for new parents to wake up in the middle of the night to make sure that their child is still breathing. *Not* being anxious when there is a helpless baby at home is not normal.

Anxiety is a broad category under which several specific disorders are classified in the DSM-5. The ones of particular importance during the postpartum period are the three that most commonly occur: generalized anxiety disorder, GAD; panic disorder, PD; and obsessive compulsive disorder, OCD. Although OCD was previously classified as an anxiety disorder in the DSM IV (American Psychiatric Association & American Psychiatric Association Task Force on DSM-5, 1994), in the recently revised DSM-5 it has been placed in a category with other disorders that are considered to have similar features of unwanted thoughts and behaviors. Due to the fact that the anxiety component of OCD is a significant feature during the postpartum period, for the purposes of this chapter it will continue to be included in the section on anxiety disorders.

Generalized Anxiety Disorder

Anxiety symptoms become problematic when they are out of control and interfere with the mother's ability to function. The psychiatric disorder GAD includes physical symptoms of chest tightness, shortness of breath, racing heart, irritability, fatigue, nausea, sweating, muscle tension or trembling, and psychological symptoms of constant worry or obsessing about small things, a sense of impending doom, and difficulty concentrating (Jiang, Gagliardi, Krishnan, & Rama, 2009). GAD is a pervasive feeling of anxiety that is present all the time, with little relief from symptoms.

This heightened sense of anxiety makes it impossible to do almost anything other than thinking about the baby and keeping it safe. Although checking the baby to make sure that it is breathing normal, having to do so over and over again is not. Mothers may stop eating, sleeping, and feel like that they are "going crazy." They may need constant reassurance that their baby is okay, and this may result in frequent calls or trips to the pediatrician. Imagining all sorts of horrible things that may occur, even if these things make no sense, is a constant worry. Any attempt to calm the fears with logic and facts makes little difference. The mother with anxiety often realizes that she is being "ridiculous" but is unable to control her thoughts.

Postpartum anxiety has received less attention than PPD, and fewer studies have been published specifically looking at the rates of and risk factors for anxiety during the postpartum period (Ross & McLean, 2006). In a recently published study, 17 % of new mothers tested scored positively for anxiety. Positive scores were associated with caesarean section, reduced duration of breastfeeding, and higher use of maternal health care in the first 2 weeks postpartum (Paul, Downs, Schaefer, Beiler, & Weisman, 2013). For women with anxiety, the symptoms can be equally as distressing and disabling as PPD.

Although diagnosed separately, anxiety and PPD often go hand in hand (Wisner, Peindl, Gigliotti, & Hanusa, 1999). A recent study found that 38 % of women diagnosed with PPD also had comorbid anxiety (Austin et al., 2010). It may be difficult to tell if depression or anxiety is the predominant symptom. This combination of symptoms can be particularly debilitating.

Panic Disorder

PD may accompany generalized anxiety or it may occur on its own. As opposed to GAD where anxiety is constant, PD is intermittent, symptoms coming out of the blue, and usually remitting within 15 min to half an hour, although some women may describe symptoms lasting longer. Classic symptoms of PD include palpitations, pounding heart, or accelerated heart rate, sweating, shaking, shortness of breath, chest pain or tightness, feeling dizzy or lightheaded, fear of losing control or going crazy, numbness or tingling, chills or hot flashes, and a fear of impending doom (American Psychiatric Association & American Psychiatric Association DSM-5 Task Force, 2013). One of the most disabling symptoms is the fear of having another panic attack that can lead to agoraphobia or fear of leaving home.

Research differs on the course of panic disorder during pregnancy. PD may be one of the few psychiatric illnesses that will improve during pregnancy. Studies show mixed results with approximately half the patients improving and the other half with no change in symptoms or worsening (Cohen, Sichel, Dimmock, & Rosenbaum, 1994). For women with preexisting PD, symptoms often worsen postpartum even with treatment during pregnancy. In some cases the first presentation of the illness is during the first months postpartum (Wisner, Peindl & Hanusa, 1996).

Obsessive-Compulsive Disorder

OCD affects about 1–2 % of the population, and symptoms can range from mild to severe (Kessler, Petukhova, Sampson, Zaslavsky, & Wittchen, 2012). At its most severe OCD is debilitating, and leading a normal life can be difficult.

According to the DSM-5, OCD is marked by obsessions, unwanted thoughts that persist despite the attempt to get rid of them, and compulsions or behaviors designed to relieve the anxiety that is generated by the obsession (American Psychiatric Association & American Psychiatric Association DSM-5 Task Force, 2013). One of the most common OCD symptoms is a fear of contamination or fear of germs. These fears become a psychiatric disorder when the fear of contamination is constant and hand washing only relieves that fear momentarily. The hand-washing behavior must be repeated over and over again as the thoughts and resultant anxiety continue. For a new mother, contamination fears and other fears that some harm will come to the baby can lead to frequent washing and checking. These thoughts and behaviors cause extraordinary anxiety, and sometimes the new mother feels that she is going "crazy."

Studies have shown that the first episode of OCD for many occurs during the postpartum period in women with no previous obsessional or compulsive symptoms (Brandes, Soares, & Cohen, 2004; Sichel, Cohen, Dimmock, & Rosenbaum, 1993; Uguz, Akman, Kaya, & Cilli, 2007). Other women with milder obsession and compulsions prior to pregnancy find that the symptoms become worse postpartum and require treatment for the first time (Altshuler, Hendrick, & Cohen, 1998). Women who had been treated for OCD prior to and throughout pregnancy may have a worsening of symptoms postpartum despite continued treatment (Chaudron & Nirodi, 2010; Forray, Focseneanu, Pittman, McDougle, & Epperson, 2010).

There are unique features during the postpartum period that have led to the label "postpartum OCD." There is no official diagnosis for OCD that occurs specifically postpartum, but there are differences in classical OCD and the disorder that occurs only during the postpartum period (McGuinness, Blissett, & Jones, 2011; Uguz et al., 2007). The obsessions almost always involve the infant, either concerns of some harm from the outside environment or fear that the mother herself will inflict harm on her baby (Uguz et al., 2007). The thoughts can be incapacitating given that they come out of the blue and are intrusive and unwanted and the mother does not want to act on them. The overwhelming fear is that she will lose control and act out the unwelcome images.

Some common intrusive thoughts or obsessions include letting go of the baby in the bathtub, dropping it down the stairs or out a window, or picking up a knife and stabbing the baby. These thoughts are horrifying, and the anxiety-relieving behavior is to avoid the baby. Mothers will stop giving the baby a bath, will not carry the baby by staircases, and will not go into the kitchen where there are knives. At worst, women shut themselves away from the infant and refuse to care for it.

These thoughts of harm are not the same as postpartum psychosis, which carries a risk of infanticide. Psychotic symptoms are delusions or hallucinations that sometimes will cause the mother to hurt her baby for some bizarre reason, such as saving the world because the baby is possessed, or to fulfill some plan of God (Sit, Rothschild, & Wisner, 2006). Women with postpartum OCD do not want to hurt their infant but are terrified that they will. They know that the intrusive thoughts make no sense and are not something they want to do. Women with postpartum OCD will not harm their babies.

Women may experience only postpartum OCD symptoms, or they may occur in the context of PPD (Wisner et al., 1999). It is not known what percentage of postpartum women will have OCD symptoms, but there are some estimates that as many as 90 % of new mothers will infrequently experience some negative and intrusive thoughts of harm to their infant at some point after delivery (Abramowitz, Khandker, Nelson, Deacon, & Rygwall, 2006). Most women will not volunteer these thoughts, given the horrible nature of them and the shame associated. Some women are afraid that if they admit these thoughts, the child will be taken away from them. When asked if a woman has ever had thoughts that something bad will happen to her baby or if she has had thoughts about harming her baby, she is usually relieved that the subject has been brought out into the open, especially when she receives reassurance that these symptoms are common and do not make her a horrible mother.

Cause

As previously mentioned, anxiety is a normal response to any stressful situation, including the birth of a new baby. When working properly, the hypothalamic-pituitary-adrenal axis, HPA axis, regulates our flight or fight response to a potentially dangerous situation (Connor & Davidson, 1998). The HPA axis controls the release of epinephrine and norepinephrine, modulates blood flow throughout the body, can sharpen our focus and attention, and can increase immediate available energy for action. Anxiety disorders have been hypothesized to be due to maladaptive over-functioning of the HPA axis resulting in a heightened sense of danger as well as the inability to calm down when the danger has disappeared or is no longer present (Slattery & Neumann, 2008). Other biologic systems and pathways have been implicated in the pathophysiology of anxiety (Connor & Davidson, 1998), but simplistically, the nervous system is "hyper alert" and ready to take action. This process explains why mothers with anxiety often need constant reassurance. Even though the danger has passed, the brain has not been able to turn off the normal response to a perceived threat.

Risk Factors

Anxiety disorders can occur in any new mother, but there is limited research on the risk factors for anxiety disorders during the postpartum period. In general women with a history of anxiety are more likely to have symptoms that reemerge or worsen postpartum (Cohen et al., 1994). Women who are used to being in control and are high achievers may find that the anxiety they felt that was useful in helping them succeed in school or at work now interferes with their ability to function in a situation they have very little control over. The unpredictability of a new baby can be particularly stressful, and the anxiety can be disabling.

Having a family history of anxiety disorders, panic attacks, or OCD makes it more likely that postpartum anxiety will occur. A history of trauma, poor social support, economic distress, or chronic illness can also increase the risk of postpartum anxiety (Misri et al., 2012). More attention needs to be paid to anxiety disorders during pregnancy and postpartum as these conditions are common and little is known about risk factors and prevention.

Treatment

There are several treatment options for anxiety and panic disorders. Many non-pharmacologic interventions have been found to have efficacy in the treatment of perinatal mood and anxiety disorders (Sutter-Dallay, Giaconne-Marcesche, Glatigny-Dallay, & Verdoux, 2004). In particular, cognitive-behavioral therapy, CBT, has proven efficacy in relieving the symptoms of anxiety, panic, and OCD during pregnancy and postpartum (Brandes et al., 2004). Focusing on maladaptive thinking patterns that can then lead to physical symptoms and behaviors and working to reframe these negative thoughts can cause a significant reduction in distress.

Exposure response prevention, ERP, is a therapy specific to OCD where the person is exposed to the distressing trigger (i.e., germs) and then is prevented from performing the behavior that decreases the anxiety, such as hand washing (Lindsay, Crino, & Andrews, 1997). The exposures become more and more intense, and the amount of time tolerating the anxiety becomes longer. With time, the offending thought no longer causes the symptoms, for example, touching a door handle no longer means that you have to wash your hands immediately. These types of behavioral therapies are effective but are time consuming and can initially cause an increase in anxiety.

SRIs as well as other antidepressants are useful agents for the treatment of depression and anxiety disorders (Kapczinski et al., 2003). Unfortunately, for both depression and anxiety, it may take 2–3 weeks to notice an improvement in symptoms and up to 6 or 8 weeks to achieve symptom remission. For this reason alternative treatments are imperative to control anxiety until the antidepressants have time to work.

Benzodiazepines can be extremely effective in the short term in decreasing anxiety and can provide almost immediate relief. These medications must be used cautiously as they can be addicting and have the potential to be abused; however, they were designed to treat the symptoms of anxiety, and when used appropriately, they are excellent medications. The goal is to use them sparingly until the antidepressants begin to cause a remission of symptoms and then to taper off. Used judiciously benzodiazepines can be of huge benefit to a mother with paralyzing anxiety. Newer literature suggests that they can be safe to use during breastfeeding and will not cause increased infant sedation (Kelly, Poon, Madadi, & Koren, 2012).

Conclusion

Pregnancy and birth can be a time of great joy and a time of new beginnings for many women, but it is also a period in a women's life where she is most vulnerable, both physically and emotionally. It is not uncommon for all new mothers to experience both positive and negative feelings after having a baby. However, some women are sensitive to the hormonal and psychological changes that occur after delivery and will develop a serious mood or anxiety disorder. It is imperative to understand the difference between normal adjustments that occur after childbirth and more serious symptoms that require intervention. With early treatment mothers can recover quickly and enjoy those first few challenging and important months with her new baby.

References

Abramowitz, J. S., Khandker, M., Nelson, C. A., Deacon, B. J., & Rygwall, R. (2006). The role of cognitive factors in the pathogenesis of obsessive-compulsive symptoms: A prospective study. *Behavior Research & Therapy, 44*(9), 1361–1374. doi:10.1016/j.brat.2005.09.011.

Altshuler, L. L., Hendrick, V., & Cohen, L. S. (1998). Course of mood and anxiety disorders during pregnancy and the postpartum period. *Journal of Clinical Psychiatry, 59*(Suppl 2), 29–33.

American Psychiatric Association., & American Psychiatric Association. DSM-5 Task Force. (2013). *Diagnostic and statistical manual of mental disorders: DSM-5* (5th ed.). Washington, DC: American Psychiatric Association.

American Psychiatric Association., & American Psychiatric Association. Task Force on DSM-IV. (1994). *Diagnostic and statistical manual of mental disorders : DSM-IV* (4th ed.). Washington, DC: American Psychiatric Association.

Austin, M. P., Hadzi-Pavlovic, D., Priest, S. R., Reilly, N., Wilhelm, K., Saint, K., et al. (2010). Depressive and anxiety disorders in the postpartum period: How prevalent are they and can we improve their detection? *Archives of Women's Mental Health, 13*(5), 395–401. doi:10.1007/s00737-010-0153-7.

Beck, C. T. (2001). Predictors of postpartum depression: An update. *Nursing Research, 50*(5), 275–285.

Beck, C. T. (2006). Postpartum depression: It isn't just the blues. *American Journal of Nursing, 106*(5), 40–50. quiz 50-41.

Birnbaum, C. S., Cohen, L. S., Bailey, J. W., Grush, L. R., Robertson, L. M., & Stowe, Z. N. (1999). Serum concentrations of antidepressants and benzodiazepines in nursing infants: A case series. *Pediatrics, 104*(1), e11.

Bloch, M., Schmidt, P. J., Danaceau, M., Murphy, J., Nieman, L., & Rubinow, D. R. (2000). Effects of gonadal steroids in women with a history of postpartum depression. *American Journal of Psychiatry, 157*(6), 924–930.

Brandes, M., Soares, C. N., & Cohen, L. S. (2004). Postpartum onset obsessive-compulsive disorder: Diagnosis and management. *Archives of Women's Mental Health, 7*(2), 99–110. doi:10.1007/s00737-003-0035-3.

Chaudron, L. H., & Nirodi, N. (2010). The obsessive-compulsive spectrum in the perinatal period: A prospective pilot study. *Archives of Women's Mental Health, 13*(5), 403–410. doi:10.1007/s00737-010-0154-6.

Cohen, L. S., Sichel, D. A., Dimmock, J. A., & Rosenbaum, J. F. (1994). Postpartum course in women with preexisting panic disorder. *Journal of Clinical Psychiatry, 55*(7), 289–292.

Connor, K. M., & Davidson, J. R. (1998). Generalized anxiety disorder: Neurobiological and pharmacotherapeutic perspectives. *Biological Psychiatry, 44*(12), 1286–1294.

Cox, J. L., Holden, J. M., & Sagovsky, R. (1987). Detection of postnatal depression. Development of the 10-item Edinburgh postnatal depression scale. *British Journal of Psychiatry, 150*, 782–786.

Dennis, C. L., & Dowswell, T. (2013). Psychosocial and psychological interventions for preventing postpartum depression. *Cochrane Database Systematic Reviews, 2*, CD001134. doi:10.1002/14651858.CD001134.pub3.

Dennis, C. L., Ravitz, P., Grigoriadis, S., Jovellanos, M., Hodnett, E., Ross, L., et al. (2012). The effect of telephone-based interpersonal psychotherapy for the treatment of postpartum depression: Study protocol for a randomized controlled trial. *Trials, 13*, 38. doi:10.1186/1745-6215-13-38.

Engineer, N., Darwin, L., Nishigandh, D., Ngianga-Bakwin, K., Smith, S. C., & Grammatopoulos, D. K. (2013). Association of glucocorticoid and type 1 corticotropin-releasing hormone receptors gene variants and risk for depression during pregnancy and post-partum. *Journal of Psychiatry Research, 47*(9), 1166–1173. doi:10.1016/j.jpsychires.2013.05.003.

Forray, A., Focseneanu, M., Pittman, B., McDougle, C. J., & Epperson, C. N. (2010). Onset and exacerbation of obsessive-compulsive disorder in pregnancy and the postpartum period. *Journal of Clinical Psychiatry, 71*(8), 1061–1068. doi:10.4088/JCP.09m05381blu.

Freeman, M. P. (2009). Complementary and alternative medicine for perinatal depression. *Journal of Affective Disorders, 112*(1–3), 1–10. doi:10.1016/j.jad.2008.06.017.

Gentile, S. (2005). The safety of newer antidepressants in pregnancy and breastfeeding. *Drug Safety, 28*(2), 137–152.

Healey, C., Morriss, R., Henshaw, C., Wadoo, O., Sajjad, A., Scholefield, H., et al. (2013). Self-harm in postpartum depression and referrals to a perinatal mental health team: An audit study. *Archives of Women's Mental Health, 16*(3), 237–245. doi:10.1007/s00737-013-0335-1.

Jiang, W., Gagliardi, J. P., Krishnan, K., & Rama, R. (2009). *Clinician's guide to psychiatric care*. Oxford: Oxford University Press.

Jonas, W., Mileva-Seitz, V., Girard, A. W., Bisceglia, R., Kennedy, J. L., Sokolowski, M., ... on behalf of the, Mavan Research Team. (2013). Genetic variation in oxytocin rs2740210 and early adversity associated with postpartum depression and breastfeeding duration. *Genes Brain Behavior, 12*(7), 681–694. doi: 10.1111/gbb.12069

Jones, I., Cantwell, R., & Nosology Working Group, Royal College of Psychiatrists Perinatal Section. (2010). The classification of perinatal mood disorders–suggestions for DSMV and ICD11. *Archives of Women's Mental Health, 13*(1), 33–36. doi:10.1007/s00737-009-0122-1.

Kapczinski F. F. K., Silva de Lima, M., dos Santos Souza, J. J. S. S., Batista Miralha da Cunha, A. A. B. C., & Schmitt, R. R. S. (2003). Antidepressants for generalized anxiety disorder. *Cochrane Database of Systematic Reviews,2* (2). http://onlinelibrary.wiley.com/doi/10.1002/14651858.CD003592/abstract doi: 10.1002/14651858.CD003592

Kelly, L. E., Poon, S., Madadi, P., & Koren, G. (2012). Neonatal benzodiazepines exposure during breastfeeding. *Journal of Pediatrics, 161*(3), 448–451. doi:10.1016/j.jpeds.2012.03.003.

Kessler, R. C., Petukhova, M., Sampson, N. A., Zaslavsky, A. M., & Wittchen, H. U. (2012). Twelve-month and lifetime prevalence and lifetime morbid risk of anxiety and mood disorders in the United States. *International Journal of Methods in Psychiatric Research, 21*(3), 169–184. doi:10.1002/mpr.1359.

Khazaie, H., Ghadami, M. R., Knight, D. C., Emamian, F., & Tahmasian, M. (2013). Insomnia treatment in the third trimester of pregnancy reduces postpartum depression symptoms: A randomized clinical trial. *Psychiatry Research, 201*(3), 901–905. doi:10.1016/j.psychres.2013.08.017.

Lindsay, M., Crino, R., & Andrews, G. (1997). Controlled trial of exposure and response prevention in obsessive-compulsive disorder. *British Journal of Psychiatry, 171*, 135–139.

Markhus, M. W., Skotheim, S., Graff, I. E., Froyland, L., Braarud, H. C., Stormark, K. M., et al. (2013). Low omega-3 index in pregnancy is a possible biological risk factor for postpartum depression. *PLoS One, 8*(7), e67617. doi:10.1371/journal.pone.0067617.

McGuinness, M., Blissett, J., & Jones, C. (2011). OCD in the perinatal period: Is postpartum OCD (ppOCD) a distinct subtype? A review of the literature. *Behavioral and Cognitive Psychotherapy, 39*(3), 285–310. doi:10.1017/s1352465810000718.

Misri, S., Albert, G., Abizadeh, J., Kendrick, K., Carter, D., Ryan, D., et al. (2012). Biopsychosocial determinants of treatment outcome for mood and anxiety disorders up to 8 months postpartum. *Archives of Women's Mental Health, 15*(4), 313–316. doi:10.1007/s00737-012-0288-9.

Moses-Kolko, E. L., Wisner, K. L., Price, J. C., Berga, S. L., Drevets, W. C., Hanusa, B. H., et al. (2008). Serotonin 1A receptor reductions in postpartum depression: A positron emission tomography study. *Fertility and Sterility, 89*(3), 685–692. doi:10.1016/j.fertnstert.2007.03.059.

Nanzer, N., Sancho Rossignol, A., Righetti-Veltema, M., Knauer, D., Manzano, J., & Palacio Espasa, F. (2012). Effects of a brief psychoanalytic intervention for perinatal depression. *Archives of Women's Mental Health, 15*(4), 259–268. doi:10.1007/s00737-012-0285-z.

Nonacs, R., & Cohen, L. S. (1998). Postpartum mood disorders: Diagnosis and treatment guidelines. *Journal of Clinical Psychiatry, 59*(Suppl 2), 34–40.

Nonacs, R., & Cohen, L. S. (2002). Depression during pregnancy: Diagnosis and treatment options. *Journal of Clinical Psychiatry, 63*(Suppl 7), 24–30.

O'Hara, M. W., & McCabe, J. E. (2013). Postpartum depression: Current status and future directions. *Annual Review of Clinical Psychology, 9*, 379–407. doi:10.1146/annurev-clinpsy-050212-185612.

O'Hara, M. W., Stuart, S., Watson, D., Dietz, P. M., Farr, S. L., & D'Angelo, D. (2012). Brief scales to detect postpartum depression and anxiety symptoms. *Journal of Women's Health (Larchmt), 21*(12), 1237–1243. doi:10.1089/jwh.2012.3612.

O'Mahen, H., Himle, J. A., Fedock, G., Henshaw, E., & Flynn, H. (2013). A pilot randomized controlled trial of cognitive behavioral therapy for perinatal depression adapted for women with low incomes. *Depression and Anxiety, 30*(7), 679–687. doi:10.1002/da.22050.

Paul, I. M., Downs, D. S., Schaefer, E. W., Beiler, J. S., & Weisman, C. S. (2013). Postpartum anxiety and maternal-infant health outcomes. *Pediatrics, 131*(4), e1218–e1224. doi:10.1542/peds.2012-2147.

Pinheiro, R. T., Coelho, F. M., Silva, R. A., Pinheiro, K. A., Oses, J. P., Quevedo Lde, A., et al. (2013). Association of a serotonin transporter gene polymorphism (5-HTTLPR) and stressful life events with postpartum depressive symptoms: A population-based study. *Journal of Psychosomatic Obstetrics & Gynaecology, 34*(1), 29–33. doi:10.3109/0167482X.2012.759555.

Reay, R. E., Mulcahy, R., Wilkinson, R. B., Owen, C., Shadbolt, B., & Raphael, B. (2012). The development and content of an interpersonal psychotherapy group for postnatal depression. *International Journal of Group Psychotherapy, 62*(2), 221–251. doi:10.1521/ijgp.2012.62.2.221.

Ross, L. E., & McLean, L. M. (2006). Anxiety disorders during pregnancy and the postpartum period: A systematic review. *Journal of Clinical Psychiatry, 67*(8), 1285–1298.

Ross, L. E., Murray, B. J., & Steiner, M. (2005). Sleep and perinatal mood disorders: A critical review. *Journal of Psychiatry Neuroscience, 30*(4), 247–256.

Shaw, E., Levitt, C., Wong, S., Kaczorowski, J., & McMaster University Postpartum Research, Group. (2006). Systematic review of the literature on postpartum care: Effectiveness of postpartum support to improve maternal parenting, mental health, quality of life, and physical health. *Birth, 33*(3), 210–220. doi:10.1111/j.1523-536X.2006.00106.x.

Sichel, D. A., Cohen, L. S., Dimmock, J. A., & Rosenbaum, J. F. (1993). Postpartum obsessive compulsive disorder: A case series. *Journal of Clinical Psychiatry, 54*(4), 156–159.

Sit, D., Rothschild, A. J., & Wisner, K. L. (2006). A review of postpartum psychosis. *Journal of Women's Health (Larchmt), 15*(4), 352–368. doi:10.1089/jwh.2006.15.352.

Skalkidou, A., Hellgren, C., Comasco, E., Sylven, S., & Sundstrom Poromaa, I. (2012). Biological aspects of postpartum depression. *Women's Health (London, England), 8*(6), 659–672. doi:10.2217/whe.12.55.

Slattery, D. A., & Neumann, I. D. (2008). No stress please! Mechanisms of stress hyporesponsiveness of the maternal brain. *Journal of Physiology, 586*(2), 377–385. doi:10.1113/jphysiol.2007.145896.

Spinelli, M. G. (2004). Maternal infanticide associated with mental illness: Prevention and the promise of saved lives. *American Journal of Psychiatry, 161*(9), 1548–1557. doi:10.1176/appi.ajp.161.9.1548.

Steiner, M., Peer, M., Macdougall, M., & Haskett, R. (2011). The premenstrual tension syndrome rating scales: An updated version. *Journal of Affective Disorders, 135*(1–3), 82–88. doi:10.1016/j.jad.2011.06.058.

Stowe, Z. N., & Nemeroff, C. B. (1995). Women at risk for postpartum-onset major depression. *American Journal of Obstetrics & Gynecology, 173*(2), 639–645.

Stuart, S. (2012). Interpersonal psychotherapy for postpartum depression. *Clinical Psychology Psychotherapy, 19*(2), 134–140. doi:10.1002/cpp.1778.

Studd, J., & Nappi, R. E. (2012). Reproductive depression. *Gynecology & Endocrinology, 28*(Suppl 1), 42–45. doi:10.3109/09513590.2012.651932.

Suda, S., Segi-Nishida, E., Newton, S. S., & Duman, R. S. (2008). A postpartum model in rat: Behavioral and gene expression changes induced by ovarian steroid deprivation. *Biological Psychiatry, 64*(4), 311–319. doi:10.1016/j.biopsych.2008.03.029.

Sutter-Dallay, A. L., Giaconne-Marcesche, V., Glatigny-Dallay, E., & Verdoux, H. (2004). Women with anxiety disorders during pregnancy are at increased risk of intense postnatal depressive symptoms: a prospective survey of the MATQUID cohort. *European Psychiatry, 19*(8), 459–463. doi:10.1016/j.eurpsy.2004.09.025.

Swanson, L. M., Pickett, S. M., Flynn, H., & Armitage, R. (2011). Relationships among depression, anxiety, and insomnia symptoms in perinatal women seeking mental health treatment. *Journal of Women's Health (Larchmt), 20*(4), 553–558. doi:10.1089/jwh.2010.2371.

Uguz, F., Akman, C., Kaya, N., & Cilli, A. S. (2007). Postpartum-onset obsessive-compulsive disorder: Incidence, clinical features, and related factors. *Journal of Clinical Psychiatry, 68*(1), 132–138.

Weissman, M. M., Prusoff, B. A., Dimascio, A., Neu, C., Goklaney, M., & Klerman, G. L. (1979). The efficacy of drugs and psychotherapy in the treatment of acute depressive episodes. *American Journal of Psychiatry, 136*(4B), 555–558.

Westberg, L., & Eriksson, E. (2008). Sex steroid-related candidate genes in psychiatric disorders. *Journal of Psychiatry Neuroscience, 33*(4), 319–330.

Wisner, K. L., Peindl, K. S., Gigliotti, T., & Hanusa, B. H. (1999). Obsessions and compulsions in women with postpartum depression. *Journal of Clinical Psychiatry, 60*(3), 176–180.

Wisner, K. L., Peindl, K. S., & Hanusa, B. H. (1996). Effects of childbearing on the natural history of panic disorder with comorbid mood disorder. *Journal of Affective Disorders, 41*(3), 173–180.

Worsley, R., Gilbert, H., Gavrilidis, E., Naughton, B., & Kulkarni, J. (2013). Breastfeeding and psychotropic medications. *Lancet, 381*(9870), 905. doi:10.1016/S0140-6736(13)60671-6.

Chronic Mental Illness in Pregnancy and Postpartum

Melissa L. Nau and Alissa M. Peterson

Introduction

The reproductive years confer the greatest risk in a woman's lifetime for the development of mental illness (Kendell, Chalmers, & Platz, 1987). In this chapter, we focus on bipolar disorder and schizophrenia, specifically as these disorders relate to puerperal periods, which include pregnancy and the postpartum period. As both bipolar disorder and schizophrenia can begin in early adulthood, women are at risk of having mood or psychotic episodes throughout their reproductive years. Additionally, because childbirth and reproductive events can be significant and stressful for women, illness episodes are often triggered during this time (Sharma & Pope, 2012). Although we focus on the entire reproductive period for this chapter, it is noteworthy that the postpartum period is widely considered a high-risk period for the onset or the exacerbation of severe mood or psychotic episodes (Sharma & Pope, 2012).

Diagnostic Categories

Bipolar Affective Disorder

Bipolar affective disorder is a chronic and episodic severe mental disorder, characterized by periods of both mania and depression. Manic episodes are characterized by a distinct period during which there is an abnormally and persistently elevated, expansive, or irritable mood (American Psychiatric Association, 2013). In contrast,

---

M.L. Nau, M.D. (✉) • A.M. Peterson, M.D.
Department of Psychiatry, University of California, San Francisco, CA, USA
e-mail: Melissa.Nau@ucsf.edu; Alissa.Peterson@ucsf.edu

depressive episodes are characterized by depressed mood or loss of interest or pleasure in nearly all activities. Bipolar I disorder is the more severe form in which manic episodes can be debilitating and can often have significant consequences for social and occupational functioning. Bipolar II is a tempered form of illness in which the hypomanic episodes are characteristically mild forms of mania but can still result in impairment in daily life. This disorder often requires ongoing pharmacologic treatment to prevent relapses or to lower the risk of suicide. Lithium, certain anticonvulsants, and antipsychotics are recommended as mood stabilizers in bipolar disorder. If left untreated, bipolar disorder is associated with high rates of morbidity and mortality (Frieder, Dunlop, Culpepper, & Bernstein, 2008).

The prevalence of bipolar disorder in the USA is 0.5–1.5 % (Yonkers et al., 2004). Its onset is typically in early adulthood; therefore, illness episodes can affect women during their childbearing years (Doyle et al., 2012).

Schizophrenia

Schizophrenia is a chronic and disabling mental disorder that affects approximately 0.3 % of the population and is characterized by disordered perceptions, disordered thought processes, and deficits in emotional response. It is also accompanied by impairment in social or occupational functioning. People who suffer from schizophrenia display characteristic signs and symptoms (both positive and negative) for at least 6 months. Positive symptoms reflect an excess or a distortion of normal functions and include auditory hallucinations, delusions (distortions in thought content), and disorganization of thought and speech. Negative symptoms reflect a diminution or a loss of functions and include restrictions in the range and intensity of emotional expression and behavior (American Psychiatric Association, 2013). Schizophrenia generally develops in early adulthood and can have a significant impact on a woman's childbearing years.

The mainstay of treatment for schizophrenia includes the use of antipsychotic medications. People who suffer from schizophrenia usually require lifetime use of pharmacologic agents to maintain stability; often, even with good medication compliance, exacerbations of severe illness occur (American Psychiatric Association, 2013).

Bipolar Affective Disorder in Pregnancy

Research has shown that women with a history of bipolar disorder have a 25–50 % risk of severe mood episodes during pregnancy and the postpartum period. In patients who discontinue mood stabilization treatment, rates of recurrence for pregnant patients are similar to rates of recurrence for nonpregnant patients (Viguera et al., 2000). However, the risk of severe mood episodes during pregnancy and the postpartum period is not thought to be due to the cessation of maintenance treatment alone. Additionally, childbirth is commonly related to the initial onset of bipolar disorder (Terp & Mortensen, 1998). Although the exact reason for this is not known, researchers have theorized that this could be related to the stress of reproductive events (Sharma & Pope, 2012).

Differential Diagnosis

When diagnosing bipolar disorder, a manic episode must first be distinguished from other possible etiologies. Mood changes or erratic behavior can also be caused by an organic illness, significant substance misuse, or other mental illnesses such as attention-deficit/hyperactivity disorder. A careful assessment is necessary before initiating treatment to ensure that the underlying cause of illness has been elucidated.

Symptoms

While prevalence of bipolar disorder is similar between the sexes, symptom presentation in men and women can be quite different (Burt & Rasgon, 2004). Rapid cycling, in which episodes of mania or depression occur at least four times yearly, occurs more frequently in women (Kilzieh & Akiskal, 1999). Mixed mania, in which symptoms of both depression and mania are present simultaneously, is also more common in women (Robb, Young, Cooke, & Joffe, 1998). Both rapid cycling and mixed mania are associated with poorer prognosis (Keller et al., 1986).

With respect to pregnancy manifestations of illness, symptoms of bipolar disorder in pregnancy are largely the same as those at other times of a woman's life. Some data suggests an increased likelihood of depressive symptoms or mixed episodes as compared to mania or hypomania (Viguera et al., 2007).

Risk Factors

The onset of bipolar disorder during pregnancy has been traced to both biological and environmental factors. A younger age at pregnancy, illness onset at an early age, obstetric or somatic complications during pregnancy, psychiatric comorbidities, and a history of prenatal or postpartum mood episodes have all been associated with childbearing-related episodes of bipolar disorder (Akdeniz et al., 2003; Doyle et al., 2012; Jones & Craddock, 2002; Viguera, Cohen, Baldessarini, & Nonacs, 2002).

Moreover, women with bipolar disorder can exhibit poor insight into their condition, which could interfere with appropriate treatment (Frieder et al., 2008).

Psychosis in Pregnancy

Women with schizophrenia often suffer from chronic psychotic symptoms and are at high risk of continuing psychosis in pregnancy. As most studies focus only on hospitalized women, the prevalence of psychosis in pregnancy, as well as the risk of pregnancy worsening psychosis for women with schizophrenia, is largely unknown. It does appear; however, that pregnancy is not protective against psychotic symptoms and that the severity of illness prior to pregnancy correlates with the severity of psychosis during pregnancy (Vigod & Ross, 2010). Additionally, women with schizophrenia who discontinue psychotropic medication during pregnancy are at high risk for relapse (Seeman, 2013).

Differential Diagnosis

The differential diagnosis of psychosis in pregnancy parallels that of psychosis in women who are not pregnant. As with bipolar disorder, one must consider organic and nonorganic possibilities. Substance intoxication as the sole cause of psychosis should be ruled out. Psychiatric illnesses that may have psychosis as a symptom include schizophrenia, schizoaffective disorder, bipolar disorder, major depressive disorder, post-traumatic stress disorder, and borderline personality disorder. For the purposes of this section, we will be focusing on schizophrenia.

Symptoms

Positive, negative, and cognitive symptoms of schizophrenia can be problematic for women in pregnancy. Delusions may arise against the fetus. Possible complications are delay in recognition of pregnancy, delay in getting prenatal care, and psychotic denial of pregnancy. Psychotic denial of pregnancy is particularly problematic as it can lead to lack of prenatal care or lack of response to signs of labor. Women with psychotic denial of pregnancy will often make delusional interpretations of the normal physiological changes of pregnancy. For example, a woman might attribute her growing abdomen to a demon inside of her (Solari, 2010). Maternal filicide is also a devastating, though rare, complication associated with denial of pregnancy (Friedman, Horwitz, & Resnick, 2005).

Risk Factors

Risk factors influencing psychotic symptoms include the rapidly changing physiology of pregnancy and medication compliance. For women who choose to take psychotropic medications, alterations in metabolism, excretion, absorption, and distribution of drugs during pregnancy can affect drug levels. The nature of these alterations is often individual and is not always predictable (Seeman, 2013). Additionally, fear of the effect of psychotropic medication on the fetus can lead to rapid lowering of dosages or discontinuation (Vigod & Ross, 2010).

Treatment of Mania and Psychosis in Pregnancy

Preconception Considerations

Unplanned pregnancies are common for women with severe, chronic mental illnesses. Women with schizophrenia are more likely to engage in risky sexual behavior and be sexually exploited than women without a psychiatric illness (Romans, 2010). Similarly, high-risk sexual behavior in women with bipolar disorder is a symptom of mania and can lead to unintended pregnancies (Frieder et al., 2008).

Ideally, the decision to conceive is made with the support of family, friends, and providers, and a clear treatment plan is developed for the pregnancy and postpartum period with a mental health specialist. This plan might include medications, psychotherapy, and social interventions, or even hospitalization if necessary (Doyle et al., 2012). All parties should be enlisted, whenever possible, to help monitor the woman's symptoms, so early signs of decompensation are detected (Robinson, 2012). This is particularly important for women who struggle with poor insight or impulse control problems in the midst of an illness episode (Frieder et al., 2008).

Risk of Non-treatment

Untreated bipolar disorder or schizophrenia carries significant risks to both mother and fetus; these risks must be balanced against the potential teratogenic risks of medication. Pregnancy complications linked to untreated bipolar disorder and schizophrenia include slightly increased risk of preterm birth, higher risk of postpartum psychiatric illness, increased rate of substance abuse, lower participation in prenatal care, and giving birth to small, for gestational age, infants (Burt & Rasgon, 2004; Lee & Lin, 2010). Women who are untreated during pregnancy are subject to increased rates of impulsive and self-injurious behavior, substance abuse, inattention to perinatal care, and unfavorable hormonal environment for child development (Doyle et al., 2012). If acute emergency treatment is required, then the fetus is often exposed to high doses of multiple psychotropic drugs in an effort to rapidly stabilize a woman in crisis.

There is also a high risk of recurrence of chronic mental illness in pregnancy if treatment is discontinued abruptly (Viguera et al., 2002). In a study by Viguera and colleagues focusing on bipolar disorder, women who discontinued mood stabilization treatment spent over 40 % of their pregnancy in an illness episode versus 8.8 % of pregnancy for those who continued treatment (Viguera et al., 2000).

Emergency Interventions

A woman who presents in an acute manic, depressed, or psychotic episode while pregnant must immediately be evaluated for the need of psychiatric hospitalization. Untreated mania or psychosis can lead to irrational and impulsive behavior that can be dangerous for both mother and fetus. Clinicians should perform careful suicide and violence risk assessments and should also weigh the possibility of involuntary commitment in severe cases.

Pharmacologic Treatment

Mania and psychosis are most commonly treated with mood-stabilizing medications and antipsychotics. Due to ethical constraints, there are no randomized, controlled studies of medications in pregnancy, which makes safety data limited.

One general principle for use of psychotropics in pregnancy is to use the least amount of medications at the lowest effective dosage(s). Ideally, this would mean management of symptoms with only one medication, which is possible given the dual use of antipsychotic agents for mood stabilization and psychotic symptoms. Another recommendation is close monitoring throughout pregnancy with fetal surveillance, drug level monitoring (where applicable), and appropriate laboratory tests based on medication side effect profiles (Gentile, 2010; Sharma & Pope, 2012).

Below is a brief overview of psychotropic use in the severely mentally ill pregnant woman. Please see chapter "The Role of Reproductive Psychiatry in Women's Mental Health" for an in-depth look at psychotropic medications in the reproductive years.

Mood Stabilizers and Lithium

Mood stabilizers are often used in the treatment of mania. The most commonly used mood stabilizers are lithium, valproic acid, lamotrigine, and carbamazepine. Unfortunately, all four have a risk of fetal malformation in pregnancy, to varying degrees, necessitating a clear risk–benefit analysis before starting or continuing one of these medications.

Antipsychotics

Antipsychotics are used to treat both psychotic and manic symptoms. Research does not point to any particular antipsychotic as being "safest" in pregnancy (Coverdale, McCullough, & Chervenak, 2010). When working with a pregnant woman already stabilized on a particular antipsychotic agent, the first recommendation is to continue on that agent to avoid the risk of destabilization (Gentile, 2010).

If a woman is antipsychotic naïve, it is recommended that an agent with the highest amount of reassuring data and lowest evidence of fetal malformation be chosen.

Electroconvulsive Therapy

Electroconvulsive therapy (ECT) is a highly effective treatment for both mania and psychosis. ECT has been found to be safe throughout pregnancy and works more quickly than medications (Saatcioglu & Tomruk, 2011). The electrical current from ECT does not pass through the uterus; therefore, no seizure activity is induced in the fetus. Rare, adverse events for the fetus include fetal bradyarrhythmia and premature labor (Anderson & Reti, 2009). Despite the safety profile of ECT in pregnancy, it is generally reserved for women with life-threatening symptoms, such as low oral intake, suicidality, or catatonia, or for patients who are refractory to medications (Saatcioglu & Tomruk, 2011).

Psychotherapy and Social Interventions

In treatment planning for pregnant women with bipolar disorder and schizophrenia, consideration should be given to a woman's social supports. Partner involvement in treatment planning should occur from the outset. In instances where partner involvement is not possible and/or the degree of disability from bipolar disorder or schizophrenia is severe, thought should be given to disability benefits as well as other interventions to minimize stress and maximize self-care, such as regular sleep and healthy eating habits.

Additionally, women and their social supports should be counseled regarding the risks and benefits of medication and a long-term approach considered, including careful thought about breastfeeding and postpartum management. Frequent clinical contact with mental health providers and obstetric clinicians is recommended, and brief supportive interventions can be incorporated into such visits. Examples of such interventions are education on the normal physiologic changes of pregnancy and beginning discussions about parenting (Miller, 2010; Robinson, 2012). Cognitive behavioral therapy, motivational interviewing, and social skill therapy have all been shown to benefit patients with schizophrenia and are likely to be helpful for pregnant women with psychosis (Miller, 2010). Ideally, psychotherapy, medications, and social interventions are utilized simultaneously.

Ethical and Legal Considerations

A woman's pregnancy raises questions of ethics and the law in regard to her treatment. As physicians, our goal is to provide care that is within medical, ethics-related, and legal standards in every case (Nau, McNiel, & Binder, 2012). A woman must be carefully evaluated for the need for acute psychiatric intervention. When considering forced psychiatric treatment for a woman with an intrauterine pregnancy, clinicians must be mindful that their goal is to treat the patient, with attention to her goals and preferences. That said, consideration for the welfare of the fetus is necessary, provided that it does not conflict with the welfare of the mother. The laws regarding intervention in this type of scenario vary from state to state, and physicians should be aware of the laws in the area in which they practice.

Chronic Mental Illness in the Postpartum Period

It has long been recognized that the postpartum period is a time of high risk for the onset of severe episodes of mental illnesses in women (Viguera et al., 2002; Viguera & Cohen, 1998). The early postpartum period is strongly associated with an elevated risk of major affective or psychotic episodes, with most occurring within the first 2 weeks of delivery (Viguera et al., 2002).

Differential Diagnosis

As is the case with presentations of mental illness during pregnancy, organic disease processes and other psychiatric disorders must be considered in the evaluation of postpartum psychosis and mania. A review of the patient's medical history, physical and mental status exams, laboratory and imaging studies, and current medications is essential to rule out any potential organic cause of symptoms. Trauma, endocrine disorders, structural lesions, toxins, infections, autoimmune disorders, electrolyte imbalances, and metabolic substrate deficiencies must all be considered (Seyfried & Marcus, 2003). Finally, as with pre-pregnancy mania and psychosis, the effects of substances should be ruled out before treatment is initiated.

The term postpartum psychosis is broadly defined as psychotic symptoms occurring in a woman following childbirth; therefore, postpartum psychosis can be associated with a variety of psychiatric diagnoses. Using the Diagnostic and Statistical Manual of Mental Disorders, 5th Edition (DSM-V), postpartum psychosis is diagnosed as a major depressive disorder with psychotic features, brief psychotic disorder, or bipolar affective disorder with psychotic features. Diagnosis includes an additional specifier stating the onset of symptoms must be during pregnancy or within 4 weeks of delivery (American Psychiatric Association, 2013).

In the literature, postpartum psychosis is generally recognized as a distinct syndrome, most commonly linked with cyclic mood disorders such as bipolar affective disorder or schizoaffective disorder. One large, retrospective database study found that 72–80 % of postpartum psychosis cases were associated with diagnoses of bipolar or schizoaffective disorder and only 12 % with schizophrenia (Kendell et al., 1987).

Symptoms

A postpartum exacerbation of mania in a woman with bipolar disorder appears largely the same as in the non-childbearing period (Colom et al., 2010; Harlow et al., 2007; Manber, Blasey, & Allen, 2008; Munk-Olsen et al., 2009). Most commonly, women present with elation, mood lability, distractibility, and increased activity (Seyfried & Marcus, 2003). Given the high risk for development of postpartum psychosis in women with postpartum mania, clinicians should be vigilant about watching for the development of psychotic symptoms.

The onset of postpartum psychosis is rapid, usually between 2 days and 2 weeks of delivery. The first symptoms often resemble manic episodes with sleep disturbance and mood lability, but these symptoms are followed by delusions, auditory hallucinations, disorganization, and sometimes catatonia (Sharma, 2008). Rare types of hallucinations, such as visual, olfactory, and tactile, are more common in postpartum than non-postpartum psychosis. Cognitive symptoms resembling delirium, such as confusion and disorientation are also more frequently present (Wisner, Peindl, & Hanusa, 1994). As above, episodes with these distinct clinical features appear to be most often associated with a history of or a new diagnosis of a cyclic mood disorder.

Conversely, postpartum psychotic symptoms in women with schizophrenia can occur weeks to months after delivery and resemble episodes of their pre-pregnancy illness, though delusions and hallucinations might reflect the mother's new social circumstances and involve the child (Vigod & Ross, 2010); therefore, it is possible that these episodes are relapses of the primary psychotic illness and only coincidentally related in time to childbirth.

Risk Factors

The severity of mental illness prior to pregnancy has been shown to correlate with the severity of symptoms in the postpartum period. Likewise, discontinuation of medications places a woman at increased risk for relapse of mental illness in the postpartum period (Vigod & Ross, 2010).

The risk of relapse in the postpartum period is higher for bipolar disorder than other forms of mental illness (Doyle et al., 2012). Although exact numbers vary, studies report that 40–70 % of women with bipolar disorder experience a postpartum mood episode within 1 month of delivery (Burt & Rasgon, 2004; Freeman et al., 2002; Munk-Olsen et al., 2009). Doyle et al. conducted a study on the risk factors for postpartum relapse in women with bipolar disorder. They found that a younger age at delivery, an unplanned pregnancy, and being unwell at referral were significantly associated with risk of postpartum mood and/or psychotic symptoms (Doyle et al., 2012).

A severe form of relapse is postpartum psychosis. The incidence of postpartum psychosis is 1–2/1,000 deliveries (Vigod & Ross, 2010), and etiology is unclear, though it is thought to be related to the abrupt drop in maternal progesterone and estrogen at delivery (Spinelli, 2009).

There are several identified biologic risk factors associated with the development of postpartum psychosis. The most significant of these is a personal history of bipolar disorder or postpartum psychosis. A recent study showed that over 50 % of women with a previous episode of postpartum psychosis will experience another (Blackmore et al., 2013). Other important biologic risk factors are a family history of postpartum psychosis, a family history of bipolar disorder, and a personal history of psychotic symptoms prior to or during pregnancy.

There are also a number of clinical and demographic risk factors specifically associated with the development of postpartum psychosis. A long labor and a night-time delivery have been shown to increase the risk. These variables may precipitate sleep loss, a known risk factor for the development of mania in those with bipolar disorder (Sharma, Smith, & Khan, 2004). Other associations include primiparity, complications during delivery, and an unmarried status (Sharma, 2008).

Treatment of Mania and Psychosis in the Postpartum Period

Emergency Interventions

Postpartum mania, or psychosis, is a severe illness that often requires hospitalization and should be considered a psychiatric emergency. A careful suicide and violence risk assessment should be performed with attention to safety of the infant. Although the incidence of infanticide is low, clinicians should be aware that this is possible and should also note that women suffering from postpartum mania or psychosis are at an increased risk for self-harm.

Pharmacologic

Pharmacologic treatment of postpartum psychosis or mania depends on several factors including patient preference, prior trials, medication side effect profiles, and the mother's choice regarding breastfeeding. As in pregnancy, the mainstay of treatment is mood stabilizers and antipsychotics; however, there is limited literature on the effectiveness of these agents in the treatment of postpartum psychosis or mania.

In non-breastfeeding, postpartum women, clinicians generally focus solely on effective treatment of the underlying diagnosis or symptoms (Sharma, 2008). The decision for the breastfeeding mother can be more complicated. As in pregnancy, randomized controlled trials of psychotropic medications in breastfeeding are not available and data is limited. The benefits of taking a medication for the mother and the benefits of breastfeeding for the baby must be weighed against the risk to the infant of medication exposure (American Academy of Pediatrics, 2012); however, data on concentrations of psychotropic medications in breastfed infants show that exposure is much lower during breastfeeding than in utero (Sit, Rothschild, & Wisner, 2006). LactMed, an Internet-accessed source published by the National Library of Medicine/National Institutes of Health, is considered an excellent source of information on medication safety in breastfeeding (American Academy of Pediatrics, 2012).

According to a recent meta-analysis, a drug can be considered compatible with breastfeeding when, based on the available literature, there are no adverse effects reported in infants exposed through breast milk and the relative infant dosage is <10 % of the maternal dosage (Fortinguerra, Clavenna, & Bonati, 2009). As in pregnancy, it is recommended to use the lowest effective dose and fewest medications possible in order to treat the mother's symptoms. Additionally, medication can be given in divided doses throughout the day to decrease peak serum (and thus breast milk) concentration (Sit et al., 2006). Some highly motivated women may even choose to "pump and dump" at peak serum concentration times throughout the day. The pediatrician should be aware of medications the breastfeeding mother is taking so that the infant can be monitored closely for side effects or signs of toxicity (Sit et al., 2006).

There is limited data available on the effects of infant exposure to antipsychotics in breast milk. A recent meta-analysis deemed olanzapine and quetiapine viable options given the low excretion in breast milk and minimal evidence of adverse effects for the infant (Klinger, Stahl, Fusar-Poli, & Merlob, 2013). Clozapine is contraindicated in breastfeeding due to the risk of agranulocytosis in the infant (Fortinguerra et al., 2009). Most antipsychotic drugs are sedating, and therefore, breastfed infants should be monitored for lethargy (Fortinguerra et al., 2009).

Mood stabilizers can also be used in the treatment of postpartum psychosis and mania. They should, along with atypical antipsychotics, be considered in women with preexisting or a family history of bipolar disorder (Sharma, 2008). Both carbamazepine and valproic acid are thought to be compatible with breastfeeding (Sharma, Burt, & Ritchie, 2009). Lamotrigine is difficult to evaluate given limited data, though there is some evidence that plasma concentrations of this drug are relatively high in exposed infants (Liporace, Kao, & D'Abreu, 2004). One recent study showed no long-term cognitive effects in children previously exposed in utero with further exposure to lamotrigine, valproic acid, or carbamazepine through breastfeeding (Meador et al., 2010).

Lithium is highly effective in the treatment of bipolar mania. Several small studies have demonstrated a benefit of lithium treatment in postpartum psychosis (Doucet et al., 2011). Lithium use has been controversial in breastfeeding due to concerns about high concentration in breast milk and the risk of infant toxicity (Sharma et al., 2009); however, one recent study demonstrated no adverse effects on infants from lithium exposure in breast milk (Viguera et al., 2007). Given the need to monitor drug levels, renal function, and thyroid function in adults, it is advisable to do the same in the breastfed infant (Viguera et al., 2007).

Electroconvulsive Therapy

ECT is an excellent treatment option for women who cannot tolerate medications, have failed multiple medication trials, or have severe symptoms threatening safety and requiring a rapid resolution (Sit et al., 2006). Women with postpartum psychosis have been shown to respond more robustly to ECT than those with non-postpartum psychosis (Reed, Sermin, Appleby, & Faragher, 1999). One recent study showed only transient maternal side effects of anterograde amnesia and prolonged seizure responsive to an additional dose of a barbiturate anesthetic. The same study showed no side effects for the breastfed infants, making ECT a nice alternative for mothers concerned about infant exposure to medications (Babu, Thippeswamy, & Chandra, 2013).

Psychotherapeutic and Social Interventions

In the case of a postpartum mania or psychosis, the need for hospitalization should be carefully considered. In addition, local child protective services should be involved, when appropriate, to evaluate the situation at home and to ensure the safety of the infant. Whenever possible, family should be included in treatment planning and safety measures. Psychoeducation for the patient, partner, and family is crucial, especially as postpartum symptoms may signal a developing chronic mental illness (Sit et al., 2006). It is important to recognize that postpartum mania and psychosis are treatable conditions that usually resolve with appropriate pharmacologic interventions. The mere presence of bipolar disorder and schizophrenia does not in and of itself deem a woman unfit to parent; the ultimate goal of treatment should be to reunite the mother and child in a safe and healthy environment.

As with medications, it is helpful to consider which psychotherapeutic interventions have helped the mother manage her symptoms in the past. Supportive psychotherapy begun immediately, perhaps even prior to hospital discharge, is one possible intervention. A focus on bonding with the newborn and learning how to parent should be included in the therapy. If symptoms do not interfere, more advanced therapies requiring organized thinking such as interpersonal therapy or cognitive behavioral therapy can be considered (Sit et al., 2006).

Prognosis and Postpartum Psychosis

Prognosis for the Mother

The prognosis for a woman with postpartum psychosis is favorable when, if symptoms do occur, the woman seeks help within 1 month of delivery (Robling, Paykel, Dunn, Abbott, & Katona, 2000). Previous levels of social and occupational functioning can be regained or preserved with appropriate treatment (Pfuhlmann, Stoeber, & Beckmann, 2002).

Women who experience postpartum mood and psychotic symptoms are at risk for further episodes and ongoing psychiatric illness. One recent study showed a 54 % risk of recurrence of postpartum psychosis after an initial episode. This same study found that 69 % of women diagnosed with postpartum psychosis had a later non-puerperal episode of mania or depression and, subsequently, met the criteria for a diagnosis of bipolar affective disorder (Blackmore et al., 2013).

Women who experience postpartum psychiatric disorders are also at an increased risk for suicide. Studies show suicide rates of approximately 4 % for women with postpartum psychosis (Pfuhlmann et al., 2002).

Prognosis for the Baby

Paranoia, stigma, and poor insight can prevent mothers from obtaining postpartum parenting support from family, friends, or providers (Solari, Dickson, & Miller, 2009). It is important that services such as parenting classes, support groups, and parenting coaching are established early to help promote successful parenting and mother–infant bonding (Solari et al., 2009). In addition to symptoms interfering with a woman's ability to parent, poor preparation for parenting places her at risk of losing custody of her child (Solari, 2010). Infant abuse and neglect are also concerns. It has been shown that maternal insight into mental illness functions as a protective factor against child physical abuse and neglect, adding further support for psychoeducation and aggressive treatment of maternal symptoms (Mullick, Miller, & Jacobsen, 2001).

Maternal neonaticide (killing of an infant within the first 24 h of life) and infanticide (killing of an infant less than 12 months) are further rare, yet devastating, events (Porter & Gavin, 2010). Characteristics of women who kill their children are challenging to determine given the low incidence of this occurrence (Ostler & Kopels, 2010). For women with chronic psychotic disorders, auditory hallucinations or delusions surrounding the infant and psychotic denial of pregnancy are risk factors (Ostler & Kopels, 2010). Other characteristics often shown to be associated with mothers who commit neonaticide are low socioeconomic status, young age (late teens to twenties), lack of partner, and lack of prenatal care (Friedman & Resnick, 2009). Clinicians should be aware of such risk factors in women with severe mental illness and monitor both mother and infant closely and frequently after delivery.

There are few long-term outcome studies on children of mothers with severe postpartum illness; however, it has been shown that children of mothers who experienced a severe postpartum psychiatric episode versus children whose mothers had only non-puerperal episodes are at higher risk for subsequent mental health problems in adulthood (Abbott, Dunn, Robling, & Paykel, 2004). This suggests a further environmental contribution from maternal postpartum psychiatric symptoms on child development.

Conclusions

Chronic mental illness affects men and women across the life-span but can be particularly destabilizing for women during the reproductive years. Although women with bipolar disorder and schizophrenia are at high risk for exacerbation of their illness during this time, appropriate treatment can allow for a healthy pregnancy and postpartum period, with maximum benefit to the infant and family.

Women who suffer from mental illness often feel stigmatized, which in turn can be a deterrent from seeking help (Dolman, Jones, & Howard, 2013). Research has shown that the stigma associated with a psychiatric diagnosis can be reinforced by also being a parent (Wilson & Crowe, 2009). Women can feel doubly stigmatized because their capacity to be a "good mother" can be automatically doubted in the face of a mental illness diagnosis (Dolman et al., 2013). Additionally, women with severe mental illness often experience feelings of guilt around their need for treatment during pregnancy, postpartum, and beyond, and suffer from chronic fears of custody loss due to their mental illness (Dolman et al., 2013). Access to treatment is also often difficult, whether due to misdiagnosis, need for assistance with childcare during a crisis, or perceived or actual bias among healthcare providers (Dolman et al., 2013).

The mental health practitioner should be mindful that women who suffer from chronic mental illness might have difficulty seeking help during this time. A proactive, thoughtful approach to the pregnancy and postpartum period can have lasting implications for both the patient and her family. In particular, ensuring that a mother with severe mental illness has sufficient information about her illness, parenting resources, and places to obtain peer support can assist with feelings of isolation and reticence to seek help (Dolman et al., 2013).

References

Abbott, R., Dunn, V. J., Robling, S. A., & Paykel, E. S. (2004). Long-term outcome of offspring after maternal severe puerperal disorder. *Acta Psychiatric Scandinavcia, 110*(5), 365–373. doi:10.1111/j.1600-0447.2004.00406.x.

Akdeniz, F., Vahip, S., Pirildar, S., Vahip, I., Doganer, I., & Bulut, I. (2003). Risk factors associated with childbearing-related episodes in women with bipolar disorder. *Psychopathology, 36*(5), 234–238. doi:73448.

American Academy of Pediatrics. (2012). Breastfeeding and the use of human milk. *Pediatrics, 129*(3), e827–e841. doi:10.1542/peds.2011-3552.

American Psychiatric Association. (2013). *Diagnostic and statistical manual of mental disorders* (5th ed.). Author: Washington, DC.

Anderson, E. L., & Reti, I. M. (2009). ECT in pregnancy: A review of the literature from 1941 to 2007. *Psychosomatic Medicine, 71*(2), 235–242. doi:10.1097/PSY.0b013e318190d7ca.

Babu, G. N., Thippeswamy, H., & Chandra, P. S. (2013). Use of electroconvulsive therapy (ECT) in postpartum psychosis—A naturalistic prospective study. *Archives of Women's Mental Health, 16*(3), 247–251. doi:10.1007/s00737-013-0342-2.

Blackmore, E. R., Rubinow, D. R., O'Connor, T. G., Liu, X., Tang, W., Craddock, N., et al. (2013). Reproductive outcomes and risk of subsequent illness in women diagnosed with postpartum psychosis. *Bipolar Disorder, 15*(4), 394–404. doi:10.1111/bdi.12071.

Burt, V. K., & Rasgon, N. (2004). Special considerations in treating bipolar disorder in women. [Research Support, Non-U.S. Gov't Review]. *Bipolar Disorder, 6*(1), 2–13.

Colom, F., Cruz, N., Pacchiarotti, I., Mazzarini, L., Goikolea, J. M., Popova, E., ... Vieta, E. (2010). Postpartum bipolar episodes are not distinct from spontaneous episodes: Implications for DSM-V. [Research Support, Non-U.S. Gov't]. *Journal of Affective Disorders, 126*(1-2), 61–64. doi: 10.1016/j.jad.2010.02.123.

Coverdale, J., McCullough, L., & Chervenak, F. (2010). Ethical issues in managing the pregnancies of patients with schizophrenia. *Current Women's Health Reviews, 6*(1), 63–67.

Dolman, C., Jones, I., & Howard, L. M. (2013). Pre-conception to parenting: A systematic review and meta-synthesis of the qualitative literature on motherhood for women with severe mental illness. [Meta-Analysis Review]. *Archives of Women's Mental Health, 16*(3), 173–196. doi:10.1007/s00737-013-0336-0.

Doucet, S., Jones, I., Letourneau, N., Dennis, C. L., & Blackmore, E. R. (2011). Interventions for the prevention and treatment of postpartum psychosis: A systematic review. *Archives of Women's Mental Health, 14*(2), 89–98. doi:10.1007/s00737-010-0199-6.

Doyle, K., Heron, J., Berrisford, G., Whitmore, J., Jones, L., Wainscott, G., et al. (2012). The management of bipolar disorder in the perinatal period and risk factors for postpartum relapse. [Comparative Study]. *European Psychiatry, 27*(8), 563–569. doi:10.1016/j.eurpsy.2011.06.011.

Fortinguerra, F., Clavenna, A., & Bonati, M. (2009). Psychotropic drug use during breastfeeding: A review of the evidence. *Pediatrics, 124*(4), e547–e556. doi:10.1542/peds.2009-0326.

Freeman, M. P., Smith, K. W., Freeman, S. A., McElroy, S. L., Kmetz, G. E., Wright, R., et al. (2002). The impact of reproductive events on the course of bipolar disorder in women. [Comparative Study]. *Journal of Clinical Psychiatry, 63*(4), 284–287.

Frieder, A., Dunlop, A. L., Culpepper, L., & Bernstein, P. S. (2008). The clinical content of preconception care: Women with psychiatric conditions. *American Journal of Obstetrics & Gynecology, 199*(6 Suppl 2), S328–S332. doi:10.1016/j.ajog.2008.09.001.

Friedman, S. H., Horwitz, S. M., & Resnick, P. J. (2005). Child murder by mothers: A critical analysis of the current state of knowledge and a research agenda. *American Journal of Psychiatry, 162*(9), 1578–1587. doi:10.1176/appi.ajp.162.9.1578.

Friedman, S. H., & Resnick, P. J. (2009). Neonaticide: Phenomenology and considerations for prevention. *International Journal of Law Psychiatry, 32*(1), 43–47. doi:10.1016/j.ijlp.2008.11.006.

Gentile, S. (2010). Antipsychotic therapy during early and late pregnancy: A systematic review. *Schizophrenia Bulletin, 36*(3), 518–544. doi:10.1093/schbul/sbn107.

Harlow, B. L., Vitonis, A. F., Sparen, P., Cnattingius, S., Joffe, H., & Hultman, C. M. (2007). Incidence of hospitalization for postpartum psychosis and bipolar episodes in women with and without prior prepregnancy or prenatal psychiatric hospitalizations. [Comparative Study Research Support, Non-U.S. Gov't]. *Archives of General Psychiatry, 64*(1), 42–48. doi:10.1001/archpsyc.64.1.42.

Jones, I., & Craddock, N. (2002). Do puerperal psychotic episodes identify a more familial subtype of bipolar disorder? Results of a family history study. [Comparative Study Research Support, Non-U.S. Gov't]. *Psychiatric Genetics, 12*(3), 177–180.

Keller, M. B., Lavori, P. W., Coryell, W., Andreasen, N. C., Endicott, J., Clayton, P. J., ... Hirschfeld, R. M. (1986). Differential outcome of pure manic, mixed/cycling, and pure depressive episodes in patients with bipolar illness. [Comparative Study]. *Journal of the American Medical Association, 255*(22), 3138–3142.

Kendell, R. E., Chalmers, J. C., & Platz, C. (1987). Epidemiology of puerperal psychoses. *British Journal of Psychiatry, 150*, 662–673.

Kilzieh, N., & Akiskal, H. S. (1999). Rapid-cycling bipolar disorder: An overview of research and clinical experience. [Review]. *Psychiatric Clinics of North America, 22*(3), 585–607.

Klinger, G., Stahl, B., Fusar-Poli, P., & Merlob, P. (2013). Antipsychotic drugs and breastfeeding. *Pediatric Endocrinology Reviews, 10*(3), 308–317.

Lee, H. C., & Lin, H. C. (2010). Maternal bipolar disorder increased low birth weight and preterm births: A nationwide population-based study. [Research Support, Non-U.S. Gov't]. *Journal of Affective Disorders, 121*(1–2), 100–105. doi:10.1016/j.jad.2009.05.019.

Liporace, J., Kao, A., & D'Abreu, A. (2004). Concerns regarding lamotrigine and breast-feeding. *Epilepsy & Behavior, 5*(1), 102–105.

Manber, R., Blasey, C., & Allen, J. J. (2008). Depression symptoms during pregnancy. [Comparative Study Research Support, N.I.H., Extramural Research Support, U.S. Gov't, P.H.S.]. *Archives of Women's Mental Health, 11*(1), 43–48. doi:10.1007/s00737-008-0216-1.

Meador, K. J., Baker, G. A., Browning, N., Clayton-Smith, J., Combs-Cantrell, D. T., Cohen, M., … Group, N. S. (2010). Effects of breastfeeding in children of women taking antiepileptic drugs. *Neurology, 75*(22), 1954–1960. doi: 10.1212/WNL.0b013e3181ffe4a9

Miller, L. J. (2010). Psychotherapy for pregnancy women with schizophrenia. *Current Women's Health Reviews, 6*(1), 39–43.

Mullick, M., Miller, L. J., & Jacobsen, T. (2001). Insight into mental illness and child maltreatment risk among mothers with major psychiatric disorders. *Journal of Psychiatric Services, 52*(4), 488–492.

Munk-Olsen, T., Laursen, T. M., Mendelson, T., Pedersen, C. B., Mors, O., & Mortensen, P. B. (2009). Risks and predictors of readmission for a mental disorder during the postpartum period. [Research Support, Non-U.S. Gov't]. *Archives of General Psychiatry, 66*(2), 189–195. doi:10.1001/archgenpsychiatry.2008.528.

Nau, M. L., McNiel, D. E., & Binder, R. L. (2012). Postpartum psychosis and the courts. *Journal of the American Academy of Psychiatry Law, 40*(3), 318–325.

Ostler, T., & Kopels, S. (2010). Schizophrenia and filicide. *Current Women's Health Reviews, 6*(1), 58–62.

Pfuhlmann, B., Stoeber, G., & Beckmann, H. (2002). Postpartum psychoses: Prognosis, risk factors, and treatment. *Current Psychiatry Reports, 4*(3), 185–190.

Porter, T., & Gavin, H. (2010). Infanticide and neonaticide: A review of 40 years of research literature on incidence and causes. *Trauma, Violence & Abuse, 11*(3), 99–112. doi:10.1177/1524838010371950.

Reed, P., Sermin, N., Appleby, L., & Faragher, B. (1999). A comparison of clinical response to electroconvulsive therapy in puerperal and non-puerperal psychoses. *Journal of Affective Disorders, 54*(3), 255–260.

Robb, J. C., Young, L. T., Cooke, R. G., & Joffe, R. T. (1998). Gender differences in patients with bipolar disorder influence outcome in the medical outcomes survey (SF-20) subscale scores. *Journal of Affective Disorders, 49*(3), 189–193.

Robinson, G. E. (2012). Treatment of schizophrenia in pregnancy and postpartum. *Journal of Popular Therapy Clinical Pharmacology, 19*(3), e380–e386.

Robling, S. A., Paykel, E. S., Dunn, V. J., Abbott, R., & Katona, C. (2000). Long-term outcome of severe puerperal psychiatric illness: A 23 year follow-up study. *Psycholical Medicine, 30*(6), 1263–1271.

Romans, S. (2010). Sexuality in women with schizophrenia. *Current Women's Health Reviews, 6*(1), 3–11.

Saatcioglu, O., & Tomruk, N. B. (2011). The use of electroconvulsive therapy in pregnancy: A review. *Israel Journal of Psychiatry & Related Sciences, 48*(1), 6–11.

Seeman, M. V. (2013). Clinical interventions for women with schizophrenia: Pregnancy. *Acta Psychiatrica Scandinavica, 127*(1), 12–22. doi:10.1111/j.1600-0447.2012.01897.x.

Seyfried, L. S., & Marcus, S. M. (2003). Postpartum mood disorders. [Research Support, U.S. Gov't, P.H.S. Review]. *International Review of Psychiatry, 15*(3), 231–242. doi:10.1080/0954 026031000136857.

Sharma, V. (2008). Treatment of postpartum psychosis: Challenges and opportunities. *Current Drug Safety, 3*(1), 76–81.

Sharma, V., Burt, V. K., & Ritchie, H. L. (2009). Bipolar II postpartum depression: Detection, diagnosis, and treatment. *American Journal of Psychiatry, 166*(11), 1217–1221. doi:10.1176/appi.ajp.2009.08121902.

Sharma, V., & Pope, C. J. (2012). Pregnancy and bipolar disorder: A systematic review. *Journal of Clinical Psychiatry, 73*(11), 1447–1455. doi:10.4088/JCP.11r07499.

Sharma, V., Smith, A., & Khan, M. (2004). The relationship between duration of labour, time of delivery, and puerperal psychosis. *Journal of Affective Disorders, 83*(2–3), 215–220. doi:10.1016/j.jad.2004.04.014.

Sit, D., Rothschild, A. J., & Wisner, K. L. (2006). A review of postpartum psychosis. *Journal of Women's Health (Larchmt), 15*(4), 352–368. doi:10.1089/jwh.2006.15.352.

Solari, H. (2010). Psychotic denial of pregnancy. *Current Women's Health Reviews, 6*(1), 22–27.

Solari, H., Dickson, K. E., & Miller, L. (2009). Understanding and treating women with schizophrenia during pregnancy and postpartum—Motherisk Update 2008. *Canadian Journal of Clinical Pharmacology, 16*(1), e23–e32.

Spinelli, M. G. (2009). Postpartum psychosis: Detection of risk and management. *American Journal of Psychiatry, 166*(4), 405–408. doi:10.1176/appi.ajp.2008.08121899.

Terp, I. M., & Mortensen, P. B. (1998). Post-partum psychoses. Clinical diagnoses and relative risk of admission after parturition. [Research Support, Non-U.S. Gov't]. *British Journal of Psychiatry, 172,* 521–526.

Vigod, S., & Ross, L. (2010). Epidemiology of psychotic symptoms during pregnancy and postpartum in women with schizophrenia. *Current Women's Health Reviews, 6*(1), 17–21.

Viguera, A. C., & Cohen, L. S. (1998). The course and management of bipolar disorder during pregnancy. [Review]. *Psychopharmacology Bulletin, 34*(3), 339–346.

Viguera, A. C., Cohen, L. S., Baldessarini, R. J., & Nonacs, R. (2002). Managing bipolar disorder during pregnancy: Weighing the risks and benefits. [Comparative Study Research Support, Non-U.S. Gov't Research Support, U.S. Gov't, P.H.S. Review]. *Canadian Journal of Psychiatry, 47*(5), 426–436.

Viguera, A. C., Newport, D. J., Ritchie, J., Stowe, Z., Whitfield, T., Mogielnicki, J., ... Cohen, L. S. (2007). Lithium in breast milk and nursing infants: Clinical implications. *American Journal of Psychiatry, 164*(2), 342–345. doi: 10.1176/appi.ajp.164.2.342.

Viguera, A. C., Nonacs, R., Cohen, L. S., Tondo, L., Murray, A., & Baldessarini, R. J. (2000). Risk of recurrence of bipolar disorder in pregnant and nonpregnant women after discontinuing lithium maintenance. [Comparative Study Research Support, Non-U.S. Gov't Research Support, U.S. Gov't, P.H.S.]. *American Journal of Psychiatry, 157*(2), 179–184.

Wilson, L., & Crowe, M. (2009). Parenting with a diagnosis bipolar disorder. *Journal of Advanced Nursing, 65*(4), 877–884. doi:10.1111/j.1365-2648.2008.04954.x.

Wisner, K. L., Peindl, K., & Hanusa, B. H. (1994). Symptomatology of affective and psychotic illnesses related to childbearing. *Journal of Affective Disorders, 30*(2), 77–87.

Yonkers, K. A., Wisner, K. L., Stowe, Z., Leibenluft, E., Cohen, L., Miller, L., ... Altshuler, L. (2004). Management of bipolar disorder during pregnancy and the postpartum period. [Review]. *American Journal of Psychiatry, 161*(4), 608–620.

Does Psychiatric Diagnosis Affect Fertility Outcomes?

Dorette Noorhasan

Introduction

Infertility affects many women in the USA. According to the Center for Disease Control and Prevention's (CDC) report in July 2012, utilizing Key Statistics from the National Survey of Family Growth (2006–2010), there are 10.9 % (6.7 million) women aged 15–44 in the USA with impaired fecundity (CDC, 2012). The prevalence numbers are generally workable estimates but are not always an accurate approximation since many women who have problems conceiving do not seek treatment or report to a general data bank regarding their fertility issues. Thoma et al. (2013) demonstrated that the prevalence of infertility might actually be higher (15.5 %) using the estimation time to pregnancy model rather than the traditional constructed model. The traditional constructed model derives data from responses to questions on contraceptive use, surgical sterilization, sexual activity, relationship status, duration of partnership, and current or recent pregnancy. All married and cohabiting respondents were considered infertile if they have had sexual activity each month for 12 months without contraception and without conceiving. The estimation time to pregnancy model derives data from all these parameters but also documents whether or not the couple had an intention to conceive and the number of months/years they were trying to get pregnant. By adding these two other parameters, infertility prevalence is higher than previously reported (Thoma et al., 2013).

According to the American Society for Reproductive Medicine (ASRM), infertility is defined as "no evidence of conception after 1 year of trying in a couple where the female partner is less than age 35, and after 6 months of trying when the female partner is age 35 and older (ASRM, 2008a)." Primary infertility is defined as

D. Noorhasan, M.D. (✉)
Dallas, TX, USA

infertility in a woman who has never been pregnant, whereas secondary infertility is defined as infertility in a woman who has been pregnant in the past (ASRM, 2013a).

Most, if not all, of us know someone who is struggling with infertility. The ability to reproduce is a privilege that is frequently taken for granted, like the ability to walk, see, and speak. Unsuccessful attempts at conception are likely to have a huge negative psychological impact. The repeated disappointment and discouragement inevitably create stress, which often leads to relational and occupational problems as well as difficulties interacting with a marital partner, family, and friends; this frequently leaves a woman feeling isolated and alone. Infertility affects self-esteem, and self-confidence, causing disturbances in sleep along with mood swings, irritability, and a myriad of other emotions including shock, guilt, anger, frustration, grief, anxiety, and depression. One study found that infertile women have global symptom scores equivalent to cancer patients (Domar, Zuttermeister, & Friedman, 1993). Hence, the problem is very real.

Anxiety and depression are commonly linked to infertility outcomes (Cousineau & Domar, 2007; Ramezanzadeh et al., 2004). Although unclear whether it is depression that affects these outcomes or whether poor outcomes lead to depression, it seems more likely that these mood disorders and infertility outcomes are delicately intertwined as each exacerbates the other in a vicious cycle. In this chapter, the biopsychosocial relationship between stress and psychiatric diagnoses and infertility outcomes is reviewed. Subsequently, ways to manage stress in an effort to improve infertility outcomes are addressed.

Causes of Infertility

The rise in infertility is a result of a variety of factors, including waiting to have children at an older age after establishing a successful career, increase in tubal disease, increase in sterilization procedures, and an increase in second marriages. The ASRM reports that approximately one-third of the causes of infertility are identified in the woman, one-third in the man, and one-tenth in both partners, and in 10–20 % the cause is unknown (ASRM, 2008b).

Impact of Stress

Anecdotally, the couple trying for years to conceive is a familiar story. Following multiple treatment cycles they decide to adopt and then become pregnant shortly after bringing home their adopted child. Or the couple that tried for years to conceive and had multiple treatment procedures until one finally worked. Soon after the first child is born, they conceive a second child. It appears in some cases of infertility when expectations and the pressure to conceive are eliminated, a couple becomes fertile.

Stress related to infertility affects a woman's marriage, intimacy, and sexual health (Valsangkar, Bodhare, Bele, & Sai, 2011). One study compared marital satisfaction and their subjective quality of life between 18 couples diagnosed with infertility to 12 couples that had no problems conceiving. The findings indicated that women diagnosed with infertility had significantly lower marital adjustment test scores ($P=0.01$) and a trend toward lower quality-of-life scores ($P=0.09$) when compared to controls (Monga, Alexandrescu, Katz, Stein, & Ganiats, 2004).

A study by Andrews, Abbey, and Halman (1991) also evaluated the effects of infertility stress on marriage and life quality. This study found that infertility stress leads to increased marital conflict and decreased sexual self-esteem as well as decreased satisfaction with one's own sexual performance and decreased frequency of sexual intercourse. Couples also reported a decrease in positive evaluations of their lives as a whole.

There are multiple factors that contribute to growing tension in the relationship. One factor is culpability, where the partner without fertility issues may feel cheated out of his/her chance to have a child had he/she married someone else. This results in constant reminders and comments to the infertile partner. Furthermore, something as intimate as their sexual lives is now being controlled by a practice that dictates to them when and how frequently to have intercourse. Men worry about their potency, and women worry about their sexuality and whether or not their husbands still find them sexually attractive. Lovemaking that previously may have felt spontaneous and playful now becomes a chore and an obligation. Since women are often ready for children earlier than men, this may lead to increased conflict as to when to have a child. Generally, men tend to be more relaxed about seeking treatment and often give up earlier on treatments than women do. This often results in additional tension regarding their readiness to start a family.

Fertility and Cultural Implications

There are many social and cultural influences on fertility stress. In many Asian cultures, family is the most important unit. For women in these cultures, childbearing is important to keep the marriage stable and to improve relationships with the in-laws (Wiersema et al., 2006). In Nigeria and many parts of Africa, polygamy and sexually transmitted infections resulting in tubal factor infertility are not uncommon (Upkong & Orji, 2006). Women are often unfairly blamed for their perceived inability to produce children. Adoption in this culture is not acceptable, and there are medical, ethical, and legal implications regarding fertility treatments (Upkong & Orji, 2006). In the Muslim culture there are social pressures to reproduce immediately after marriage. This culture also values a male offspring more than a female offspring (Ashkani, Akbari, & Heydari, 2006). As a result, females learn early in childhood that they are the less desired gender. In the Muslim culture, women are often forced to agree to polygamy so that their husbands can have their desired children (Ashkani et al., 2006).

Fertility and Religious Concerns

In addition to culture, certain religious practices create moral contradictions that can also be a source of stress which potentially affect fertility outcomes. Catholicism encourages procreation but disapproves of most fertility treatments. How a woman navigates the dictates of her faith has a profound impact on her sense of freedom regarding physical intimacy, her choices about contraception, and the extent to which she will seek out the available advancements in reproductive technology. When in vitro fertilization (IVF) is a recommended course of treatment, she may find herself confronting a crisis of faith—choosing between loyalty to the church and her longing for a child. Additionally, women who have had elective abortions previously may believe that their infertility is a punishment from God, which in turn intensifies their guilt for past decisions. It is often not discussed for fear of future blame from both religious leaders and themselves.

Fertility and the Career Woman

Women of advanced reproductive age often feel guilty for focusing on their careers before finding a husband and/or starting a family. Often, they are highly dedicated successful women who believe that if you work hard at anything, you will achieve it; however, that is not necessarily the case for fertility. Consequently, these women are often devastated that they have no control over their childbearing potential. This often affects self-esteem and evokes a sense of failure in women who are accustomed to achieving success and fulfillment in other areas of their lives.

Additionally, working women who undergo infertility treatments often have to take multiple hours off work to visit the infertility clinic. Invariably, they may have to let their employers know why they are missing so many days or risk losing their jobs. Co-workers may notice them coming in to work late many mornings, which can be a source of gossip. This pressures women to disclose something as private as their infertility.

The Impact of Finances on Stress and Fertility

Infertility testing and subsequent treatments are costly. In the USA, as of this writing, only 11 states have mandated fertility coverage (ASRM, 2013b), meaning that insurance companies are required to cover some level of infertility care. Even in many of these states, there are certain prerequisites before insurance assumes any reimbursement for IVF. Many couples take out loans and second mortgages to finance their treatments. The financial burden of paying for infertility treatment without any guarantee of success adds even more stress, anxiety, and depression to an already stressed out couple. Financial stress is often more pronounced in less educated, less affluent women as well as women who are single by choice, in that both populations tend to have less access to available resources (So-hyun & Grable, 2004).

Gender Differences: Women are Disproportionately Affected

Psychiatric disorders are frequently more pronounced in the female partner than the male partner since she is the one who often bears both the physiological and psychological burden of infertility. Wichman, Ehlers, Wichman, Weaver, and Coddington (2011) compared multiple psychological distress (depression, anxiety, infertility-specific distress, and general perceived stress) measures between men and women preparing for IVF. They found that women consistently scored higher on multiple measures of psychological distress than their male partners in the context of preparing for IVF. Findings from other studies indicate that infertile women have significantly higher rates of depressive symptoms than their fertile counterparts (Cwikel, Gidron, & Sheiner, 2004).

Freeman (1985) did a psychological evaluation of 200 couples consecutively seen at a pretreatment consultation in an IVF program using the Minnesota Multiphasic Personality Inventory (MMPI) and found that 20 % of their sample scored high on scales that would indicate unusually high emotional distress and/or personality deficits. They found that 50 % of the women and 15 % of the men reported that infertility is the most upsetting experience of their lives. Another study, which looked at the psychological profile of women diagnosed with unexplained infertility undergoing IVF, found no clinically significant differences in personality or levels of depression and anxiety between this group of women and another group where the source of their infertility had been identified (Romano et al., 2012). Based on the administration of the MMPI, however, the latter group appeared to have more well-developed defensive systems which enabled them to manage stress more effectively.

Timing of Depression in Relation to Fertility

The onset of depression when there is infertility varies, but one study suggests that it occurs after living with infertility for 2–3 years when comparing couples who have dealt with infertility for one year or more than 6 years (Cousineau & Domar, 2007; Domar, Broome, Zuttermeister, Seibel, & Friedman, 1992). Many couples try to conceive on their own for a year before eventually seeking medical assistance, at which time a resurgence of hope generally occurs. They then see the doctor, when a resurgence of hope occurs. After trying treatments with the physician for another year or two, putting in time, money, and emotional energy to only receive negative outcomes each month, eventually leads to depression 2–3 years after the onset of infertility (Domar, Broome, Zuttermeister, Seibel, & Friedman, 1992).

While undergoing treatment, the 2-week interval from the end of the treatment to the pregnancy test is one of the most psychologically challenging time periods. Women described waiting to see if they were pregnant and the dreaded onset of the next period as unbearably stressful and anxiety provoking (Baram, Tourtelot, Muechler, & Huang, 1988; Boivin & Lancastle, 2010; Callan & Hennessey, 1988; Connolly et al., 1993; Lancastle & Boivin, 2008).

Infertility-specific distress can affect women with both primary and secondary infertility. The longing to achieve pregnancy and being unable to do so is what leaves women vulnerable to the onset of depressive episodes and increased anxiety. Greil, Shreffler, Schmidt, and McQuillan (2011) evaluated women with primary and secondary infertility. They found that both types of infertility were associated with fertility-specific distress.

Psychiatric Diagnoses and Negative IVF Fertility Outcomes

Psychiatric diagnoses can have a negative impact on IVF outcomes. A pilot study of 106 consecutive women, undergoing their first cycle of IVF/ICSI, demonstrated a significant negative association between depression/anxiety and pregnancy rate (Sohrabvand, Abedinia, Pirjani, & Jafarabadi, 2008). Similarly, in a prospective sample of 330 women, depressed women exhibited a lower pregnancy rate for the first treatment cycle than non-depressed women (Thiering, Beaurepaire, Jones, Saunders, & Tennant, 1993). However, an additional study by Lintsen, Verhaak, Eijkemans, Smeenk, and Braat (2009) looking at any correlation between anxiety and depression levels before and after treatment (even when anxiety levels increased just before oocyte retrieval) and pregnancy rates in a sample of 783 women saw no significant impact on rates of pregnancy.

Verhaak (2007) found that when IVF resulted in pregnancy, the negative emotions disappeared, indicating that treatment-induced stress is considerably related to threats of failure. While stress, anxiety, and depression are generally resolved when a woman conceives, research looking at long-term emotional responses to unsuccessful IVF treatments showed that in the 6 months following treatment, 20 % of the women interviewed continued to experience symptoms of anxiety and depression (Verhaak, Smeenk, van Minnen, Kremer, & Kraaimaat, 2005), The researchers found, however, that personality traits, cognitive factors, and social support influence women's adjustments to treatment failure. A Danish study (Baldur-Felskov et al., 2013) that utilized a sample of over 98,000 women in order to investigate any association between treatment outcome and vulnerability to psychiatric illness found that among those women with psychiatric disorders who did not succeed in giving birth there was an increased risk of hospitalization for all mental disorders compared with those women who did give birth.

In concert with these and other studies, Hammarberg, Astbury, and Baker (2001) found that women who did not have a baby were more critical about their IVF treatment experience when compared to women who had a baby resulting from IVF treatment. Findings from another study that looked at women's experiences of infertility treatment had similar results, noting that overall satisfaction with treatment was directly related to the subsequent birth of a baby following treatment (Malin, Hemminki, Räillönen, Sihvo, & Perälä, 2001).

Infertility-related psychiatric diagnoses often present as physical symptoms that include chronic pelvic pain and gastrointestinal problems such as irritable bowel disease; there may be memory loss, concentration difficulties, frequent headaches, and intractable myalgia. These physical conditions adversely affect a woman's interactions with family, friends, and co-workers. Often the physical manifestations of emotional stress are treated medically or even surgically yet there is no resolution of symptoms. Their symptoms only resolve after their infertility is identified and treated as the source. It is only when stress and its psychological ramifications are addressed that the physical ailments are resolved.

Studies have suggested that stress may actually induce a biochemical milieu that is not conducive to conception. Smeenk et al. (2005) conducted a multicenter prospective cohort study of 168 women undergoing their first cycle of IVF/ICSI. Nocturnal urinary adrenaline, noradrenaline, and cortisol levels were measured pretreatment, before oocyte retrieval, and before embryo transfer. Additionally, two questionnaires were administered before the start of treatment to measure anxiety and depression. There was a positive correlation between urinary adrenaline concentrations at baseline and at embryo transfer with the scores of the depression scale. Women with successful IVF outcomes had lower concentrations of adrenaline at oocyte retrieval and lower concentrations of adrenaline and noradrenaline at embryo transfer compared to those women with unsuccessful outcomes. These higher concentrations of stress-induced biological markers provide additional evidence of the direct effect of stress on fertility outcomes. Before ultrasound-guided oocyte aspirations, oocyte retrievals were done via laparoscopy. When compared with women who were having laparoscopy for routine gynecological reasons, women who were having laparoscopy for infertility had elevated levels of the stress hormones serum prolactin and cortisol (Harlow, Fahy, Talbot, Wardle, & Hull, 1996).

Similarly, Demyttenaere, Nijs, Evers-Kiebooms, and Koninckx (1992) found that women with high anticipatory-state anxiety levels and high anticipatory cortisol concentrations had lower IVF pregnancy rates. Another study administered a psychological questionnaire and compared the stress markers and cortisol and prolactin concentrations among both fertile and infertile women. They found that infertile women had significantly higher scores of suspicion, guilt, and hostility as well as elevated levels of cortisol and prolactin when compared to fertile women (Csemiczky, Landgren, & Collins, 2001).

The research remains unclear as to whether stress affects the secretion of gonadotropins, as seen in women with anorexia nervosa and other hypothalamic amenorrheic disorders. However, generally, hypothalamic amenorrheic causes of infertility can be curtailed with exogenous gonadotropin use. Additional, although not well studied, theories on the biological effects of stress on infertility include stress-induced catecholamines as having a local effect on the uterus and on the functions of the fallopian tubes. Those stress-induced biomarkers can create a breakdown in a woman's immune system and decrease or eliminate the immunological markers involved in implantation (Anderheim, Holter, Bergh, & Moller, 2005).

Stress and Behavior

In addition to the direct effect of stress on biomarkers and infertility, there are many indirect effects of stress, such as stress-influenced behaviors including addiction and sexual problems. Women who already have a known prior or current addiction to cigarettes can relapse or their behavior can worsen with stress. Many of these women find that smoking lowers their anxiety; however, ovarian follicular fluid in smokers contains nicotine and most studies conclude that follicular fluid nicotine levels adversely affect egg quantity and quality in addition to overall pregnancy rate (ASRM, 2012).

Alcohol use is another behavior that many people utilize to manage worry and anxiety. Some studies find a negative relationship between alcohol use and fertility rates (Eggert, Theobald, & Engfeldt, 2004). An early study by Jensen et al. (1998) performed an earlier cohort study of 430 couples by evaluating the chances of conception over six menstrual cycles. They found that a woman's alcohol intake had a negative association with her chances of conception.

The Infertile Woman We Do Not See

Although profound sadness, and even clinical depression, that results from the emotional challenges surrounding infertility commonly show up in the physician's office, there is another group of women that many clinicians may never see. These women are so psychologically immobilized by their depression that they do not have the physical capacity to seek out medical advice for infertility concerns. Herbert, Lucke, and Dobson (2010) reported that compared to infertile women who sought medical advice, those who had not sought medical advice had significantly higher odds of self-reported depression and other mental health problems. Consequently, the relationship between depression and infertility may be underestimated (Ramezanzadeh et al., 2004). In addition to the group of women receiving fertility treatments and the group who are too psychologically immobilized to see the clinician, there is a third group of women. This is the group of women who became overwhelmed and stopped seeing the clinician after the new patient visit, after the diagnostic evaluation, before starting treatment, and/or after realizing how much everything will cost without a 100 % guarantee of success. Therefore, there are a large number of women who are not seeking appropriate level of care because of their psychological symptoms and financial concerns.

Miscarriages

The relationship between psychiatric diagnoses and infertility outcomes may be influenced both by the lack of conception and by miscarriages. The ASRM defines recurrent pregnancy loss (RPL) as a disease distinct from infertility where a woman has had two or more failed pregnancies (ASRM, 2005; 2008a). A cause for RPL is found in approximately 25–50 % of couples (ASRM, 2005). There appears to be no explanation for the remaining 50–75 % (ASRM, 2005). Various studies have evaluated the relationship between stress and unexplained RPL with mixed results. Li, Newell-Price, Jones, Ledger, and Li (2012) studied stress status in 45 women with RPL and 40 fertile women. The study found that women with RPL had significantly higher scores on the Fertility Problem Inventory Scale, Perceived Stress Scale, and the Negative Affect Scale. The RPL group also had significantly lower scores on the Positive Affect Scale stress-related biochemical markers that are being assessed as a source of RPL. Craig (2001) suggested that elevated levels of the "abortive" cytokine tumor necrosis factor-alpha (TNF-α, released from T cells, macrophages, and mast cells) and depressed levels of the "anti-abortive" cytokine transforming growth factor-P2 (TGF-P2) may be related to RPL. Another study demonstrated that RPL is associated with elevated levels of the stress marker malondialdehyde (Baban, 2010). Many more studies are investigating other oxidative stress biomarkers and free radicals and their possible association with RPL. However, we currently do not have any compelling evidence to recommend a surplus of antioxidant vitamins to all women with RPL (Gupta, Agarwal, Jashoman, & Alvarez, 2007). The topic of recurrent pregnancy loss is explored in detail in Chap. 9 of this book.

Traditional Medical Management of Anxiety and Depression

Since anxiety and depression are observed in women with infertility problems, an automatic response is to treat these women with antidepressant drugs including selective serotonin reuptake inhibitors (SSRIs). SSRIs are a large group of antidepressant drugs that, to date, has the most data regarding its impact on pregnancy. Approximately 11 % of women take an antidepressant and 13.4 % of pregnant women take an antidepressant during part or all of their pregnancy (Barber, 2008; Cooper, Willy, Pont, & Ray, 2007). Many believe that if antidepressants help with depression and there is no harm to the pregnancy, then the benefits outweigh the risks. Although it is very clear that antidepressants help with severe depression, it is still controversial as to whether or not it helps with mild-to-moderate depression (Urato, 2011). It is also unclear if there is a placebo effect in those with mild-to-moderate depression since women feel like they are doing something by taking a pill. Additionally, it is difficult to classify women who take antidepressants for only part of the pregnancy into the treatment or the control groups. Therefore, obtaining an accurate assessment of antidepressant safety and efficacy in pregnancy is quite difficult. Domar, Moragianni, Ryley, and Urato (2013) did a thorough review of the literature regarding the safety and efficacy of SSRI in pregnant women. The review found that SSRI use has been associated with elevated risks of miscarriages, birth defects (particularly with the use of paroxetine), preterm birth, newborn behavioral syndrome, prolonged QT syndrome on neonatal electrocardiographs, preeclampsia (particularly if SSRIs were taken after the first trimester), and possible long-term neurobehavioral effects on the neonate. Thus far, there has been no evidence of improved pregnancy outcome with SSRI usage in women with mild-to-moderate depression, but there is a benefit for SSRI use in women with severe depression (Domar et al., 2013). However, the data regarding SSRI usage in pregnancy is not black and white. Stewart (2011) agrees that antidepressant medications are indicated for severe depression; however, she (2011) advocates the use of antidepressants in women with mild-to-moderate depression if these women:

- Prefer medication for treatment
- Do not have access or have a poor response to cognitive behavioral therapy or interpersonal psychotherapy
- Have an inability to perform their usual activities
- Have a history of severe depression
- Had a response to a previous antidepressant therapy

Stewart (2011) notes that untreated depression during pregnancy has been linked to increased risks of suicide, miscarriage, preterm birth, poor fetal growth, and impaired fetal and postnatal development. She recommends a multidisciplinary care approach involving the physician, psychiatrist/psychologist/other mental health professionals, psychotherapy, and/or antidepressant medications. Additionally, Koren and Nordeng (2012) suggest that congenital abnormalities may be overly diagnosed in women taking SSRI. Women with anxiety and depression go to the emergency room more frequently than the general population. They are more likely to have an echocardiogram, and their infants are more likely to be seen by a pediatrician and to also have an echocardiogram (Koren & Nordeng, 2012). Because they present to the health care provider more frequently, they are more likely to have abnormalities detected than the general population who do not see the physician as frequently. Hence the data surrounding antidepressant use in pregnancy, as well as for infertile women who may be pregnant soon, is unclear. All of the information to date is based on observational studies, and presently there are no randomized control trials done. Based on all the information presented thus far regarding SSRI use and pregnancy, it is clear that untreated depression can result in maternal and fetal morbidity and mortality, and a multidisciplinary approach entailing psychotherapy and/or antidepressant use is recommended to curb the effects of depression on pregnancy. Proper counseling regarding the benefits and risks of SSRI should be given to all women contemplating SSRI use to determine those who are good candidates.

Alternative Treatments for Stress, Anxiety, and Depression

Acupuncture is a very common mode of treatment used to decrease stress in women with infertility problems. Many studies have demonstrated a benefit, while other studies have refuted this. In a non-blinded, prospective, randomized study of 160 patients undergoing IVF, where the treatment group received 25 min of acupuncture before and after embryo transfer and the control group received no supportive care, the treatment group had a statistically significant higher pregnancy rate (42.5 % vs.

26.3 %, $P=0.03$) (Paulus, Zhang, Strehler, El-Danasouri, & Sterzik, 2002). Another study with a prospective randomized trial of 273 women undergoing IVF demonstrated that acupuncture on the day of embryo transfer significantly improved IVF success when compared to the control group (Westergaard et al., 2006). The acupuncture group was then compared to another group of women who received another session of acupuncture 2 days following embryo transfer; however, no benefit was found to this addition. A meta-analysis of 23 randomized controlled studies evaluating the effects of acupuncture on IVF outcome showed that the acupuncture group had a significantly higher clinical pregnancy rate than the control group; however, there was no difference in the live birth rate between both groups (Zheng, Huang, Zhang, & Wang, 2012). Yet, not all studies have demonstrated a benefit to acupuncture. Smith, Coyle, and Norman (2006) did a single, blind, randomized controlled trial in 228 women undergoing IVF where one group received acupuncture and the control group received noninvasive sham acupuncture. They found no difference in the pregnancy rates. There was a trend toward higher ongoing pregnancy rate in the treatment group at 18 weeks of gestation, but this trend did not reach statistical significance. A prospective, randomized, controlled, single blind trial of 150 women randomized to acupuncture 25 min before and after embryo transfer showed no significant difference in pregnancy rates between the two groups (Domar, Mesay, Kelliher, Alper, & Powers, 2009). Similarly, another prospective randomized controlled trial of 160 women demonstrated no difference in the chemical or the clinical pregnancy rates between the group of women who received 25 min of acupuncture before and after embryo transfer when compared to controls (Moy et al., 2011). Essentially, the benefits of acupuncture for fertility remain controversial based on the studies cited.

Hypnosis has been around for centuries. One study evaluated the impact of hypnosis during embryo transfer on the outcome of IVF. This was a case–control study evaluating 98 IVF cycles where the women underwent hypnosis at the time of embryo transfer compared to 96 IVF cycles where they did not receive any form of treatment at the time of embryo transfer. They demonstrated a 53.1 % clinical pregnancy rate in the hypnosis group compared to 30.2 % in the control group; however, this study had multiple limitations including small sample size, groups being different at baseline, and different IVF protocols (Levitas et al., 2006). Therefore, further studies are necessary to determine if there is a benefit to hypnosis at the time of embryo transfer.

Current research seems to indicate that yoga and massage have beneficial effects with regard to stress reduction (Smith et al., 2010). It has been reported that women who practice yoga have markedly higher scores in life satisfaction and lower scores in excitability, aggressiveness, openness, emotionality, and somatic complaints (Schell, Allolio, & Schonecke, 1994). Additionally, there are many reports of the benefits of yoga on pregnancy. A review study indicated that pregnant women who practiced yoga had a significant reduction in rates of preterm labor, intrauterine growth restriction, low birth weight, pregnancy discomforts/pain, perceived sleep disturbances, perceived stress, and improved quality of life (Babbar, Parks-Savage, & Chauhan, 2012). However, many of the randomized trials assessed in this review study were poorly done. A very limited cohort study demonstrated that pregnant women who practiced a yoga-focused prenatal program had statistical improvements in stress, anxiety, labor pain, and labor confidence (Shim & Lee, 2012). An additional study demonstrated that pregnant women who underwent 12 weeks of yoga twice weekly or massage therapy had a greater decrease in depression, anxiety, and back and leg pain and a greater increase in a relationship scale when compared to controls (Field et al., 2012). Theory proposes that yoga increases vagal activity, which in turn decreases cortisol, increases serotonin, and decreases substance P, a neuropeptide that functions as a neurotransmitter especially in the transmission of pain impulses; this ultimately leads to decreased pain (Field, 2012). These are very limited studies and therefore further evaluation will need to be done to evaluate the effects of yoga on psychiatric diagnoses and infertility.

There have been multiple studies demonstrating the benefits of a mind–body program, which teaches stress reduction techniques, on infertility-related stress, whether simply deep breathing and relaxation techniques or meditation and guided imagery of peaceful past locations or events. In a prospective, randomized, controlled study involving 143 women undergoing IVF, a 10-session mind–body (MB) group was compared to a control group. Only 9 % of MB subjects attended MB sessions during their first IVF cycle. There was no difference in the pregnancy rate in the MB group compared to the controls in their first IVF cycle; 76 % of the MB subjects attended the program during their second cycle, and pregnancy rates for cycle number 2 were 52 % in the MB group and 20 % in the control group (Domar et al., 2011). Hence, with good attendance to the MB program, IVF success was improved.

There are some studies that demonstrate a benefit to exercise for relieving mild-to-moderate depression (Daley, 2008; Dunn, Trivedi, Kampert, Clark, & Chambliss, 2005). Generally, exercise provides good medical benefits including weight loss, lower risk for diabetes, hypertension, and hypercholesterolemia. Additionally, exercise makes women feel healthy and improves their self-esteem. A meta-analysis of 30 studies revealed a decrease (although marginal) in depression in the exercise group (Rimer et al., 2012). Other researches that examined physical fitness in relation to reproductive health found that exercise was associated with a reduction in infertility as an outcome of problems with ovulatory functioning (Rich-Edwards et al., 2002). Overall there is a benefit to exercise reduction of stress. However, it is equally counterproductive to do excessive exercise since this can also have negative fertility outcomes.

Cognitive and Behavioral Approaches to Reducing Stress

Cognitive restructuring is the process of positive thinking, which in turn yields a positive emotional state and physical health. Consultation with a professional to discuss the stresses brought on by infertility and restructuring the thought process has been shown to be beneficial for infertility (Terzioglu, 2001). Terzioglu (2001) conducted an experimental study where couples undergoing artificial reproductive techniques (ART) were assigned to either counseling sessions (experimental group) or no counseling sessions (control group). The study found that the couples undergoing counseling during ART had lower anxiety and depression scores as well as higher life satisfaction scores and pregnancy rates. Similarly, McNaughton-Cassill, Bostwick, Arthur, Robinson, and Neal (2002) assigned couples undergoing IVF to either biweekly support group counseling sessions (experimental group) or no support sessions (control group). They found that women who attended the group sessions were significantly less anxious after the IVF treatment than they were before the cycle, while the control group had no reduction in stress. In a prospective, controlled, single, blind, randomized study, 184 women with infertility were randomized to a 10-session cognitive-behavioral group (cognitive restructuring, relaxation training, methods of emotional expression, nutritional and exercise information), a standard-support group (support group where infertile women shared their stories regarding the impact of infertility on their lives), or routine-care control group. These women were followed for 1 year. The group sizes were small, and therefore the study results did not reach statistical significance. However, there was a trend with the cognitive-behavioral group conceiving spontaneously and therefore requiring less assisted reproductive technologies (Domar et al., 2000). Another randomized control study comparing the efficacy of cognitive-behavioral therapy versus fluoxetine in the treatment of depression and anxiety in infertile women found CBT to be a reliable alternative to medication and actually superior to fluoxetine in reducing depression and anxiety in this population (Faramarzi et al., 2008).

Third-Party Reproduction and Other Alternatives

Donor egg, donor sperm, donor embryo, adoption, and living a happy childless life are alternatives for infertile women. Many women with diminished ovarian reserve will try utilizing their own eggs for many cycles and will fail to conceive. For some of these women, having a genetic child is important. Recurring negative treatment cycles often leave women feeling discouraged and, in many cases, emotionally consumed by their need to become pregnant. Quite often, professional counseling becomes an integral part of the treatment plan as many women begin to consider donor eggs. Many women will be able to move forward with an alternative mode of treatment after counseling. Counseling allows a woman to grieve the loss of the genetically connected child that she longed for.

Resources and Support

There are many other methods of alleviating stress. First and foremost is support. Whether it is family, friends, and/or support groups, having someone to talk to becomes a critical part of managing the undue psychological and emotional stress imposed by infertility. Online websites that many women find helpful for support include www.Resolve.org and www.FertilityFriend.com. The ASRM (www.asrm.org) is a resource for patients seeking information and professional assistance on fertility and its often associated psychiatric problems. The National Institute of

Mental Health (www.nimh.nih.gov) is a source for mental health disorders. The Mind/Body Institute (www.mindbodyinfertility.com) is a resource for information and allows access to professionals who can help women struggling with the psychiatric and emotional aspects of infertility. Some women find multiple benefits to keeping a journal or a diary of their experiences. Others find that engaging in activities they find personally enjoyable and meaningful alleviates some of the emotional intensity of the treatment process.

Is There an Association Between Psychiatric Diagnoses and Fertility Outcomes?

There seems to be a negative correlation between psychiatric diagnoses and infertility outcomes as described in the studies cited thus far; however, there are also studies that suggest that there is no association between psychiatric diagnoses and infertility outcomes. A meta-analysis of 14 prospective psychosocial studies with 3,583 infertile women undergoing a cycle of infertility treatment concluded that emotional distress caused by infertility problems or other life events co-occurring with treatment did not compromise the chance of becoming pregnant (Boivin, Griffiths, & Venetis, 2011) Zaig, (2012), evaluated the effects of baseline psychiatric diagnoses and situational psychiatric symptoms on several biological outcome factors of IVF treatments. They found that women diagnosed with a mood or an anxiety disorder prior to the onset of IVF treatment had similar (actually non-statically significant trend higher) pregnancy rates compared with women without such diagnoses (Zaig, 2012). However, this study is limited since they evaluated women who already had a mood or an anxiety disorder prior to the onset of IVF treatment and did not focus on women who may have developed clinically recognized psychiatric diagnoses due to their fertility problems. A prospective longitudinal study of 166 women undergoing IVF evaluated the effect of psychological stress before and during IVF treatment on the outcome of IVF, controlling for known physiological predictors (Anderheim et al., 2005). They found no evidence of psychological stress based on IVF success (Anderheim et al., 2005). As discussed in this chapter, the majority of the evidence thus far points toward a more difficult conception process in the presence of psychiatric diagnoses, but additional research is needed to better understand and characterize this relationship.

Conclusion

As mentioned in this chapter's introduction, stress and infertility are intertwined in a tumultuous cycle. While stress is not the only reason that a woman is infertile, it can have a negative impact on her infertility treatments. The recurring theme of this book is the impact of reproductive events on a woman's mental health across her life-span. The childbearing years are a particularly challenging time physically as well as psychologically as a woman makes = the transition from daughter to mother. Many women are faced with difficulties in regard to fertility when they are ready to conceive. These fertility problems have associated psychiatric diagnoses that were explored in this chapter. Fortunately, most women who have fertility problems do not meet the clinical threshold for depression and eventually become a parent by some means. Through medical care; communicating with their partner, family, friends, and support groups; and seeing a counselor, many women learn to manage stress, anxiety, and depression and, as a result, turn negative fertility outcomes into positive ones.

References

American Society for Reproductive Medicine (ASRM). (2005). Retrieved from http://www.asrm.org/Recurrent_Pregnancy_Loss/

American Society for Reproductive Medicine (ASRM). (2008a). Definitions of Infertility and recurrent pregnancy loss. *Supplement to Fertility and Sterility, 2008 Compendium of Practice Committee Reports, 90*, S60.

American Society for Reproductive Medicine (ASRM). (2008b). Retrieved from https://www.asrm.org/detail.aspx?id=3018

American Society for Reproductive Medicine (ASRM). (2012). Smoking and infertility: A committee opinion. *Fertility and Sterility, 98*, 1400–1406.

American Society for Reproductive Medicine (ASRM). (2013a). Retrieved from https://www.asrm.org/Templates/SearchResults.aspx?q=primary%20and%20secondary%20infertility%20definition

American Society for Reproductive Medicine (ASRM). (2013b). Retrieved from https://www.asrm.org/insurance.aspx

Anderheim, L., Holter, H., Bergh, C., & Moller, A. (2005). Does psychological stress affect the outcome of in vitro fertilization? *Human Reproduction, 20*, 2969–2975.

Andrews, F. M., Abbey, A., & Halman, L. J. (1991). Stress from infertility, marriage factors, and subjective well-being of wives and husbands. *Journal of Health and Social Behavior, 32*, 238–253.

Ashkani, H., Akbari, A., & Heydari, S. T. (2006). Epidemiology of depression among infertile and fertile couples in Shiraz, Southern Iran. *Indian Journal of Medical Sciences, 60*, 399–406.

Baban, R. S. (2010). Oxidative stress in recurrent pregnancy loss women. *Saudi Medical Journal, 31*, 759–763.

Babbar, S., Parks-Savage, A. C., & Chauhan, S. P. (2012). Yoga during pregnancy: A review. *American Journal of Perinatology, 29*, 459–464.

Baldur-Felskov, B., Kjaer, S. K., Albieri, V., Steding-Jenssen, M., Kjaer, T ... Jensen, A. (2013). Psychiatric disorders in women with fertility problems: Results from a large Danish register-based cohort study. *Human Reproduction, 28*(3), 683–690.

Baram, D., Tourtelot, E., Muechler, E., & Huang, K. E. (1988). Psychosocial adjustment following unsuccessful in vitro fertilization. *Journal of Psychosomatic Obstetrics & Gynaecology, 9*, 181–190.

Barber, C. (2008). The medicated Americans: Antidepressant prescriptions on the rise. *Scientific American Mind*, Feb 27. Retrieved from http://www.scientificamerican.com/article.cfm?id=the-medicated-americans

Boivin, J., Griffiths, E., & Venetis, C. A. (2011). Emotional distress in infertile women and failure of assisted reproductive technologies: Meta-analysis of prospective psychosocial studies. *British Medical Journal, 342*, d223.

Boivin, J., & Lancastle, D. (2010). Medical waiting periods: Immence, emotions, & coping. *Women's Health, 6*(1), 59–69.

Callan, V. J., & Hennessey, J. F. (1988). Emotional aspects and support in in vitro fertilization and embryo transfer programs. *Journal of In Vitro Fertilization and Embryo Transfer, 5*, 290–295.

Center for Disease Control and Prevention (CDC). (2012). Infertility. Retrieved from http://www.cdc.gov/nchs/fastats/fertile.htm

Connolly, K. J., Edelmann, R. J., Bartlett, H., Cooke, I. D., Lenton, E., & Pike, S. (1993). An evaluation of counseling for couples undergoing treatment for in vitro fertilization. *Human Reproduction, 8*, 1332–1338.

Cooper, W. O., Willy, M. E., Pont, S. J., & Ray, W. A. (2007). Increasing use of antidepressants in pregnancy. *American Journal of Obstetrics and Gynecology, 196*, 544.e1–e5.

Cousineau, T. M., & Domar, A. D. (2007). Psychological impact of infertility. *Best Practice & Research Clinical Obstetrics & Gynecology, 21*(2), 293–308.

Craig, M. (2001). Stress and recurrent miscarriage. *Stress, 4*, 205–213.

Csemiczky, G., Landgren, B. M., & Collins, A. (2001). The influence of stress and state anxiety on the outcome of IVF-treatment: Psychological and endocrinological assessment of Swedish women entering IVF-treatment. *Acta Obstetricia et Gynecologica Scandinavica, 79*, 113–118.

Cwikel, J., Gidron, Y., & Sheiner, E. (2004). Psychological interactions with infertility among women. *European Journal of Obstetrics, Gynecology and Reproductive Biology, 117*, 126–131.

Daley, A. (2008). Exercise and depression: A review of reviews. *Journal of Clinical Psychology in Medical Settings, 15*(2), 140–147.

Demyttenaere, K., Nijs, P., Evers-Kiebooms, G., & Koninckx, P. R. (1992). Coping and the ineffectiveness of coping influence the outcome of in vitro fertilization through stress responses. *Psychoneuroendocrinology, 17*, 655–665.

Domar, A. D., Broome, A., Zuttermeister, P. C., Seibel, M., & Friedman, R. (1992). The prevalence and predictability of depression in infertile women. *Fertility and Sterility, 58*, 1158–1163.

Domar, A. D., Clapp, D., Slawsby, E. A., Dusek, J., Kessel, B., & Freizinger, M. (2000). Impact of group psychological interventions on pregnancy rates in infertile women. *Fertility and Sterility, 73*, 805–811.

Domar, A. D., Mesay, I., Kelliher, J., Alper, M., & Powers, R. D. (2009). The impact of acupuncture on in vitro fertilization outcome. *Fertility and Sterility, 91*, 723–726.

Domar, A. D., Moragianni, V. A., Ryley, D. A., & Urato, A. C. (2013). The risks of selective serotonin reuptake inhibitors use in infertile women: A review of the impact on fertility, pregnancy, neonatal health and beyond. *Human Reproduction, 28*, 160–171.

Domar, A. D., Rooney, K. L., Wiegand, B., Orav, E. J., Alper, M. M., Berger, B., et al. (2011). Impact of a group mind/body intervention on pregnancy rates in IVF patients. *Fertility and Sterility, 95*, 2269–2273.

Domar, A. D., Zuttermeister, P. C., & Friedman, R. (1993). The psychological impact of infertility: A comparison with patients with other medical conditions. *Journal of Psychosomatic Obstetrics and Gynaecology, 14*(Suppl), 45–52.

Dunn, A. L., Trivedi, M. H., Kampert, J. B., Clark, C. G., & Chambliss, H. O. (2005). Exercise treatment for depression: Efficacy and dose response. *American Journal of Preventive Medicine, 28*(1), 1–8.

Eggert, J., Theobald, H., & Engfeldt, P. (2004). Effects of alcohol consumption on female fertility during an 18-year period. *Fertility & Sterility, 81*(2), 379–383.

Faramarzi, M., Alipor, A., Esmaelzadeh, S., Kheirkhah, F., Poladi, K., & Pash, H. (2008). Treatment of depression and anxiety in infertile women: Cognitive behavioral therapy versus fluoxetine. *Journal of Affective Disorders, 108*(1–2), 159–164.

Field, T. (2012). Prenatal exercise research. *Infant Behavior and Development, 35*, 397–407.

Field, T., Diego, M., Hernandez-Reif, M., Medina, L., Delgado, J., & Hernandez, A. (2012). Yoga and massage therapy reduce prenatal depression and prematurity. *Journal of Bodywork and Movement Therapies, 16*, 204–209.

Freeman, E. W. (1985). Psychological evaluation and support in a program of in vitro fertilization and embryo transfer. *Fertility and Sterility, 43*, 48–53.

Greil, A. L., Shreffler, K. M., Schmidt, L., & McQuillan, J. (2011). Variation in distress among women with infertility: Evidence from a population-based sample. *Human Reproduction, 26*, 2101–2112.

Gupta, S., Agarwal, A., Jashoman, B., & Alvarez, J. G. (2007). The role of oxidative stress in spontaneous abortion and recurrrent pregnancy loss: A systematic review. *Obstetrical & Gynecological Survey, 62*, 335–347.

Hammarberg, K., Astbury, J., & Baker, H. W. G. (2001). Women's experience of IVF: A follow-up study. *Human Reproduction, 16*, 374–383.

Harlow, C. R., Fahy, U. M., Talbot, W. M., Wardle, P. G., & Hull, M. G. (1996). Stress and stress-related hormones during in-vitro fertilization treatment. *Human Reproduction, 11*, 274–279.

Herbert, D. L., Lucke, J. C., & Dobson, A. J. (2010). Depression: An emotional obstacle to seeking medical advice for infertility. *Fertility and Sterility, 94*, 1817–1821.

Jensen, T. K., Hjollund, N. H. I., Henriksen, T. B., Scheike, T., Kolstad, H., Giwercman, A., ... Olsen, J. (1998). Does moderate alcohol consumption affect fertility? Follow up study among couples planning first pregnancy. *British Medical Journal, 317*, 505–510.

Koren, G., & Nordeng, H. (2012). Antidepressant use during pregnancy: The benefit-risk ratio. *American Journal of Obstetrics and Gynecology, 207*, 157–163.

Lancastle, D., & Boivin, J. (2008). A feasibility study of a brief coping intervention (PRCI) for the waiting period before a pregnancy test during fertility treatment. *Human Reproduction, 23*(10), 2299–2307.

Levitas, E., Parmet, A., Lunenfeld, E., Bentov, Y., Burstein, E., Friger, M., et al. (2006). Impact of hypnosis during embryo transfer on the outcome of in vitro fertilization—embryo transfer: A case control study. *Fertility and Sterility, 85*, 1404–1408.

Li, W., Newell-Price, J., Jones, G. L., Ledger, W. L., & Li, T. C. (2012). Relationship between psychological stress and recurrent miscarriage. *Reproductive Biomedicine Online, 25*, 180–189.

Lintsen, A. M. E., Verhaak, C. M., Eijkemans, M. J. C., Smeenk, J. M. J., & Braat, D. D. M. (2009). Anxiety and depression have no influence on the cancellation and pregnancy rates of a first IVF or ICSI treatment. *Human Reproduction, 24*(5), 1092–1098.

Malin, M., Hemminki, E., Räillönen, O., Sihvo, S., & Perälä, M.-L. (2001). What do women want? Women's experiences of infertility treatment. *Social Science and Medicine, 53*(1), 123–133.

McNaughton-Cassill, M. E., Bostwick, J. M., Arthur, N. J., Robinson, R. D., & Neal, G. S. (2002). Efficacy of brief couples support groups developed to manage the stress of in vitro fertilization treatment. *Mayo Clinic Proceedings, 77*, 106–1066.

Monga, M., Alexandrescu, B., Katz, S. E., Stein, M., & Ganiats, T. (2004). Impact of infertility on quality of life, marital adjustment, and sexual function. *Urology, 63*, 126–130.

Moy, I., Milad, M. P., Barnes, R., Confino, E., Kazer, R. R., & Zhang, X. (2011). Randomized controlled trial: Effects of acupuncture on pregnancy rates in women undergoing in vitro fertilization. *Fertility and Sterility, 95*, 583–587.

Paulus, W. E., Zhang, M., Strehler, E., El-Danasouri, I., & Sterzik, K. (2002). Influence of acupuncture on the pregnancy rate in patients who undergo assisted reproduction therapy. *Fertility and Sterility, 77*, 721–724.

Ramezanzadeh, F., Aghassa, M.M., Abedinia, N., Zayeri, F., Khanafshar, N., Shariat, M., ... Jafarabadi, M. (2004). A survey of relationship between anxiety, depression and duration of infertility. *BMC Women's Health, 4*(1), 9. doi: 10.1186/1472-6874-4-9

Rich-Edwards, J. W., Spiegelman, D., Garland, M., Hertzmark, E., Hunter, D. J. ... Manson, J. E. (2002). Physical activity, body mass, and ovulatory disorder infertility. *Epidemiology, 13*, 184–190.

Rimer, J., Dwan, K., Lawlor, D. A., Greig, C. A., McMurdo, M., Morley, W., et al. (2012). Exercise for Depression. *Cochrane Database of Systematic Reviews, 7*.

Romano, G. A., Ravid, H., Zaig, I., Schreiber, S., Azem, F., Shachar, I., et al. (2012). The psychological profile and affective response of women diagnosed with unexplained infertility undergoing in vitro fertilization. *Archives of Women's Mental Health, 15*(6), 403–411.

Schell, F. J., Allolio, B., & Schonecke, O. W. (1994). Physiological and psychological effects of Hatha-Yoga exercise in healthy women. *International Journal of Psychosomatics, 41*, 46–52.

Shim, C. S., & Lee, Y. S. (2012). Effects of a yoga-focused prenatal program on stress, anxiety, self confidence and labor pain in pregnant women with in vitro fertilization treatment. *Journal of Korean Academy of Nursing, 42*, 369–376.

Smeenk, J. M. J., Verhaak, C. M., Vingerhoets, A. J. J. M., Sweep, C. G. J., Merkus, J. M. W. M., Willemsen, S. J., … Braat, D. D. M. (2005). Stress and outcome success in IVF: The role of self-reports and endocrine variables. *Human Reproduction, 20, 991*–96.

Smith, C., Coyle, M., & Norman, R. J. (2006). Influence of acupuncture stimulation on pregnancy rates for women undergoing embryo transfer. *Fertility and Sterility, 85*, 1352–1358.

Smith, J. F., Eisenberg, M. L., Millstein, S. G., Nachtigall, R. D., Pasch, L., & Katz, P. P. (2010). The use of complementary and alternative fertility treatment in couples seeking fertility care: Data from a prospective cohort in the United States. *Fertility & Sterility, 93*(7), 2169–2174.

Sohrabvand, F., Abedinia, N., Pirjani, R., & Jafarabadi, M. (2008). Effect of anxiety and depression on ART outcome. *Iranian Journal of Reproductive Medicine, 6*, 89–94.

So-hyun, J., & Grable, J. E. (2004). An exploratory framework of the determinants of financial satisfaction. *Journal of Family and Economic Issues, 25*(1), 25–50.

Stewart, D. (2011). Depression during pregnancy. *New England Journal of Medicine, 365*, 1605–1611.

Terzioglu, F. (2001). Investigation into effectiveness of counseling on assisted reproductive techniques in Turkey. *Journal of Psychosomatic Obstetrics & Gynaecology, 22*, 133–141.

Thiering, P., Beaurepaire, J., Jones, M., Saunders, D., & Tennant, C. (1993). Mood state as a predictor of treatment outcome after in vitro fertilization/embryo transfer technology (IVF/ET). *Journal of Psychosomatic Research, 5*, 481–491.

Thoma, M. E., McLain, A. C., Louis, J. F., King, R. B., Trumble, A. C., Sundaram, R., et al. (2013). Prevalence of infertility in the United States as estimated by the current duration approach and a traditional constructed model. *Fertility and Sterility, 99*, 1324–1331.

Upkong, D., & Orji, E. (2006). Mental health of infertile women in Nigeria. *Turkish Journal of Psychiatry, 17*, 259–265.

Urato, A. C. (2011). Antidepressants and pregnancy: Continued evidence of harm-still no evidence of benefit. *Ethical Human Psychology and Psychiatry, 13*, 190–193.

Valsangkar, S., Bodhare, T., Bele, S., & Sai, S. (2011). An evaluation of the effect of infertility on marital, sexual satisfaction indices, and health-related quality of life in women. *Journal of Human Reproductive Sciences, 4*(2), 80–85.

Verhaak, C. M. (2007). Women's emotional adjustment to IVF: A systematic review of 25 years of research. *Human Reproduction, 13*, 27–36.

Verhaak, C. M., Smeenk, J. M. J., van Minnen, A., Kremer, J. A. M., & Kraaimaat, F. W. (2005). A longitudinal, prospective study on emotional adjustment before, during and after consecutive fertility treatment cycles. *Human Reproduction, 20*(8), 2253–2260.

Westergaard, L. G., Mao, Q., Krogslund, M., Sandrini, S., Lenz, S., & Grinsted, J. (2006). Acupuncture on the day of embryo transfer significantly improves the reproductive outcome in infertile women: A prospective, randomized trial. *Fertility and Sterility, 85*(1341–1346), 1368–1369.

Wichman, C. L., Ehlers, S. L., Wichman, S. E., Weaver, A. L., & Coddington, C. (2011). Comparison of multiple psychological distress measures between men and women preparing for in vitro fertilization. *Fertility and Sterility, 95*, 717–721.

Wiersema, N. J., Drukker, A. J., Tien Dung, M. B., Huynh Nhu, G., Thanh Nh, N., & Lambalk, C. B. (2006). Consequences of infertility in developing countries: Results of a questionnaire and interview survey in the south of Vietnam. *Journal of Translational Medicine, 4*, 54.

Zaig, I. (2012). Women's psychological profile and psychiatric diagnoses and the outcome of in vitro fertilization: Is there an association? *Archives of Women's Mental Health, 15*, 353–359.

Zheng, G. H., Huang, G. Y., Zhang, M. M., & Wang, W. (2012). Effects of acupuncture on pregnancy rates in women undergoing in vitro fertilization: A systematic review and meta-analysis. *Fertility and Sterility, 97*, 599–611.

The Reproductive Story: Dealing with Miscarriage, Stillbirth, or Other Perinatal Demise

Janet Jaffe

Introduction

Becoming a mother is key to many women's sense of self. Additionally, a woman's relationship with her partner and her role in her family and society at large is often defined by motherhood. Whether conscious or not, everyone has a reproductive story: the internal narrative of what we imagine it will be like when we have children and become a mother someday (Jaffe & Diamond, 2011; Jaffe, Diamond, & Diamond, 2005). The story entails all the hopes and dreams parents have for their children as well as the internalized image of what it means to be a mother. This story is so deeply woven into the very fabric of a woman's identity that it might only be recognized when it unravels, whether due to infertility, miscarriage, stillbirth, genetic termination, or other perinatal trauma. These are losses like no other; they are often misunderstood, and women suffer in silence and isolation with feelings of guilt, self-blame, grief, depression, and anxiety.

This chapter describes the concept of the reproductive story, how it develops from early childhood into adulthood, and it also explores the multiple layers of loss that occur when the story goes awry, both from theoretical and clinical perspectives. Understanding the grief process particular to reproductive loss is essential for clinicians and caregivers who work with this population. The differences in the ways men and women cope and grieve is addressed as well as issues specific to same-sex couples. Clinical interventions to help women process their losses are also discussed. Additionally, when working with a woman's intense feelings of grief, trauma, and loss, the caregiver may also feel overwhelmed, and as such, the vicarious impact on the clinician is examined in this chapter.

J. Jaffe, Ph.D. (✉)
Center for Reproductive Psychology, San Diego, CA, USA
e-mail: doctorjanetj@yahoo.com

Types of Losses: Definitions

When a woman wants to become a mother, there are no guarantees that she will become pregnant easily or that she will be able to carry a pregnancy to term and deliver a healthy baby. Pregnancy losses are often measured by the length of time a woman is pregnant. The term perinatal loss is an all-inclusive term, which includes fetal demise occurring prior to 20 weeks gestation (miscarriage and ectopic pregnancies), fetal death after 20 weeks (stillbirth), as well as the death of a newborn up to 28 days post-birth (neonatal death) (Moore, Parrish, & Black, 2011).

While the incidence of miscarriage is generally recognized to be 15–20 % (Brier, 2004; Leon, 2008; Robinson, 2011), the occurrence may be much higher. Women who have a "late" period may actually experience a very early pregnancy loss, perhaps never having their pregnancy validated. It has been speculated that the true rate of miscarriage is closer to 40–50 % of all pregnancies (Covington, 2006; Freda, Devine, & Semelsberger, 2003; Leon, 2008), and in women over 45, the rate soars to 75 % (Hemminki & Forssas, 1999; Nybo Andersen, Wohlfahrt, Christens, Olsen, & Melbye, 2000). Because miscarriage is seen as a medically common event, the impact of the loss is often minimized. Women's reactions, however, suggest that experiencing a miscarriage, or any other perinatal loss, can be devastating, with depressed mood, feelings of self-blame, anxiety, shame, anger, and intense grief (Brier, 2004, 2008; Freda et al., 2003; Robinson, 2011). Clinically, women may present with depression, panic disorder, obsessive or intrusive thoughts, or symptoms of post-traumatic stress disorder (Carter, Misri, & Tomfohr, 2007). The risk of a major depression for women miscarrying is 2.5 times higher when compared with a control group (Neugebauer et al., 1997). Similarly, there is an increased risk of anxiety with the most common diagnoses being obsessive-compulsive disorder and post-traumatic stress disorder (Brier, 2004; Carter et al., 2007).

An ectopic pregnancy occurs when the embryo implants outside of the uterus, most often in the fallopian tube. These pregnancies can become medical emergencies and potentially life threatening if not diagnosed and treated early. Ectopic pregnancies can result in a ruptured fallopian tube, which requires surgery. Thankfully the incidence of ectopic pregnancy is much more rare than miscarriage, occurring in 2–3 % of pregnancies (Covington, 2006; Leon, 2008).

Stillbirth is a fetal demise, which occurs in utero after 20 weeks gestation. The mother may be aware that fetal movement has stopped; nonetheless, she must go through labor only to deliver a baby who has died. Delivery rooms, which would normally be filled with a baby's cries and much celebration, are instead met with a chilling silence. The rates of stillbirth vary widely around the globe, ranging from 5 per 1,000 in developed countries to 32 per 1,000 in South Asia and sub-Saharan Africa (Stanton, Lawn, Rahman, Wilczynska-Ketende, & Hill, 2006). Often, the cause of the stillbirth is not known, leading to profound grief, confusion, self-blame, and loss of self-esteem (Leon, 2008; Robinson, 2011). Indeed, many mothers question their ability to produce a healthy baby and feel that their body has betrayed them.

Some pregnancies, whether viable or not, are terminated because of a genetic abnormality. The decision to terminate a desired pregnancy can be very stressful, both physically and emotionally. If the abnormality is found early, the process of termination may be a dilation and curettage, D&C; however, later in the pregnancy, a woman may require an induction and need to go through labor and delivery as in a stillbirth. The impact on the woman, her partner, and other family members can be quite traumatic and is dependent on feelings about abortion, the prognosis of the baby, and the potential long-term negative effects on the family (Robinson, 2011).

The loss of an infant within the first 28 days post-birth is referred to as neonatal death and occurs in approximately 1 % of the population in industrialized nations. These deaths may be caused by premature births, which can have any number of health issues associated with them, birth defects, or sudden infant death syndrome, SIDS (Covington, 2006). SIDS occurs unexpectedly in previously healthy infants for no discernable reason. Needless to say, these deaths are devastating to parents, siblings, other family members, and friends.

Finally, although not traditionally described as a perinatal loss, it is important to broaden the definition to include infertility and its treatment. After taking medication for treatment, a woman might feel symptomatic, take an early pregnancy test, and get a positive reading, but then her period starts. This is known as a chemical pregnancy or very early miscarriage. Similarly, with in vitro fertilization, IVF, egg and sperm are brought together in a petri dish and allowed to grow for 3–5 days, and then the resulting embryo is transferred into the woman's uterus. A preimplantation miscarriage occurs if the transfer is not successful. Additionally, more than one embryo may be transferred during IVF, although single-embryo transfer, SET, is becoming more the norm. In the event that a multiple gestation results, women may choose selective reduction, known as multi-fetal pregnancy reduction, in order to terminate a specific number of embryos. These events related to infertility treatment are also reproductive losses and can result in a grief reaction just as any other perinatal loss (Covington, 2006; Jaffe & Diamond, 2011).

Grief and Mourning: A Theoretical Overview

How does a woman grieve a pregnancy loss? How does she cope with death when there should have been life? The normal expectations of life and death are out of order; babies should not predecease their parents. "Instead of giving life as expected, parents must grapple with death and with mourning a child who, in most instances, was imbued with promise and expectation" (Bennett, Litz, Lee, & Maguen, 2005, p. 180). Because there is a primal instinct for a mother to protect her offspring, when a baby dies, she may believe that she has failed in the most fundamental way. What are the feelings involved when the unthinkable happens and a baby, imagined or real, dies? What are the societal norms in expressing this grief? Women may feel intensely depressed, anxious, guilty, angry, and traumatized, but the depth of their grief is often minimized. With little or no support from others, and few, if any, rituals or cultural norms to fall back on, women feel isolated and alienated.

In order to understand the unique aspects of a perinatal loss and the challenges that women face, it can be helpful to briefly review some of the literature on grief in general. Much of the current understanding of grief and loss has evolved from Freud's 1917 model of bereavement. He proposed that people need to hypercathect (invest intense emotion in), and then decathect (sever the bonds), with the ultimate goal of freeing oneself from the emotional attachment to the deceased (Rothaupt & Becker, 2007). Lindemann (1944) expanded on Freud's work, noting that the intensity of a grief reaction is dependent on the relationship and attachment with the deceased person, and feelings of grief may reemerge long after the death occurred. Kubler-Ross (1969) proposed a five-stage theory of grief, which would occur in this order:

1. Denial—How could this be happening?
2. Anger—Why me?
3. Bargaining—If I promise to change, then the circumstances will change.
4. Despair—Loss of hope that things will change.
5. Acceptance—This has truly happened.

These stages, however, may not be as predictable as once thought. Bereaved women have described experiencing all five stages of grief in the course of just 1 day, only to find the feelings repeating in an irregular fashion day after day. It is now recognized that grief experiences can differ in intensity, timing, and duration depending on the person and on one's culture (Zisook & Shear, 2009).

The idea that one can truly detach from the deceased has also been challenged. Current thinking is that there exists a continued emotional bond between the bereaved and the deceased. Based on Bowlby's (1969) attachment theory, it has been suggested that rather than the relationship being broken, a new connection with the deceased emerges, one built on meaningful thoughts, feelings, and memories (Capitulo, 2005). This shift in thinking coincided with the work of Kennell, Slyter, and Klaus (1970); not only did these researchers recognize the development of a parental attachment with an infant, but they also identified the pattern of grief following a perinatal loss, including an intense bonding with the child who died (Leon, 2008). Indeed, prior to the 1970s, perinatal losses were often dismissed; women were frequently told to put it behind them, get on with their lives, and have another baby (Badenhorst & Hughes, 2007; Brownlee & Oikonen, 2004; Leon, 2008). The implication was that to grieve "properly," women had to disregard their feelings.

A Silent Loss: Misunderstandings of Perinatal Grief

"You're young; you will have another" is one of the well-intentioned, but off-the-mark, comments that bereaved women hear all the time. While it may be true that a woman will conceive again and give birth to a healthy baby, this is not always the case. Additionally, a comment such as this leaves women feeling that they can just replace the pregnancy or the child that was lost and all will be well. It negates the true grief and intense emotions that are a normal reaction to a reproductive loss. A grieving process that feels unrecognized or illegitimate is known as disenfranchised grief (Doka, 1989). Women who experience infertility and/or other perinatal loss are at prime risk for disenfranchised grief. These are losses that are not widely recognized or acknowledged and consequently are minimized by society, making the task of mourning feel unsanctioned.

A disenfranchised woman may feel as if she must be silent in her grief, especially if she has suffered an early miscarriage or a failed infertility treatment cycle. Because it is customary not to announce a pregnancy until after the first trimester, the unspoken message is that these losses do not count. Indeed, a woman's social network may have had no idea she was even "trying" and thus cannot offer her the support that she needs (Brier, 2008). Women also feel alone and misunderstood if they elect to terminate a pregnancy, either due to having multiples or if genetic testing reveals an abnormality. These are heartbreaking situations and come with the added burden of not only making the decision but also with moral and societal pressures that can be quite controversial (Covington, 2006). Because most multiple pregnancies are a result of infertility treatment, multi-fetal pregnancy reductions are especially painful given the lengths to which the woman desired a family. Likewise, terminating due to a genetic anomaly can create enormous angst and guilt and leave her wondering for years to come if she made the right decision. Even if she is clear on her decision, her grief is no less intense than those suffering other perinatal losses; her longed-for baby has died (Zeanah, Dailey, Rosenblatt, & Saller, 1993).

While reduction of a multiple pregnancy is a difficult choice, the mortality risk in a twin, or higher multiple, is much greater than with singletons (Scher et al., 2002), and the higher the multiple, the greater the chance of demise (Bryan, 2002). If there are no surviving babies in a multiple pregnancy, the grief process is anticipated. If one baby in a multiple pregnancy survives and others do not, however, the emotional impact can be overpowering. Attending to a live baby while grieving the loss of another is confusing, to say the least (Withrow & Schwiebert, 2005). The loss gets subsumed in the celebration of life; women often receive little sympathy or understanding from others who may focus only on the child who has survived (Bryan, 2002).

If a woman cannot readily "move on," she may feel that there is yet something else wrong with her. These are "silent losses" in part because others feel so awkward talking about them and worry that if they do, they will make things worse (Bennett et al., 2005; Kelley & Trinidad, 2012), but a woman also may not know how to address her loss with others. How often, at social gatherings, does the question arise, "Do you have any children?" How does a bereaved mother answer this question? How awkward to admit that she has had a loss, and yet, if she avoids the topic, is she dishonoring her child and her experience? In one woman's voice who had a stillborn child, "When people ask me, do you have kids, or how many, I have to check myself. It depends on who I'm talking to, and whether they get it. If it's people comfortable with this, I say, I have three kids—two living, and a daughter who died …" (Kelley & Trinidad, 2012, p. 145).

The Reproductive Story and Attachment

The reproductive story, as previously mentioned, is defined by a woman's conscious and unconscious ideas about becoming a mother. It encompasses all the hopes and dreams that she has for a future child and the hoped for relationship that she will have with that child. Women may fantasize about concrete ideas: reading stories, playing Monopoly, attending sports activities or ballet lessons, or baking cookies. Sometimes her "story" may appear more like a "picture": watching a child play in a sandbox and seeing her child graduate from college. These internalized images of what she wants for her child are deeply ingrained in her sense of self and in fact can be traced to her own childhood. Playing house or "dress-up," nurturing a baby doll or a stuffed animal, or caring for a pet are all precursors of a woman's unique reproductive story. Likewise, the interactions and dynamics of her relationship with her own parents become internalized and shape the particulars of her parental identity (Jaffe et al., 2005; Jaffe & Diamond, 2011).

Attachment to her future child, therefore, happens way before the birth of that child. It starts early in a woman's own life with the beginnings of the reproductive story—prior to conception and pregnancy and prior even to fantasies about a romantic relationship (Jaffe & Diamond, 2011; Jaffe et al., 2005). Thus a psychological parenthood exists long before the physical reality of a pregnancy (Covington, 2006). There are periods in which a woman's connection to her child is heightened: feeling fetal movement in pregnancy, giving birth, and then the subsequent caring for the baby all create an increased sense of attachment. The bond, however, begins much earlier, with thinking about and planning for the pregnancy (Peppers & Knapp, 1980).

Advances in technology may also facilitate attachment. Women going through IVF can literally see their embryos in a Petri dish prior to transferring them into the uterus. Ultrasound allows her to peak inside her uterus and see her baby develop, thereby offering the possibility of heightened attachment (Klier, Geller, & Ritsher, 2002). These early images—pictures of embryos and ultrasounds—often become part of the baby album. Some suggest, however, that even without ultrasound, attachment can be measured by women's dreams, daydreams, and internal dialogues prior to the baby's birth (Beutel, Deckardt, von Rad, & Weiner, 1995). Indeed, by the time a baby is born, mothers feel as if they truly "know" their child (Robinson, Baker, & Nackerud, 1999).

Because the reproductive story and attachment to her child-to-be are so integral to a woman's sense of self, it becomes clear that these are critical factors in understanding the meaning and depth of her reproductive loss. While it would seem logical that the grief response would be more intense if the loss occurred later in the pregnancy, this is not necessarily so (Covington, 2006; Kersting & Wagner, 2012; Peppers & Knapp, 1980). There are many factors that predict a woman's grief reaction besides the timing of the loss: her age, the length of time it took to conceive, whether or not outside medical intervention was necessary, whether or not she has any other living children, or if she had any previous reproductive trauma and losses (Bennett et al., 2005; Conway & Valentine, 1987; Klier et al., 2002; Lasker &

Toedter, 2000). Greenfield, Diamond, and DeCherney (1988) described the grief response after a failed IVF cycle as parallel to the emotional reaction of a pregnancy loss. Likewise, Harris and Daniluk (2010) found that women who had undergone infertility treatments and then had a miscarriage in their first trimester reported similar reactions to women with a second or a third trimester loss. This suggests that a woman's response can be predicted not by the length of gestation, but by the attachment, investment, and meaning of her anticipated pregnancy (Robinson, 2011).

What Is Normal?

Grief, in general, can be thought of as occurring in two distinguishable time frames: an acute phase and an integrated, or abiding, grief. The acute phase is marked by feelings of shock, depression, anxiety, self-blame, rage, and guilt that can be overwhelming and can sometimes overtake a woman without warning. These intense emotions diminish over time, generally from 6 months to a year (Brier, 2008; Covington, 2006). This period is followed by a time in which the loss becomes integrated and assimilated into a woman's life. Whereas acute grief interferes with normal activities and preoccupies the mind, with abiding grief, thoughts about the deceased ebb and flow and become less all consuming and disruptive (Zisook & Shear, 2009).

While the reaction immediately following a reproductive loss generally follows the pattern of acute followed by integrated grief, it may also come in waves (Covington, 2006). Indeed, a grief reaction can be prolonged, be delayed, or reemerge long after the loss occurred (Lindemann, 1944). Referred to as shadow grief (Peppers & Knapp, 1980), a woman's feelings about her loss are always there and may be triggered by a subsequent pregnancy, the anniversary date of the birth, or her due date. This is an important and often misunderstood aspect of the bereavement process for women: feelings of grief actually serve as a connection to the baby. Even after the birth of another baby, feelings about the loss do not disappear and serve as a reminder of what could have been. Women, who years later feel these emotions re-erupt, should be reassured that this is a normal reaction and is a way of keeping the memories and the attachment alive.

There is much debate in the literature distinguishing "normal" or uncomplicated grief, with complicated grief, considered a more pervasive and incapacitating emotional response (Kersting & Wagner, 2012; Moore et al., 2011). Complicated grief, also described in studies as prolonged grief disorder, PGD, is proposed to be a distinct syndrome, different from normal grief, PTSD, and depression (Bennett, Ehrenreich-May, Litz, Boisseau, & Barlow, 2012). While most women's symptoms of grief abate after 6–12 months, it has been estimated that 20 % of women who have had a perinatal loss continue to have clinically significant symptoms beyond the first year and fit the qualifications of PGD (Bennett et al., 2012).

The most recent version of the *Diagnostic and Statistical Manual of Mental Disorders*, *5th edition*, describes a similar condition to PGD: persistent complex bereavement disorder, PCBD (American Psychiatric Association, 2013). This is a newly proposed diagnostic category, and, although it is not intended for clinical use at this time, further research in this area has been encouraged. Acute emotional pain, intense yearning for the deceased, intrusive thoughts about the deceased, and preoccupation with the circumstances of death characterize PCBD. Some researchers have expressed concern that this newly described disorder represents only one type of complicated grief (Rando et al., 2012). Others worry that the removal of the bereavement exclusion from the diagnosis of major depressive disorder, MDD, which had been in the previous edition of the DSM, along with the creation of PCBD, runs the risk of pathologizing a normal human reaction, grief, to a mental disorder (Thieleman & Cacciatore, 2013).

However, there are others who feel that the proposed PCBD best portrays the ongoing impact of perinatal loss (Bennett et al., 2005; Bennett, Litz, Maguen, & Ehrenreich, 2008). It is important to consider that what may appear to be "abnormal" in general grief reactions may be more understandable when the loss involves a pregnancy or a baby. For example, a psychotic-like experience, such as hearing the cries of a dead child, is not uncommon for a bereaved mother and does not necessarily indicate psychopathology (Thieleman & Cacciatore, 2013). Although it is prudent not to pathologize a "normal" reaction to a devastating event, the diagnosis of PCBD in future editions of the DSM may help women get the support they need, thus allowing their voices to be heard instead of remaining silent.

What Happens When the Reproductive Story Goes Awry?

Unlike other types of loss, perinatal demise poses unique challenges. It is a loss of the future, rather than the past; there are no memories to call upon and few, if any, rituals to facilitate grieving. It comes at a time that is usually associated with great anticipation and joy and instead becomes psychologically, and often physically, traumatic. A woman may have no time to prepare herself, as these losses are usually sudden and may constitute medical emergencies. There may be little acknowledgement or support, in fact, as in the case of an early miscarriage or a failed IVF cycle, no one outside of the woman and her partner may have known about the pregnancy or the attempt to conceive. The impact of perinatal loss can be felt like the ripples in a lake when a stone has been thrown: it affects her sense of self, her intimate relationship, her relationships with family and friends, and how she views herself in society.

Effects on the Individual

Becoming a mother is a time of enormous change and growth; as such, it has been referred to as a developmental crisis (Colarusso, 1990; Leon, 2008). The rapid physical changes in a woman's body during pregnancy mirrors the psychological changes in her sense of self, enabling her to feel more fully feminine (Leon, 2008).

Her identity gets redefined as she shifts from "child" to "parent," with a psychological move from the "kids" to the "grown-ups" table (Jaffe & Diamond, 2011). Additionally, her self-esteem may grow with the imagined idealized child she is creating—the best qualities of herself and her partner (Covington, 2006; Leon, 2008). However, with a pregnancy loss the developmental progression gets thwarted, resulting in a "crisis within a crisis," especially when it is a first pregnancy or if there are multiple reproductive losses (Leon, 2008). Indeed, in losses that occur late in pregnancy, women will produce breast milk but have no baby to feed. Having made the mental leap into parenthood without the physical evidence of a healthy baby, women feel psychologically stuck in limbo.

Pregnancy loss also affects a woman's sense of self as healthy and normal. Many women feel as if their body has failed and experience enormous shame and guilt, as if they were to blame (Cote-Arsenault & Mahlangu, 1999). One woman described her feelings: "The baby was in my body, and my body did not do its job to protect my baby. I failed at the most fundamental task. How could it not be my fault?" The sense of failure is all encompassing. Many women cannot distinguish that only part of her body is malfunctioning; rather they take on the loss as their total identity.

Effects on Intimate Relationships: The Couple's Dilemma

Couples come together with their own history, beliefs, culture, and coping strategies; in other words, they bring to the relationship their unique individuality and their own distinctive reproductive story. When a perinatal loss occurs, couples may find themselves feeling closer to each other, a coming together in a time of crisis, but sadly, relationships are often strained by the trauma. Incongruent grief refers to the different ways that men and women experience reproductive losses in terms of intensity, timing, and expectations (Peppers & Knapp, 1980). One might assume that if parents had the same loss, they would have the same grief response, but this is seldom true. Their grief may be expressed in dissimilar ways, with each person dealing with different issues at different points in the process (Gilbert, 1996; Moore et al., 2011). Incongruence in how couples grieve may result in misunderstandings, miscommunication, and more emotional distress. They may tiptoe around talking about their loss and their feelings in a misguided effort to protect each other (Bennett et al., 2005).

What are the differences in how men and women grieve, and what is the impact on women as they deal with their male partners? Women typically express grief through tears and sadness and report a higher degree of suffering. The feminine model of grief is demonstrated by the need for women to repeatedly talk about their feelings and to "process" the experience. The open expression of women's sadness is what most people expect and anticipate. Men, however, are socialized otherwise; they tend to avoid talking about their feelings and are cast in the role of stoic partner. Men's grief is not generally expressed with tears, but with anger, difficulty working and concentrating, increased use of alcohol, and withdrawal from social engagements (Covington, 2006). Men take on the role of caring for their partner, who may have just gone through birth or a medical trauma; he is the one to take care of business, make phone calls to family, and orchestrate funeral arrangements, if necessary. He may turn into a coach with the message that "We can get through this; it's going to be okay!" Men tend to use cognitive, problem-solving strategies to cope with loss (Rando, 1985); as such, his support is more instrumental (taking care of things) than emotional (Moore et al., 2011).

So how does a man's reaction affect the grieving woman? What is the impact of incongruent grief? Because he may not want to talk about the loss as much as she does, she may feel that he does not care. In an effort to protect her from becoming upset, he may avoid discussions; the irony, of course, is that she is upset because he is *not* talking. He may throw himself into work to focus on something else and regain control, giving the illusion that he is back to "normal." This may make her feel worse about herself when she cannot do the same. He may lash out in irritation, with little patience for things, and while this may be an expression of his grief, she may interpret his anger as a personal attack. He may be ready to have sex before she is. She may associate the sexual act with the loss, have a negative body image resulting in diminished libido, and feel guilty in feeling pleasure. She may construe his frustration as criticism and feel a wedge drive between them. Educating women on the typical ways that men cope with perinatal loss will help them understand behavior that would otherwise seem unacceptable.

While most of the literature on perinatal loss focuses on the differences between men and women, many of the same concepts can be applied to same-sex couples. As in heterosexual couples, similar dynamics may emerge. There are, however, specific challenges that lesbians and gay men experience in pregnancy loss. As "silent" as these losses are for heterosexual couples, gay and lesbian couples may feel that their loss is absolutely inaudible. These pregnancy attempts, by necessity, are planned; there are no accidental conceptions, and many, again by necessity, need medical assistance to conceive. Lesbian couples use either anonymous or known sperm donation; gay men must enlist the use of an egg donor plus a surrogate. Issues such as which member of the couple is genetically related to the child and, in the case of lesbian parenthood, which partner will become pregnant are beyond the scope of this chapter to discuss, but it is important to note that because many emotional challenges exist for same-sex couples *prior* to conception, the experience of loss may feel even more marginalized.

Lesbian women, although not necessarily infertile, have been compared with infertile heterosexual women because of the process of getting pregnant (Bos, van Balen, & van den Boom, 2003). Due to the investment in becoming a parent, the experience of loss is amplified for lesbian and bisexual women and seems to have a longer lasting impact than heterosexual losses (Peel, 2009; Wojnar, 2007). In an interesting parallel with heterosexual couples, it was found that women who were biologically connected (the birth mother) grieved more openly than their non-biological partner (the social mother). Social mothers felt the need to be strong for their partner and were found to be more private in their grief (Wojnar, 2007). This suggests that, regardless of sexual orientation, the experience of pregnancy loss may be similar for the nonpregnant partner.

Effects on Family and Friends

Other familial relationships may also feel the brunt of the loss. The would-be grandparents have their own reproductive story to tell; if they themselves have had a loss, the past trauma may be rekindled by the present. While they may be grieving the loss of a grandchild, they may also want to protect their adult daughter from this pain and may not know how to offer support. Additionally, if there are any other children in the family, they not only have lost a sibling but are also affected by their mother's grief (Bennett et al., 2005). One mother spoke about her angst in talking with her 4-year-old daughter: "I didn't know how to tell her that her brother had died. I tried to go on as normal for her sake, but couldn't always contain my tears. How do you reassure a child that everything will be okay when it's not?"

Pregnancy loss affects not only the family unit but work relationships and friendships as well. Women may retreat from their normal social circle, which often includes individuals and couples who are also of childbearing age. While the isolation may at first feel comforting, it ultimately provides little solace. Women often complain of not fitting in anywhere: they avoid friends who are pregnant or have young children but at the same time cannot relate to friends who have not yet made the psychological leap into parenthood. The interpersonal isolation is not just their own doing; many times they are left out of events as their social network becomes involved with children's activities (Leon, 2008). While a woman may feel terrible about her choice not to attend a baby's birthday party, she may feel even worse if she was not invited at all. The work place, too, may not feel safe as at any moment someone may announce her pregnancy, triggering feelings of grief and loss. Likewise, any number of holidays can activate negative emotional responses (i.e., Mother's Day) as reminders of the loss and how it should have been.

Interventions: The Reproductive Story in Treatment

When working with couples or individuals who have had a perinatal loss, it is important for their story to be told. Encouraging women to talk about their loss in detail, no matter at what point in the pregnancy it occurred, acknowledges that what they have experienced is real. Equally important is the discussion of how their story veered off course. Knowing what they had hoped for and what their dreams of the future looked like can help grieving women, as well as the health care provider, understand the full extent of what has been lost.

Initial Interventions

It is helpful to conceptualize treatment into two phases: first, the immediate need for "psychological first aid" in a hospital setting or when the loss first occurs, and secondary interventions, after the initial shock has worn off (Bennett et al., 2005).

When a woman first discovers that something is wrong, she may be alone in her bathroom, may be looking at an ultrasound monitor with no heartbeat, may have noticed that the baby was moving less in utero, or may be rushed into an emergency operating room. A woman may or may not be in physical pain, but for certain she will be emotionally distraught and frightened about what is happening. This is a traumatic event; her baby has died. First responders need to be trained and sensitized to the emotional distress, fear, and helplessness that she feels. Things are out of control, and everything she had hoped for is suddenly gone. The goal of psychological first aid is not to process grief, but rather to validate the loss, provide initial support, and offer resources and other information. As such, providers should be caring, respectful, and patient, understanding that the woman is most likely in shock, may not be able to take in a lot of information, and may need to hear the information repeatedly (Badenhorst & Hughes, 2007; Bennett et al., 2005).

While attachment to the unborn child may not be affected by length of time in utero, the timing of a reproductive loss does matter in terms of the kind of first-aid interventions and support provided. There are more culturally sanctioned rituals with a neonatal loss or a stillbirth than with a miscarriage, ectopic pregnancy, termination, or failed fertility cycle. With a stillbirth or a neonatal demise, mothers usually name the baby and will have a funeral or a memorial service involving their support network. As painful as this is, there is more recognition of the loss as "real." With earlier losses, however, there are no formal rituals, few if any memories, and those that do exist—hospitalization, a medical emergency, and a negative pregnancy test—tend to be painful reminders of what feels "unreal."

In the past, a stillborn or a neonatal demise had the potential to feel illusory as well. The baby would be whisked away, and women would be given tranquilizers to ease the emotional pain (Covington, 2006; Leon, 2001). The message was to "get over it," creating an emotional disconnect between a woman's true feelings of grief, sadness, and loss and how she was expected to feel. Nowadays as part of the psychological first aid in hospitals, it is common for parents to spend time with and hold their stillborn child. It is also standard practice to provide a memory box with hand and footprints, photographs, and perhaps a lock of the baby's hair, thereby making the loss tangible (Bennett et al., 2005; Covington, 2006). While mothers may initially reject the idea of holding their deceased baby, when reflecting back, they are usually appreciative of having had the opportunity. One study suggested that this practice might cause higher rates of depression and PTSD (Hughes, Turton, Hopper, & Evans, 2002). Other research has suggested that mothers who did *not* have the opportunity to see their child had dreams that the baby was a monster; what they imagined was far worse than reality (Kroth et al., 2004). While more research would help clarify best practice, it may be that a one-size-fits-all approach is not in the best interest of all patients.

With earlier perinatal demise, when there is no physical evidence of a baby, the loss may feel even more unrecognized and illegitimate. Some feel particularly disenfranchised if health care professionals minimize the loss by treating it as a medical event (Kelley & Trinidad, 2012; Lang et al., 2011). Validation of the loss and recognition that her hoped-for baby has died appears to be one of the most important early interventions (Bennett et al., 2005). It seems that what women crave is simple: human compassion and understanding (Kelley & Trinidad, 2012). When a woman can tell her story, can vent her thoughts and feelings, and knows that she is being heard, she can better regulate her distress, decrease self-blame, and decrease intrusive thoughts (Brier, 2004). In addition, it has been proposed that protocols used in stillbirth be adapted to miscarriage, for example, naming the baby or holding a memorial service (Robinson, 2011).

Secondary Interventions

After the initial shock, the process of bereavement sets in. In this phase, secondary interventions are important to facilitate grieving and restore a sense of equilibrium. Both cognitive-behavioral and psychodynamic approaches have been identified as helping women through their grief. Not only is it helpful to normalize their feelings and offer concrete advice to improve coping and communication, but it is also important to find out the meaning of the perinatal loss in the context of the woman's life (Covington, 2006; Leon, 2008). Knowing a woman's individual story, which may include past losses, previous relationships, current interactions (with parents, siblings, friends), and how she copes, provides the backdrop to understanding what this pregnancy, and loss, means to her (Leon, 2008).

Validation can come in the form of psycho-education. Teaching a woman about the grief process will help her realize that she is not "going crazy." By labeling the multitude of losses that are part of this trauma—including the loss of her imagined or real baby, the loss of self-worth, the loss of connections with others, and the loss of feeling healthy and normal—a woman can confirm for herself that a significant trauma has occurred. Reminding her of the unique nature of her experience—this is not a loss of the past, but of the future—can help a woman see her grief in a new light. Exploration of her original reproductive story and how it went awry allows the possibility of rewriting her story to include this painful chapter and use it as a vehicle for growth (Jaffe & Diamond, 2011).

Rituals can play an important role in resolving grief. Finding a ritual that is meaningful—either a one-time event or something that continues for years—is a way of building memories when none exist. If a bereaved mother is at a loss of what to do, clinicians can make concrete suggestions to see what makes sense to her. Some women find that writing a letter or a poem to their unborn child is helpful, while others have released balloons, planted a garden, or donated to a charity in honor of their baby. Oftentimes, the anticipated due date becomes a time of reflection and may be an opportunity for her to retell her story; this, too, can help to acknowledge the reality of what was lost.

Adjuncts to Psychotherapy

The use of antidepressants or other psychotropic medications for perinatal loss is controversial. Should a woman be treated with medication if the intense emotions she is having are normal? On the other hand, if she is overcome with anxiety or depression, should not she be able to get some relief? Clearly, if severe depression, anxiety, or suicidal ideation is present, medication should be considered as part of her treatment (Carter et al., 2007). A history of depression or other mental health issues, or a history of trauma other than the current loss, may truly overwhelm her. Medication alone, however, will not fix the problem; bereaved women must grieve the loss in order to heal. It has been suggested that a course of short-term psychotherapy, focusing on the perinatal loss and grief, is the best intervention (Leon, 2008).

Perinatal Loss Groups

Support groups are often recommended; they provide a venue for grieving women and their partners to talk about their pain, anger, and sadness with others who have dealt with similar losses (Brier, 2008; Carter et al., 2007). Indeed, poor social support has been associated with complicated grief reactions; when perception of support is higher, scores of perinatal grief have been lower (Kersting & Wagner, 2012; Toedter, Lasker, & Janssen, 2001). Because of the isolation that many mothers feel after a perinatal loss, support groups can provide new social connections; they quickly realize that they are not alone. Veteran group members who are farther along in the grief process can act as role models for newer members, helping them understand that over time the intensity of their feelings will diminish. While many women find these groups to be helpful, clinical observation suggests that they are not right for everyone. Some people, who are private by nature, may feel uncomfortable sharing with a group; others have stated that they feel overwhelmed by hearing other member's stories (Jaffe & Diamond, 2011). A difficult situation can arise in the group if someone becomes pregnant, with a multitude of positive and negative feelings colliding (Covington, 2006). Working through these feelings within the group, however, can help women cope with pregnancies that occur in life outside of the group.

Subsequent Pregnancies

Subsequent pregnancies may trigger a host of feelings, with symptoms of depression, anxiety, PTSD, and anticipation of another loss (Bennett et al., 2012; Born, Soares, Phillips, Jung, & Steiner, 2006; Hughes et al., 2002). Even the idea of trying again can set off an unsettling emotional upheaval. Sometimes women try not to attach to their next pregnancy in an attempt to protect themselves from experiencing another trauma (Cote-Arsenault, Bidlack, & Humm, 2001; Reid, 2007).

Validating these feelings and confirming that anxiety and detachment are not only common reactions, but to be expected, can be extremely helpful. Women may feel that they are abandoning their previous baby for the new one; giving "permission" to love both can alleviate their guilt.

It is normal to be guarded, especially up to and around the time of the previous loss. To avoid feelings of PTSD, women often switch doctors or medical facilities, not wanting to expose themselves to triggers from their previous loss. They also may decide to rent a Doppler ultrasound machine to assure themselves that the fetus' heartbeat is functioning well. Women should be reassured that this is similar to using a baby monitor after a child is born and that these actions are justified if they help to reduce anxiety.

Although it may be a stressful time, pregnancy following a perinatal loss can facilitate healing, as fears can be overcome and resolved (Leon, 2008). The resultant birth of a healthy child, while it does not erase the past, can greatly reduce grief and increase overall functioning. Indeed, subsequent pregnancies offer the opportunity for women and their partners to add a new chapter to their reproductive story, one that hopefully has a happy ending.

Impact on Clinicians

Caregivers are not immune to the emotional turmoil of perinatal loss. Although it can be quite fulfilling to help patients heal, these losses often take a toll on clinicians and other caregivers. Those who counsel women post-loss must be able to tolerate intense sadness, anger, and rage. The stories women tell are full of raw emotion; they are difficult to tell and just as difficult to hear. Giving women the opportunity to discuss the darkest parts of their trauma is an essential part of the healing process. Likewise, encouraging women to use their baby's name (if they named the child), or having them share pictures, a memory box, or an ultrasound, makes what feels intangible a reality.

A study that compared women's experiences of stillbirths with their physician's experience found that doctors' reactions made a huge difference in how they felt. Physicians had a difficult time offering emotional support, noting a shift in their role from that of doctor to grief counselor. Finding an answer as to why the loss occurred was more comfortable for physicians than dealing with the women's emotional needs. For women, however, the most meaningful interactions were when doctors and nurses were the most human, when they sat with them, expressed empathy, and even cried (Kelley & Trinidad, 2012).

The physicians described above felt that it was their duty to find out what went wrong and why, in a sense trying "to fix" the problem, but there are not always answers to these questions. Working with the bereaved is emotionally draining, may create a sense of helplessness, and may vicariously traumatize clinicians and therapists. Hearing stories of multiple losses and intense psychological pain, clinicians need to address their own feelings as well. Just as a woman may need to tell her reproductive story over and over again, so, too, do the medical staffs and counselors who work with them.

Conclusion

The loss of a much-desired baby is like no other. The grief process is complicated because of the nature of this loss: this is a loss of the future, not of the past. Helping women through their grief and restoring a sense of equilibrium in their lives are the goals; as such, it is essential for clinicians and caregivers to understand the depth and breadth of these losses.

Women readily grasp the concept of the reproductive story: it provides them with deeper understanding of their loss and allows them to view it in the broader context of their lives. With support and understanding, a woman can begin to grieve, incorporate her perinatal loss into her life story, and envision how her story might unfold in the future.

References

American Psychiatric Association. (2013). *Diagnostic and statistical manual of mental health disorders* (5th ed.). Arlington, VA: American Psychiatric Association.

Badenhorst, W., & Hughes, P. (2007). Psychological aspects of perinatal loss. *Best Practice & Research Clinical Obstetrics and Gynaecology, 21*, 249–259.

Bennett, S. M., Ehrenreich-May, J., Litz, B. T., Boisseau, C. L., & Barlow, D. H. (2012). Development and preliminary evaluation of a cognitive-behavioral intervention for perinatal grief. *Cognitive and Behavioral Practice, 19*, 161–173.

Bennett, S. M., Litz, B. T., Lee, B. S., & Maguen, S. (2005). The scope and impact of perinatal loss: Current status and future directions. *Professional Psychology, Research and Practice, 36*, 180–187.

Bennett, S. M., Litz, B. T., Maguen, S., & Ehrenreich, J. T. (2008). An exploratory study of the psychological impact and clinical care of perinatal loss. *Journal of Loss and Trauma, 13*, 485–510.

Beutel, M., Deckardt, R., von Rad, M., & Weiner, H. (1995). Grief and depression after miscarriage: Their separation, antecedents, and course. *Psychosomatic Medicine, 57*, 517–526.

Born, L., Soares, C. N., Phillips, S. D., Jung, M., & Steiner, M. (2006). Women and reproductive-related trauma. *Annals of the New York Academy of Sciences, 1071*, 491–494.

Bos, H. M. W., van Balen, F., & van den Boom, D. C. (2003). Planned lesbian families: Their desire and motivation to have a child. *Human Reproduction, 18*, 2216–2224.

Bowlby, J. (1969). *Attachment, separation and loss*. New York, NY: Basic Books.

Brier, N. (2004). Anxiety after miscarriage: A review of the empirical literature and implications for clinical practice. *Birth, 31*, 138–142.

Brier, N. (2008). Grief following miscarriage: A comprehensive review of the literature. *Journal of Women's Health, 17*, 451–464.

Brownlee, K., & Oikonen, J. (2004). Toward a theoretical framework for perinatal bereavement. *British Journal of Social Work, 34*, 517–529.

Bryan, E. M. (2002). Loss in higher multiple pregnancy and multifetal pregnancy reduction. *Twin Research, 5*, 169–174.

Capitulo, K. L. (2005). Evidence for healing interventions with perinatal bereavement. *MCN: The American Journal of Maternal/Child Nursing, 30*, 389–396.

Carter, D., Misri, S., & Tomfohr, L. (2007). Psychological aspects of early pregnancy loss. *Clinical Obstetrics and Gynecology, 50*, 154–165.

Colarusso, C. A. (1990). The third individuation: The effect of biological parenthood on separation-individuation processes in adulthood. *The Psychoanalytic Study of the Child, 45,* 179–194.

Conway, P., & Valentine, D. (1987). Reproductive losses and grieving. *Journal of Social Work and Human Sexuality, 6,* 43–64.

Cote-Arsenault, D., Bidlack, D., & Humm, A. (2001). Women's emotions and concerns during pregnancy following perinatal loss. *MCN: The American Journal of Maternal/Child Nursing, 26,* 128–134.

Cote-Arsenault, D., & Mahlangu, N. (1999). Impact of perinatal loss on the subsequent pregnancy and self: Women's experiences. *Journal of Obstetric, Gynecologic, and Neonatal Nursing, 28,* 274–282.

Covington, S. N. (2006). Pregnancy loss. In S. N. Covington & L. H. Burns (Eds.), *Infertility counseling: A comprehensive handbook for clinicians* (2nd ed., pp. 290–304). New York, NY: Cambridge University Press.

Doka, K. J. (1989). Disenfranchised grief. In K. J. Doka (Ed.), *Disenfranchised grief: Recognizing hidden sorrow* (pp. 3–11). New York, NY: Lexington Books.

Freda, M. C., Devine, K. S., & Semelsberger, C. (2003). The lived experience of miscarriage after infertility. *MCN: The American Journal of Maternal/Child Nursing, 28,* 16–23.

Gilbert, K. R. (1996). "We've had the same loss, why don't we have the same grief?" Loss and differential grief in families. *Death Studies, 20,* 269–283.

Greenfield, D. A., Diamond, M. P., & DeCherney, A. H. (1988). Grief reactions following in-vitro fertilization treatment. *Journal of Psychosomatic Obstetrics and Gynaecology, 8,* 169–174.

Harris, D. L., & Daniluk, J. C. (2010). The experience of spontaneous pregnancy loss for infertile women who have conceived through assisted reproduction technology. *Human Reproduction, 25,* 714–720.

Hemminki, E., & Forssas, E. (1999). Epidemiology of miscarriage and its relation to the reproductive events in Finland. *American Journal of Obstetrics & Gynecology, 18,* 396–401.

Hughes, P. M., Turton, P., Hopper, E., & Evans, C. D. H. (2002). Assessment of guidelines for good practice in psychosocial care of mothers after stillbirth: A cohort study. *Lancet, 360,* 114–118.

Jaffe, J., & Diamond, M. O. (2011). *Reproductive trauma: Psychotherapy with infertility and pregnancy loss clients.* Washington, DC: American Psychological Association.

Jaffe, J., Diamond, M. O., & Diamond, D. J. (2005). *Unsung lullabies: Understanding and coping with infertility.* New York, NY: St. Martin's Press.

Kelley, M. C., & Trinidad, S. B. (2012). Silent loss and the clinical encounter: Parents' and physicians' experiences of stillbirth – A qualitative analysis. *BMC Pregnancy and Childbirth, 12,* 137–151.

Kennell, J. H., Slyter, H., & Klaus, M. (1970). The mourning response of parents to the death of a newborn infant. *New England Journal of Medicine, 283,* 344–349.

Kersting, A., & Wagner, B. (2012). Complicated grief after perinatal loss. *Dialogues in Clinical Neuroscience, 14,* 187–194.

Klier, C. M., Geller, P. A., & Ritsher, J. B. (2002). Affective disorders in the aftermath of miscarriage: A comprehensive review. *Archives of Women's Mental Health, 5,* 129–149.

Kroth, J., Garcia, M., Hallgren, M., LeGrue, E., Ross, L. M., & Scalise, J. (2004). Perinatal loss, trauma, and dream reports. *Psychological Reports, 94,* 877–882.

Kubler-Ross, E. (1969). *On death and dying.* New York, NY: Macmillan.

Lang, A., Fleiszer, A. R., Duhamel, F., Sword, W., Gilbert, K. R., & Corsini-Munt, S. (2011). Perinatal loss and parental grief: The challenge of ambiguity and disenfranchised grief. *Omega, 63,* 183–196.

Lasker, J. N., & Toedter, L. J. (2000). Predicting outcomes after pregnancy loss: Results from studies using the Perinatal Grief Scale. *Illness, Crisis, & Loss, 8,* 350–372.

Leon, I. G. (2001). Perinatal loss. In N. Stotland & D. Stewart (Eds.), *Psychological aspects of women's health care: The interface between psychiatry and obstetrics and gynecology* (2nd ed., pp. 141–173). Washington, DC: American Psychiatric Press.

Leon, I. G. (2008). Helping families cope with perinatal loss. *The Global Library of Women's Medicine*. Retrieved April 10, 2013, from http://www.glowm.com/resources/glowm/cd/pages/v6/v6c081.html?SESSID=jgaqktv9i4dbmtadq07trmo5b0

Lindemann, E. (1944). Symptomatology and management of acute grief. *The American Journal of Psychiatry, 101*, 141–148.

Moore, T., Parrish, H., & Black, B. P. (2011). Interconception care for couples after perinatal loss: A comprehensive review of the literature. *Journal of Perinatal Neonatal Nursing, 26*, 44–51.

Neugebauer, R., Kline, J., Shrout, P., Skodol, A., O'Connor, P., Geller, P. A., Stein, Z., & Susser, M. (1997). Major depressive disorder in the 6 months after miscarriage. *JAMA The Journal of the American Medical Association, 277*, 383–388.

Nybo Andersen, A. M., Wohlfahrt, J., Christens, P., Olsen, J., & Melbye, M. (2000). Maternal age and fetal loss: Population based register linkage study. *British Medical Journal, 320*, 1708–1712.

Peel, E. (2009). Pregnancy loss in lesbian and bisexual women: An online survey of experiences. *Human Reproduction, 25*, 721–727.

Peppers, L. G., & Knapp, R. J. (1980). *Motherhood and mourning: Perinatal death*. New York, NY: Praeger.

Rando, T. A. (1985). Bereaved parents: Particular difficulties, unique factors, and treatment issues. *Social Work, 30*, 19–23.

Rando, T. A., Doka, K. J., Fleming, S., Franco, M. H., Lobb, E. A., Parkes, C. M., & Steele, R. (2012). A call to the field: Complicated grief in the DSM-5. *Omega, 65*, 251–255.

Reid, M. (2007). The loss of a baby and the birth of the next infant: The mother's experience. *Journal of Child Psychotherapy, 33*, 181–201.

Robinson, G. E. (2011). Dilemmas related to pregnancy loss. *The Journal of Nervous and Mental Disease, 199*, 571–574.

Robinson, M., Baker, L., & Nackerud, L. (1999). The relationship of attachment theory and perinatal loss. *Death Studies, 23*, 257–270.

Rothaupt, J., & Becker, K. (2007). A literature review of Western bereavement theory: From decathecting to continuing bonds. *The Family Journal, 15*, 6–15.

Scher, A. I., Petterson, B., Blair, E., Ellenberg, J. H., Grether, J. K., Haan, E., … Nelson, K. B. (2002). The risk of mortality or cerebral palsy in twins: A collaborative population-based study. *Pediatric Research, 52*, 671–681.

Stanton, C., Lawn, J. E., Rahman, H., Wilczynska-Ketende, K., & Hill, K. (2006). Still birth rates: Delivering estimates in 190 countries. *The Lancet, 367*, 1487–1494.

Thieleman, K., & Cacciatore, J. (2013). When a child dies: A critical analysis of grief-related controversies in DSM-5. *Research on Social Work Practice, 24*, 114–122.

Toedter, L. J., Lasker, J. N., & Janssen, H. J. (2001). International comparison of studies using the perinatal grief scale: A decade of research on pregnancy loss. *Death Studies, 25*, 205–228.

Withrow, R., & Schwiebert, V. L. (2005). Twin loss: Implications for counselors working with surviving twins. *Journal of Counseling and Development, 83*, 21–28.

Wojnar, D. (2007). Miscarriage experiences of lesbian couples. *Journal of Midwifery and Women's Health, 52*, 479–485.

Zeanah, C. H., Dailey, J. V., Rosenblatt, M., & Saller, D. N. (1993). Do women grieve after terminating pregnancies because of fetal anomalies? A controlled investigation. *Obstetrics and Gynecology, 82*, 270–275.

Zisook, S., & Shear, K. (2009). Grief and bereavement: What psychiatrists need to know. *World Psychiatry, 8*, 67–74.

Birth Trauma: The Causes and Consequences of Childbirth-Related Trauma and PTSD

Kathleen Kendall-Tackett

Introduction

> The birth of a child, especially a first child, represents a landmark event in the lives of all involved. For the mother particularly, childbirth exerts a profound physical, mental, emotional, and social effect. No other event involves pain, emotional stress, vulnerability, possible physical injury or death, permanent role change, and includes responsibility for a dependent, helpless human being. Moreover, it all generally takes place within a single day. It is not surprising that women tend to remember their first birth experiences vividly and with deep emotion (Simkin, 1992, p. 64)

More than two decades ago, Penny Simkin documented that women accurately remember details of giving birth 15–20 years later (Simkin, 1991, 1992). Some 20 years after the publication of Simkin's research, our understanding of women's experiences of birth has grown. But this now sizeable body of literature mirrors the results of Simkin's work: for better or worse, a woman's experience giving birth can influence how she feels about herself as a woman and as a mother.

Giving birth can be tremendously empowering, helping women realize the strengths they never knew they had. Conversely, birth can be devastating, shattering a woman's view of who she is, and as a result, this can lead to post-traumatic stress disorder (PTSD) and other symptoms of psychological trauma, such as depression. Rarely is giving birth a neutral event. The goal of this chapter is to summarize recent research on the trauma of childbirth, detail the implications of this research, and give suggestions on how practitioners can intervene.

K. Kendall-Tackett, Ph.D., I.B.C.L.C., F.A.P.A. (✉)
Texas Tech University School of Medicine, Amarillo, TX, USA
e-mail: kkendallt@gmail.com

What Is Psychological Trauma?

In colloquial speech, "traumatic" is often synonymous with "bad" and is used to describe everything from a bad haircut to a serious car accident. "Traumatic" also has a more concise clinical meaning: symptoms of psychological trauma or PTSD as defined by the criteria established in the *Diagnostic and Statistical Manual, DSM*. The *DSM* has recently been revised, with some changes to the criteria that must be present in order to use a diagnosis of PTSD. Before discussing the studies on traumatic childbirth, it is important to review the current criteria for PTSD, which will be helpful in understanding whether a woman has been traumatized by giving birth. Many of these symptoms are ones that women frequently report, even though some of them may not seem like trauma symptoms. However, it is important to consider the entire range of symptoms women experience before making a judgment about whether they meet the criteria for a diagnosis of PTSD.

DSM-V Diagnostic Criteria for PTSD

The majority of people exposed to a traumatic event do not go on to meet full criteria for PTSD; however, someone can also have symptoms of PTSD without meeting full criteria or can be affected by other trauma sequelae, such as depression or anxiety. The criteria for PTSD has recently been revised, as described in the *Diagnostic and Statistical Manual-V*, and in order for a diagnosis of PTSD, an individual must meet these criteria.

Exposure to Traumatic Events

Criterion A, the exposure criteria, is the first that must be met. To meet full criteria for PTSD, an individual has to have been exposed to a traumatic event. A traumatic event is defined as death or threatened death, actual or threatened injury, or actual or threatened sexual violation (Friedman, Resick, Bryant, & Brewin, 2011). Many aspects of birth fit this criterion well. Women often report that they were worried that they, or their babies, might die. This can occur even if there is not an actual life-threatening event. If women believe that they are in peril, regardless if it is medically "true," they may experience posttraumatic symptoms or meet the criteria for PTSD, as Ayers (2007) describes.

> Women's thoughts of death were usually in response to complications with labor or with the infant, but some women thought that they would die without any preceding complication.

There are a number of ways that someone could be exposed to a traumatic event. They may have experienced the event directly or may have been a witness to the event. Partners and birth attendees, such as labor-and-delivery nurses or doulas, can also be traumatized by a birth. Even learning about a traumatic birth that was experienced by a close relative or friend can also cause trauma (Friedman et al., 2011).

In addition to the experiencing criteria, a diagnosis of PTSD includes symptoms that must be present in four clusters: intrusion, avoidance, negative alterations in cognitions and mood, and alterations in arousal and reactivity. These are described below.

Intrusion Symptoms

Intrusion symptoms are the most commonly thought of symptoms as being related to PTSD. Women must experience one or more of these in order to meet full criteria:

- There are involuntary and intrusive memories of the traumatic event that reoccur. These can be experienced as nightmares or flashbacks, where something triggers a memory and immediately the individual is reliving the event (Friedman et al., 2011). Intrusion symptoms are common among women who have experienced traumatic births. They will often report things like "every time I close my eyes, I am re-experiencing my birth." One mother in Ayers (2007) study reported, "I just kept thinking about it all the time and I felt like I had some sort of car crash or something. I kept getting flashbacks all the time and I found it really upsetting" (p. 261).
- Women may also experience intense or prolonged psychological distress after being exposed to something that resembles the traumatic event.
- They might also experience marked physiological reactions to reminders of the traumatic event. Reminders of their births can include smells, sights, sounds, or feelings that put them right back in their birth experiences. These symptoms can cause them to feel upset or can cause a physiological stress reaction.

Intrusion symptoms can lead to the next category of symptoms: avoidance symptoms.

Avoidance Symptoms

The avoidance symptoms include avoidance of all things that remind them of the birth, such as thoughts or feelings of conversations associated with the stressor. These symptoms also include avoidance of things associated with the traumatic event, such as activities, places, or people. Women must have at least one symptom in this cluster to meet full criteria (Friedman et al., 2011).

Avoidance symptoms are also common following a traumatic birth. Women may avoid everything that reminds them of their traumatic births, including not returning for medical appointments, and avoiding their doctors, medical offices, or the hospital where their births occurred.

Negative Alterations in Cognitions and Mood

One of the new categories in the DSM-V criteria is negative change in cognitions and mood. The changes must have either begun or worsened after the traumatic event, and women must have three or more of the following symptoms to meet full criteria.

- An inability to remember an important aspect of the traumatic event.
- A persistent or an exaggerated negative expectation about themselves, others, or the world.
- A persistent, distorted blame of self or others about the cause or the consequences of the traumatic event. These negative beliefs can include a pervasive negative emotional state, such as fear, horror, anger, guilt, or shame.
- A markedly diminished interest and participation in significant activities.
- A feeling of detachment or estrangement from others.
- A persistent inability to experience positive emotions (Friedman et al., 2011).

This symptom cluster has considerable overlap with depression: negative expectations of self or others, negative emotional state, and anhedonia. These beliefs can directly impact a woman's feelings and beliefs about their babies and their partners, possibly setting the stage for long-term problems in both relationships. In one study, Ayers, Eagle, and Waring (2006) found that women who had traumatic births described rejecting behavior towards their babies immediately after birth. Many reported eventually bonding with their babies in 1–5 years, with avoidant or overanxious attachment styles being the most common. This mother described her first reaction to her baby, which reflected her belief that her baby was viewing her negatively.

> In God's name why are you giving me a baby … I'm dying, why would I want a baby? I had no connection between … that it was my baby … the baby had one eye open, one closed, and he looked at me and there was this scowl on his face as if to say, "where am I and in God's name don't tell me you're my mother" (Ayers et al., 2006, p. 395).

Changes in Arousal and Reactivity

Changes in arousal and reactivity are perhaps the most characteristic symptoms of PTSD. These changes in reactivity must have begun or worsened after the traumatic event in order to be specifically related to birth trauma. A woman must have three or more of the following symptoms:

- An increase in anger, irritability, or aggressive behavior
- Reckless or destructive behavior
- Hypervigilance
- Exaggerated startle response
- Problems with concentration
- Sleep problems, more specifically, difficulty falling or staying asleep or having restless sleep

Sleep problems can be one of the most telling symptoms about a woman's psychological state. Asking mothers how many minutes it takes for them to go to sleep will tell you much about how they are doing. If it takes mothers more than 25 min to fall asleep, the mother is at high risk for depression (Goyal, Gay, & Lee, 2009). This long period of sleep latency (time to fall asleep) may also indicate posttraumatic stress, PTS, or PTSD. Angry or irritable behavior may be directed towards the woman's partner, her baby, or her care provider. A mother may also be hypervigilant about her baby and the possibility of danger.

Duration and Impairment Criteria

In order to meet full criteria, 1 month must have elapsed since exposure to the traumatic event. If there are symptoms prior to 1 month, acute stress disorder (the precursor syndrome) can be diagnosed. If the symptoms persist past 1 month, it may be PTSD. The symptoms must also cause significant impairment in daily life.

Prevalence of Traumatic Birth

Unfortunately, the prevalence of trauma following childbirth is quite high in many parts of the world, including the USA. For example, Childbirth Connections' Listening to Mothers' Survey II (Beck, Gable, Sakala, & Declercq, 2011) included a nationally representative sample of 1,573 mothers in the USA. The survey found that 9 % of those mothers met full criteria for PTSD following their births, and an additional 18 % had posttraumatic symptoms, PTS (Beck et al., 2011). These findings also varied by ethnic group: an astounding 26 % of non-Hispanic black mothers had PTS. The most common symptoms included difficulty falling asleep (14 %), anger and irritability (11 %), and difficulty concentrating (8 %).

If the number of women meeting full criteria does not seem high, compare it to another number: in the weeks following September 11, 2001, 7.5 % of residents of lower Manhattan met full criteria for PTSD (Galea et al., 2003). This means that in at least one large study the rates of full-criteria PTSD in the USA following childbirth are now *higher* than those following a major terrorist attack. Beck and colleagues (Beck et al., 2011) noted the following regarding their findings from Listening to Mothers II.

> In these two national surveys, mothers spoke out loudly and clearly about PTS symptoms from which they were suffering. The high percentage of mothers with elevated PTS symptoms is a sobering statistic.

Another US prospective study of 933 mothers found that 3.6 % of women met full criteria for PTSD at 4–6 weeks, 6.3 % at 12 weeks, and 5.8 % at 24 weeks (Alcorn, O'Donovan, Patrick, Creedy, & Devilly, 2010). Although the rate of PTSD is lower than the rates reported in the Listening to Mothers' Survey, 45.5 % of these mothers described their births as traumatic according to the DSM-IV criteria (Alcorn et al., 2010). Although PTSD rates were lower than Beck et al. (2011), the rates of other postpartum mood and anxiety disorders, PMADs, are quite high. Rates for depression were 66 % at 4–6 weeks, 47 % at 12 weeks, and 57 % at 24 weeks. Clinically significant rates of anxiety were also high: 74 % at 4–6 weeks, 58 % at 12 weeks, and 63 % at 24 weeks.

In a sample from Great Britain, 2.5 % of a community sample ($N=502$), and 21 % of an online sample ($N=921$), met full criteria for PTSD (Ayers, Harris, Sawyer, Parfitt, & Ford, 2009). In these samples sexual trauma interacted with delivery type, which indicated that cesarean deliveries were more traumatic for women who experienced this type of trauma, most likely due to prior vulnerability. The rates of sexual trauma were 23 % in the community sample and 33 % in the online sample. Exposure to prior traumatic events in general ranged from 56 to 59 %.

In a meta-ethnography of ten qualitative studies, women with PTSD were more likely to describe their births negatively if they felt "invisible and out of control" (Elmir, Schmied, Wilkes, & Jackson, 2010). The women used phrases, such as "barbaric, inhumane, intrusive, horrific, and degrading" to describe the mistreatment they received from health care professionals.

Some might argue that these negative effects are unavoidable and that birth is hard, and, in some cases, life threatening, and as a result, we should expect trauma responses. To counter this argument, it is imperative to examine the rates of birth trauma in countries where birth is treated as a normal event, where there are fewer interventions, and where women have continuous labor support. Sweden is one such country, and the rate of PTSD following birth is substantially lower. In a prospective study ($N=1,224$), 1.3 % of mothers from Sweden had PTSD, and 9 % described giving birth as traumatic (Soderquist, Wijma, Thorbert, & Wijma, 2009). The strongest predictors are depression in early pregnancy, severe fear of childbirth, and stress in later pregnancy (Soderquist et al., 2009).

Similarly, in a study of 907 women in the Netherlands, which is another country where birth is treated as a normal event and women have continuous labor support, researchers found that 1.2 % had PTSD and 9 % identified giving birth as traumatic (Stramrood et al., 2011). The women in this study did have other PMADs: 23 % had clinically significant anxiety, and 14 % had clinically significant depression, but their rate of PTSD is substantially lower than in the USA. This may be attributable to lower rates of birth interventions. The rate for cesarean sections in the Netherlands is 15–17 %, and the rate of instrumental deliveries is 9–10 %. Of the women who delivered in secondary tertiary care 12 % described their births as traumatic vs. 3 % of women who delivered in primary care. This indicates that birth trauma is likely due to birth complications that are unavoidable and would be the same in any sample.

In contrast, the rate for birth-related PTSD is much higher in a country where attitudes towards women are generally poor and where women are restricted and discriminated against. Researchers in a study of 400 women in Iran found that 218 reported traumatic births at 6–8 weeks postpartum, and 20 % met full criteria for PTSD (Modarres, Afrasiabi, Rahnama, & Montazeri, 2012). The risk factors for

PTSD are similar to those seen in other countries and include gestational age at delivery, number of prenatal care visits, pregnancy complications, pregnancy intervals, labor duration, and mode of delivery.

Traumatic Birth and Breastfeeding

Not surprisingly, birth experiences can also impact breastfeeding. A national survey of 5,332 mothers in England at 3 months postpartum found that women who had forceps-assisted births or an unplanned cesarean section had the poorest health and well-being and as a result may not have the option to breastfeed (Rowlands & Redshaw, 2012). Women in these two groups had the highest rates of PTS, depression, and anxiety.

Beck and Watson's study (2008) describe how women who have been traumatized in childbirth often felt like victims of rape. When practitioners handled their breasts without their permission, or pushed their babies onto their chests, they felt like their breasts were one more thing to be violated. Breastfeeding also triggered flashbacks, as described by these mothers:

> The flashbacks to the birth were terrible. I wanted to forget about it and the pain, so stopping breastfeeding would get me a bit closer to my "normal" self again (Beck, 2011, p. 306).

> I had flashbacks to the birth every time I would feed him. When he was put on me in the hospital, he wasn't breathing and he was blue. I kept picturing this and could still feel what it was like. Breastfeeding him was a similar position as to the way he was put on me (Beck, 2011, p. 306).

For other mothers, breastfeeding was hard to manage after a traumatic birth, as this mother describes:

> I hated breastfeeding because it hurt to try and sit to do it. I couldn't even seem to manage lying down. I was cheated out of breastfeeding. I feel that I have been cheated out of something exceptional (Beck & Watson, 2008, p. 234).

Another mother describes how breastfeeding allowed her to have some connection to her baby, however tenuous it might be:

> The first five months of my baby's life (before I got help) are a virtual blank. I dutifully nursed him every two to three hours on demand, but I rarely made eye contact with him and dumped him in his crib as soon as I was done. I thought that if it were not for breastfeeding, I could go the whole day without interacting with him at all (Beck & Watson, 2008, p. 235).

Conversely, breastfeeding can also be enormously healing. With gentle assistance, a mother can be successful at breastfeeding even after the most difficult birth. For some mothers in Elmir et al.'s (2010) study, breastfeeding provided women an opportunity to overcome the trauma of their birth experiences and prove their potential as mothers, as described here:

> Breastfeeding was a timeout from the pain in my head. It was a "current reality"—a way to cling onto some "real life," whereas all the trauma that continued to live on in me, live on in my head, belonged to the past, even though I couldn't seem to keep it there (Beck, 2011, p. 307).

> Breastfeeding became my focus for overcoming the birth and proving to everyone else, and mostly myself, that there was something I could do right. It was part of my crusade, so to speak, to prove myself as a mother (Beck & Watson, 2008, p. 233).

> My body's ability to produce milk, and so the sustenance to keep my baby alive, also helped to restore my faith in my body, which at some core level, I felt had really let me down, due to a terrible pregnancy, labor, and birth. It helped build my confidence in my body and as a mother. It helped me heal and feel connected to my baby (Beck & Watson, 2008, p. 233).

One potentially negative aspect of a difficult or a traumatic birth is the potential delay in lactogenesis II. In a study from Guatemala (Grajeda & Perez-Escamilla, 2002), cortisol levels were measured in 136 women both before and after birth. High levels of cortisol were related to delays in lactogenesis II, the time after birth when milk production becomes more abundant and is frequently referred to as "milk coming in." Abnormally low levels of cortisol can also delay lactogenesis II. Unfortunately, low cortisol levels are characteristic of PTSD. If women have PTSD before their births, not only they are more vulnerable to it in relation to their births, but they may also have significant delays in lactogenesis II, which can also lead to a spiral of interventions for mother and baby, including re-hospitalization of the baby for dehydration, jaundice, or failure to thrive (Kendall-Tackett, 2000).

Risk Factors for Traumatic Birth Experiences

A number of factors have been related to traumatic birth. In the Listening to Mothers Survey II (Beck et al., 2011), factors that increased the risk of PTS symptoms included low partner support, postpartum depression symptoms, more physical problems since birth, and fewer health-promoting behaviors. Some other factors that differentiated between women who had PTS vs. those with no PTS included no private health insurance, an unplanned pregnancy, pressure to have an induction or an epidural, a planned cesarean birth, not breastfeeding as long as wanted, not exclusively breastfeeding for 1 month, and not consulting a clinician since the birth.

Actions of Health Care Providers

The behavior of the women's health care providers had a significant impact on their perception of their births. In a longitudinal study of women from the UK, minimal support from health care providers during labor predicted PTS, and women with a history of trauma were especially vulnerable. Women who had more interventions were more likely to show long-term effects of minimal support during labor (Ford & Ayers, 2012). Lack of support from health care providers was also a factor in a qualitative study from Sweden (Tham, Ryding, & Christensson, 2010). Women with PTS more than likely had nervous or non-interested midwives, intense fear or shame during delivery, lack of postnatal follow-up, long-term postpartum fatigue, and inadequate help from partners. In addition, one-third reported being fearful for their babies' lives.

A meta-ethnography of ten qualitative studies found that women are often traumatized as a result of the actions, or the inactions, of midwives, nurses, and doctors (Elmir et al., 2010). The care received was sometimes described as dehumanizing, disrespectful, and uncaring. Women were also distressed when people were invited to watch their births without their consent. Women felt out of control, powerless, vulnerable, and unable to make informed decisions about their care, and they felt that their health care providers betrayed them. Some found themselves coerced into having procedures they did not want, such as epidurals and vacuum extractions, in an attempt to end the trauma they were experiencing.

Prior Perinatal Loss

Prior perinatal loss and high-risk deliveries also increase a woman's vulnerability to PTS and PTSD. In a study of 36 couples, those who experienced a prior perinatal loss were at an increased risk for PTSD, depression, or anxiety with a subsequent birth (Armstrong, Hutti, & Myers, 2009). Levels of depression, anxiety, and PTS decreased from the third trimester to 8 months postpartum. Both mothers and fathers had similar rates of PTS. Similarly, in a study of 21 mothers who had very-low-birth-weight infants, 23 % were in the clinical range for PTSD (Feeley et al., 2011). The more severe the infant's illness, the higher the mother's symptoms.

History of Abuse or Prior Trauma

A woman who has experienced previous sexual abuse, or other types of trauma, is also at a higher risk for PTSD in relation to delivery. A study of 308 women from Montreal found that those who had anxiety in pregnancy as well as a history of sexual trauma were more likely to develop PTSD after childbirth (Verreault et al., 2012). In this study, 5.6 % met full criteria for PTSD, while an additional 12 % met partial criteria, and sexual abuse survivors were three times more likely to develop PTSD following birth.

Not every study found a relationship between child sexual abuse, CSA, and birth-related PTSD. A study of 837 pregnant women from Israel compared three groups of women: CSA survivors, women who had experienced other types of trauma, but no CSA, and women with no trauma history (Lev-Wiesel, Daphna-Tekoah, & Hallak, 2009). Overall, there was no increase in birth trauma for CSA survivors, but they did experience higher intrusion and arousal symptoms.

Ethnicity

In a national study of 1,581 pregnant women, African American women were more likely to have experienced trauma than their white counterparts (Seng, Kohn-Wood, McPherson, & Sperlich, 2011). There was more lifetime PTSD and trauma exposure for black women, and current prevalence of PTSD was four times higher for black vs. white women. The rates did not differ by socioeconomic status, SES, but was explained by greater trauma exposure.

Vicarious Traumatization

Caregivers can also be traumatized. A recent study of a random sample of 464 labor-and-delivery nurses reported moderate-to-severe secondary trauma from being exposed to traumatic births (Beck & Gable, 2012). Ten percent reported high secondary traumatic stress and 14 % reported severe secondary stress. There were six themes related to vicariously traumatic births:

- Magnifying the exposure to traumatic births
- Struggling to maintain a professional role while dealing with traumatized patients
- Agonizing over what should have been done
- Mitigating the aftermath of exposure to traumatic births
- Haunted by secondary traumatic stress symptoms
- Considering foregoing careers in labor and delivery

One nurse described her experience as follows:

> The physician violated her. A perfect delivery turned violent. I felt like an accomplice to a crime. The doctor treated her like a piece of dirt. After the birth of the baby, he proceeded to put his hand inside her, practically halfway up his arm, to start pulling the placenta out…I felt like I was watching a rape (Beck & Gable, 2012, p. 8).

Another nurse described the sounds that still haunt her:

> Whenever I hear a patient screaming, I will flashback to a patient who had an unmedicated (not even local) cesarean section and to the wailing of a mother when we were coding her baby in the delivery room. I feel like I will never get these sounds/images out of my head even though they occurred more than 10 years ago (Beck & Gable, 2012, p. 11).

In examining one of the themes—"agonizing over what should have been done"—the researchers observed five sub-themes. The nurses reported that:

- They felt powerless because the person in authority was causing unnecessary trauma.
- They felt frustrated and angry at the physician for not listening.
- They felt like they failed their patients.
- They should have tried to stop the physician.
- Their patients were counting on them to protect them.

Beck and Gable (2012) noted that unavoidable medical emergencies were much less likely to cause PTSD in nursing staff than incidents where medical staffs were thoughtless and arrogant and the problems they caused were avoidable. Beck and Gable (2012) described their findings as follows:

> Traumatic deliveries are much easier to handle and cope with when they are unavoidable. The cause of anxiety and stress to the nursing staff is when they feel powerless and helpless because another person in authority is causing unnecessary trauma to the patient and infant. (p. 10)

Posttraumatic Growth

The literature on birth trauma paints a fairly bleak picture, but fortunately, this is not the whole story. One bright spot in the trauma field has been the study of posttraumatic growth, PTG. PTG describes the experiences of individuals who have grown in the wake of traumatic events and whose development has surpassed what was present before the crisis occurred (Tedeschi & Calhoun, 2004). Not only have they survived the traumatic event, but they have also experienced positive changes that are viewed as important and that go beyond the previous status quo. People who have experienced PTG are not necessarily free of PTS; rather growth occurs through the struggle. People with the highest levels of PTS are often those with the highest levels of growth (Joseph, 2011).

In the wake of trauma, those who have experienced PTG report changes that include a greater appreciation of life, warmer and more intimate relationships, a greater sense of personal strength, recognition of new possibilities or paths for one's life, and spiritual development (Tedeschi & Calhoun, 2004). People who experience growth have found ways to make sense of the experiences they have suffered and have been able to form a coherent story about their experiences. Sometimes their very personalities have been changed in many positive ways by the traumatic events (Joseph, 2011).

After a frightening delivery and numerous postpartum complications, Jess, a mother who shared her story with me, developed severe postpartum depression and anxiety. After her traumatic birth, she became a birth and postpartum doula, so that she could provide to others the support that she so desperately needed but did not receive. She describes how her difficult birth transformed her life by strengthening her relationship with her husband and even changing her career path.

> Things got better, but it took years. It took six years for me to start working towards being functional. By the grace of God my husband and I made it. We are best friends, war buddies, and love each other more every day. We deserve it. My son is 11 and is awesome. I am a birth and postpartum doula now, and I have learned to let go of my birth pregnancy and birth victimization, and I've become a survivor. I'm healthy enough to support other families, in the hopes that they don't have to go where we went.

Summarizing the research on PTG, Joseph (2011) noted the following:

> … posttraumatic growth is not simply about coping, or about the things that people say about themselves; it refers to changes that cut to the very core of our way of being in the world. Posttraumatic growth has to do with the way we greet the day as we wake in the morning, the way we brush our teeth and put on our shoes, it reflects our attitude about life itself and our place in the world. Indeed, posttraumatic growth is deeply rooted in our personalities (p. 135).

Intervention

Fortunately, there are many things that people who work in perinatal health can do to help mothers heal in the wake of traumatic births. Intervention can make a difference in the lives of these mothers and must be attempted for the sake of both mother and baby.

Recognize Symptoms

Depending on the field, it may not be within everyone's scope of practice to diagnose or treat PTSD, but even if it is not, there needs to be someone who can listen to a mother's story. That alone can be healing. If a woman is believed to have PTS, PTSD, or other sequelae of trauma, such as depression or anxiety, she can be treated, referred to specialists, or provided information about resources that are available (see below). Trauma survivors often believe that they are going "crazy." Knowing that posttraumatic symptoms are both predictable and quite treatable can reassure them. According to Joseph (2011):

> Most crucial of all is the extent to which clients perceive themselves to be valued, listened to, and understood—in such a way as to support their basic psychological needs for autonomy, competence, and relatedness. A therapeutic relationship that meets this objective provides clients with a forum in which their intrinsic drive toward growth is given a free rein. (p. 147)

Resources

If not treating mothers directly, refer them to resources for diagnosis and treatment. There are a number of short-term treatments for trauma that are effective and are widely available. Eye-movement desensitization and reprocessing, EMDR, http://emdr.com/, is a highly effective type of psychotherapy and is considered a frontline treatment for PTSD. Journaling about a traumatic experience is also helpful, http://www.apa.org/monitor/jun02/writing.aspx. If more information is needed in regard to trauma, the National Center for PTSD has many resources including a PTSD 101 course for providers, http://www.ptsd.va.gov/professional/ptsd101/course-modules/course-modules.asp, and even a free app for patients called the PTSD Coach, http://www.ptsd.va.gov/public/pages/ptsdcoach.asp. The site, www.HelpGuide.com (http://helpguide.org/mental/emotional_psychological_trauma.htm), also has many great resources including a summary of available treatments, lists of symptoms, and possible risk factors.

Help mothers anticipate possible breastfeeding problems before they occur. As mentioned earlier in this chapter, breastfeeding can be an important part of the process of healing from birth trauma. Even those who are not lactation consultants can help mothers be alert for possible breastfeeding difficulties. Work with the mother to develop a plan to counter it, involving lactation specialists where needed. Some strategies for this include increasing skin-to-skin contact if she can tolerate it and/or possibly beginning a pumping regimen until lactogenesis II has begun. She may also need to briefly supplement with formula, but this will not be necessary in all cases.

Recognize that breastfeeding can be healing for trauma survivors, but also respect the mothers' boundaries. Some mothers may be too overwhelmed to initiate or continue breastfeeding, although sometimes, with gentle encouragement, a mother may be able to handle it. However, if she cannot, this must be respected. If a mother decides not to breastfeed, she must be gently encouraged to connect with her baby in other ways, such as skin-to-skin contact, baby-wearing, or infant massage.

Helping a mother breastfeed following a traumatic birth is one way you can make a difference in lessening the impact of birth trauma. You might also want to help make changes on a wider scale and help stop birth trauma before it starts. Fortunately, there are things you can do, such as partnering with other groups and organizations that want to change the way birth happens in the USA and abroad. Rates of PTS and PTSD following birth are scandalously high in the USA. Organizations, such as Childbirth Connection, http://transform.childbirthconnection.org/, are working to reform birth in the USA. There are some hopeful signs, such as a large upswing in the number of hospitals starting the process to become baby friendly, which will encourage better birthing practices, http://www.youtube.com/watch?v=N9KptD3t110. Hopefully, more hospitals will implement practices recommended by the Mother-Friendly Childbirth Initiative, http://www.motherfriendly.org/MFCI.

There is also a major push among organizations, such as the March of Dimes, to discourage high-intervention procedures, such as elective inductions, as they increase the rate of complications babies must endure. This movement away from induction will also be helpful for mothers due to the fact that induced labors are often very difficult for mothers and frequently involve many interventions, including cesarean deliveries, http://www.marchofdimes.com/pregnancy/vaginalbirth_inducing.html.

In addition, hospitals with high cesarean rates are under scrutiny, and there is pressure from many different directions to lower the scandalously high rate of cesarean births in the USA. Change may be on the way. Childbirth educator, Amy Romano, describes it this way:

> As we begin 2013, it is clear from my vantage point at the Transforming Maternity Care Partnership that the transformation is underway. In Childbirth Connection's nearly century-long history, we've never seen so much political will from leaders, so much passion from grassroots advocates, and so much collaboration among clinicians and other stakeholders. This new landscape presents many new opportunities for educators and advocates. http://www.scienceandsensibility.org/?p=6026&utm_source=feedburner&utm_medium=email&utm_campaign=Feed%3A+science-sensibility+%28Science+%26+Sensibility%29

Conclusion

In summary, childbirth in the USA can be a difficult and potentially traumatizing experience for new mothers. It may be time for mothers and health care providers to stand together and declare that the high rate of traumatic births is not acceptable, and it is time to do something about it. Change may indeed be in the wind, and that would be a good thing for both mothers and babies. In the meantime, practitioners who work with new mothers need to be aware that women they see may not be only suffering from postpartum depression and anxiety; they may also meet the criteria for birth-related PTSD. Early identification and treatment can potentially save mothers and their families years of anguish.

References

Alcorn, K. L., O'Donovan, A., Patrick, J. C., Creedy, D., & Devilly, G. J. (2010). A prospective longitudinal study of the prevalence of post-traumatic stress disorder resulting from childbirth events. *Psychological Medicine, 40*, 1849–1859.

Armstrong, D. S., Hutti, M. H., & Myers, J. (2009). Parents' psychological distress after the birth of a subsequent healthy infant. *Journal of Obstetric, Gynecologic, and Neonatal Nursing, 38*, 654–666.

Ayers, S. (2007). Thoughts and emotions during traumatic birth: A qualitative study. *Birth, 34*(3), 253–263.

Ayers, S., Eagle, A., & Waring, H. (2006). The effects of childbirth-related post-traumatic stress disorder on women and their relationships: A qualitative study. *Psychology, Health & Medicine, 11*(4), 389–398.

Ayers, S., Harris, R., Sawyer, A., Parfitt, Y., & Ford, E. (2009). Posttraumatic stress disorder after childbirth: Analysis of symptom presentation and sampling. *Journal of Affective Disorders, 119*, 200–204.

Beck, C. T. (2011). A metaethnography of traumatic childbirth and its aftermath: Amplifying causal looping. *Qualitative Health Research, 21*(3), 301–311. doi:10.1177/1049732310390698.

Beck, C. T., & Gable, R. K. (2012). A mixed methods study of secondary traumatic stress in labor and delivery nurses. *Journal of Obstetric, Gynecologic, and Neonatal Nursing, 41*(6), 747–760. doi:10.1111/j.1552-6909 2012.01.386x.

Beck, C. T., Gable, R. K., Sakala, C., & Declercq, E. R. (2011). Posttraumatic stress disorder in new mothers: Results from a two-stage U.S. national survey. *Birth, 38*(3), 216–227.

Beck, C. T., & Watson, S. (2008). Impact of birth trauma on breast-feeding. *Nursing Research, 57*(4), 228–236.

Elmir, R., Schmied, V., Wilkes, L., & Jackson, D. (2010). Women's perceptions and experiences of a traumatic birth: A meta-ethnography. *Journal of Advanced Nursing, 66*(10), 2142–2153.

Feeley, N., Zelkowitz, P., Cormier, C., Charbonneau, L., Lacroix, A., & Papgeorgiou, A. (2011). Posttraumatic stress among mother of very low birthweight infants 6 months after discharge from the neonatal intensive care unit. *Applied Nursing Research, 24*, 114–117.

Ford, E., & Ayers, S. (2012). Support during birth interacts with prior trauma and birth intervention to predict postnatal post-traumatic stress symptoms. *Psychology & Health, 26*(12), 1553–1570.

Friedman, M. J., Resick, P. A., Bryant, R. A., & Brewin, C. R. (2011). Considering PTSD for DSM-5. *Depression and Anxiety, 28*, 750–769.

Galea, S., Vlahov, D., Resnick, H., Ahern, J., Susser, E., Gold, J., … Kilpatrick, D. (2003). Trends of probable post-traumatic stress disorder in New York City after the September 11 terrorist attacks. *American Journal of Epidemiology, 158*, 514–524.

Goyal, D., Gay, C. L., & Lee, K. A. (2009). Fragmented maternal sleep is more strongly correlated with depressive symptoms than infant temperament at three months postpartum. *Archives of Women's Mental Health, 12*, 229–237.

Grajeda, R., & Perez-Escamilla, R. (2002). Stress during labor and delivery is associated with delayed onset of lactation among urban Guatemalan women. *Journal of Nutrition, 132*, 3055–3060.

Joseph, S. (2011). *What doesn't kill us: The new psychology of posttraumatic growth.* New York, NY: Basic Books.

Kendall-Tackett, K. A. (2000). Physiological correlates of childhood abuse: Chronic hyperarousal in PTSD, depression, and irritable bowel syndrome. *Child Abuse & Neglect, 24*, 799–810.

Lev-Wiesel, R., Daphna-Tekoah, S., & Hallak, M. (2009). Childhood sexual abuse as a predictor of birth-related posttraumatic stress and postpartum posttraumatic stress. *Child Abuse & Neglect, 33*, 877–887.

Modarres, M., Afrasiabi, S., Rahnama, P., & Montazeri, A. (2012). Prevalence and risk factors of childbirth-related post-traumatic stress symptoms. *BMC Pregnancy and Childbirth, 12*, 88. http://www.biomedcentral.com/1471-2393/12/88.

Rowlands, I. J., & Redshaw, M. (2012). Mode of birth and women's psychological and physical wellbeing in the postnatal period. *BMC Pregnancy and Childbirth, 12*, 138. http://www.biomedcentral.com/1471-2393/12/138.

Seng, J. S., Kohn-Wood, L. P., McPherson, M. D., & Sperlich, M. A. (2011). Disparity in posttraumatic stress disorder diagnosis among African American pregnant women. *Archives of Women's Mental Health, 14*(4), 295–306.

Simkin, P. (1991). Just another day in a woman's life? Women's long-term perceptions of their first birth experience. Part I. *Birth, 18*(4), 203–210.

Simkin, P. (1992). Just another day in a woman's life? Part II: Nature and consistency of women's long-term memories of their first birth experiences. *Birth, 19*(2), 64–81.

Soderquist, I., Wijma, B., Thorbert, G., & Wijma, K. (2009). Risk factors in pregnancy for posttraumatic stress and depression after childbirth. *British Journal of Obstetrics & Gynecology, 116*, 672–680.

Stramrood, C. A., Paarlberg, K. M., Huis in 'T Veld, E. M., Berger, L. W. A. R., Vingerhoets, A. J. J. M., Schultz, W. C. M. W., & Van Pampus, M. G. (2011). Posttraumatic stress following childbirth in homelike and hospital settings. *Journal of Psychosomatic Obstetrics & Gynecology, 32*(2), 88–97.

Tedeschi, R. G., & Calhoun, L. G. (2004). Posttraumatic growth: Conceptual foundations and empirical evidence. *Psychological Inquiry, 15*(1), 1–18.

Tham, V., Ryding, E. L., & Christensson, K. (2010). Experience of support among mothers with and without post-traumatic symptoms following emergency caesarean section. *Sexual & Reproductive Healthcare, 1*, 175–190.

Verreault, N., Da Costa, D., Marchand, A., Ireland, K., Banack, H., Dritsa, M., & Khalife, S. (2012). PTSD following childbirth: A prospective study of incidence and risk factors in Canadian women. *Journal of Psychosomatic Research, 73*, 257–263.

Part III
The Later Years

Babies After 40: Is the "Biological Clock" Really Ticking?

Nurit Winkler

Introduction

The popular term "biological clock" refers to the age-related decline in fertility. Infertility is defined as the inability to conceive after 1 year of regular unprotected intercourse (Practice Committee of the ASRM, 2013; Pfeifer et al., 2013a). While there are many reasons couples are unable to conceive, the aging of the female reproductive system is one of the most common (Practice Committee of the ASRM, 2008; Leridon et al., 2004). Within the last decade, there appears to be a worldwide decrease in the fertility rate and an increase in the demand for infertility services. According to the National Survey of Family Growth (Chandra, Martinez, Mosher, Abma, & Jones, 2005), in the USA alone, up to 47 % of women after age 35 will face infertility. Every year approximately six to seven million women use infertility services (Hamilton & Sutton, 2013). While there are many theories as to why infertility is on the rise, advance maternal age is becoming one of the most common causes of infertility is attributed to advanced maternal age. A recent survey conducted by the Center for Disease Control indicated that one in every five women in the USA is having her first baby at age 35 or older (Hamilton, Martin, & Ventura, 2012), and while women in the early 1950s were having first babies in their early twenties, the average age for primigravida today is between 27 and 30 years old (Mathews & Hamilton, 2009). When trying to understand why more contemporary women are attempting pregnancy at an older age, it becomes important to look into socioeconomic changes and their overall effect on reproduction.

The divorce rate is significantly higher now than in past years, and more women are re-marrying later, hoping to build a family with their new partners, but at an age in which natural fertility has significantly diminished. More women are also choosing to advance their careers before starting a family. The media also influences some of the reproductive decisions in our society. The increased access to social media

---

N. Winkler, M.D. (✉)
Center for Fertility and Gynecology, Tarzana, CA, USA
e-mail: drwinkler@center4fertility.com

and the increased publicity about infertility create more "openness" about infertility making it more culturally acceptable for couples or singles to seek treatment. While the media has enhanced public understanding and perceptions about infertility, they have also created unrealistic expectations and a false sense of security for many women due to the fact that they are flooded with success stories of women who appear to conceive much later in their reproductive lives. However, those stories frequently omit critical information related to the success of fertility treatments, such as the fact that the pregnancy was achieved with the use of donated oocytes (eggs) from much younger women. In fact, the vast majority of pregnancies in women over the age of 45 are conceived with the use of an egg donor (Practice Committee of the ASRM, 2008; De Brucker et al., 2013).

For a better understanding of the underlying mechanisms that influence the biological clock, one has to look into the natural progression of changes in fertility as women age. This chapter discusses the physiological changes of the female reproductive system that occurs in women of advanced maternal age as well as the impact of these changes on fertility.

What Is the Biological Clock?

The possible effects of the biological clock were first studied in a population called the Hutterites. The Hutterites are a communal religious community that lives primarily in the upper Great Plains of the USA and in the neighboring Prairie Provinces of Canada (Tietze, 1957). They live a relatively healthy lifestyle working as farmers, and with regard to their biblical teachings, they are prohibited from using contraception. When studying the natural pregnancy rate in this population, researchers observed that the pregnancy and delivery rate declined significantly as women aged. The pregnancy rate was 50–60 % per year in women younger than age 35 and then declined to approximately 10 % in women over the age of 40. The study confirmed that natural fertility does decline significantly with age and that the decline begins in the early 30s. An additional finding stemmed from the national success rate of in vitro fertilization (IVF), which is now considered to be one of the most efficient infertility treatments (SART, National Data Summary Report, 2012), although even with its success, pregnancy rates using this procedure decline significantly with age; for women aged 35 or younger, the rate of positive outcomes is approximately 40 % and then drops to less than 8 % in women over the age of 42 (Hull, Fleming, Hughes, & McDermott, 1996; Liu & Case, 2011).

Why does a woman's fertility change so much over time, and is there a way of slowing down the biological clock? In order to answer these questions, it is helpful to understand how the female reproductive system changes over the reproductive life-span. These changes can be divided into four main categories:

- Decline in the number of oocytes
- Decline in the quality of the oocytes
- Increased risk of miscarriage
- Anatomical changes in the female reproductive system

Decline in the Number of Oocytes

Women produce eggs only once in their lifetime, and this is as a fetus in utero, in contrast to men who produce sperm all of their lives. From the time a woman is born until she reaches menopause, she is continually losing oocytes. The decline in this number is responsible for the changes in her menstrual cycle as well as her decline in fertility.

At approximately 6 weeks gestation, the original germinal cells that give rise to the oocytes undergo active multiplication reaching about six to seven million by 20 weeks gestation. From that point onward, the majority of those eggs are lost to a phenomenon of programmed cell death called apoptosis, a phenomenon that is not completely understood. From six to seven million eggs at 20 weeks gestation only about one million of them remain in the ovaries at birth, which means that women lose the majority of their eggs before birth. The loss of eggs continues from birth until menopause, when only a few hundred eggs are left. While the loss of eggs is a continuum phenomenon, there appear to be two timelines in which the loss of eggs is more accelerated. The first pick is noted in their early 30s and followed by a second pick, even more pronounced than the first, around the age of 40. Those two picks correspond to the observed decline in fertility in this age group. As a result of the decline in the number of eggs the female menstrual cycle also begins to change. In the earlier stage of declining fertility the menstrual cycle shortens, and that usually occurs around their late 30s. This period is followed by a gradual prolongation of the menstrual cycle during the perimenopausal years in which the menstrual cycle becomes scattered and unpredictable until a woman reaches menopause and a complete cessation of menstruation from a clinical perspective. Women that used to have a 30-day menstrual cycle will notice in their late 30s that their menstrual cycle is shortened to approximately 26–27 days and will then gradually change to unpredictable cycles of 40–60 days or longer until reaching menopause.

While there are certain medical conditions and environmental factors that can accelerate the loss of eggs, such as the use of tobacco or chemotherapy and radiation treatments, a decline in the number of oocytes, as well as the age of onset for menopause, is generally genetically predetermined (Wood and Rajkovic, 2013). Even though healthy lifestyle, diet, and relaxation techniques are certainly beneficial for the overall health and well-being of women, current scientific studies have failed to prove that those factors have any significant influence on how rapidly the oocyte numbers decline (Broekmans, Soules, & Fauser, 2009).

Decline in Quality of Eggs

Although the loss of eggs is a primary contributing factor to the decline in fertility as women age, the most prominent change is the decline in the quality of the oocytes. Since women produce oocytes only in the uterus, they remain in the female reproductive tract until menopause. During those years the oocytes are exposed to different environmental and internal factors that can affect their quality, such as the detrimental effect of free radicals on the oocyte known as "oxidative stress." Those free radicals are produced by the different cells, including the oocytes (Yamada-Fukunaga et al., 2013). Another common "internal factor" that affects the oocyte quality is the telomeres, which are small segments of genetic material that protect the cell from the aging process. Shortening of those telomeres, which happen as women age, leads to cell senescence and death (Kalmbach et al., 2013).

With longer exposure to those damaging factors, the oocyte's internal mechanism, which is responsible for the division of the genetic material, becomes less effective, as a result "Many ovulated eggs contain abnormal numbers of chromosomes, either too many or too few, and if fertilized by a sperm, the resulting embryos will be genetically abnormal. Those embryos have lower chances of implantation and a higher risk of miscarriage and if born will produce a child with chromosomal abnormalities, such as Down's syndrome. The decline in oocyte quality is one of the most difficult obstacles to overcome, even with the assistance of fertility treatments; it is the most frequent reason for treatment failure in women of advanced maternal age and the main culprit for the increased risk of miscarriage as women get older (Liu & Case, 2011; Qiao et al., 2013).

Increased Risk of Miscarriage

The risk of miscarrying also increases significantly with age, and while there are many reasons for miscarriages, abnormal number of chromosomes within the embryo, referred to as aneuploidy, is the most common one (Angell, 1994). Approximately 15 % of all pregnancies result in miscarriages, and the risk increases significantly with age. In women younger than age 35, there is less than a 10 % risk; however, the risk increases to 50 % by age 43 and 80 % or more after age 45 (Munne, 2012).

Changes in the Female Reproductive Tract

When discussing the female biological clock, most of the attention is given to the changes in the oocytes, but there are also changes in other parts of the female reproductive system that can affect a woman's overall ability to conceive and/or carry a healthy pregnancy to term. Women that conceive after the age of 35 are at increased risk for a number of different pregnancy complications, including intrauterine growth retardation, preterm labor, gestational diabetes, and preeclampsia. In addition, there is a heightened risk for complications during the delivery of the baby and in the postpartum, such as caesarean section, instrumental delivery, and postpartum hemorrhage (Franz & Husslein, 2010; Montan, 2007).

Pathology of the Uterus

While the function of the uterus does not appear to change significantly over time, as women age, there is an increased risk of developing many pathological processes, such as uterine leiomyoma, adenomyosis, and uterine polyps that can affect the uterus and ultimately decrease the chances of conceiving or carrying a healthy pregnancy to term.

Uterine leiomyoma, also known as uterine fibroids, are benign tumors that arise from the overgrowth of the smooth muscle of the uterus. The risk of developing uterine leiomyoma increases with age from an incidence of less than 10 % at 30 years of age to approximately 30 % at age 40 and older (Baird, Dunson, Hill, Cousins, & Schectman, 2003; Wise, Palmer, Stewart, & Rosenberg, 2005). While many uterine leiomyomas go unnoticed, in some women these can cause symptoms such as pelvic pain, pelvic pressure, and abnormal uterine bleeding. Uterine leiomyomas can also interfere with the implantation of the embryo and, as a result, can increase the risk of miscarriage and pregnancy complications, such as premature contractions and preterm labor. These tumors can be easily diagnosed with a pelvic ultrasound sonogram and can be successfully treated either medically or surgically.

Adenomyosis refers to the abnormal presence of uterine glands within the muscle of the uterus. Similar to the presence of uterine leiomyoma, the presence of adenomyosis can also go unnoticed; however, it can also cause pelvic pain, pressure, and abnormal uterine bleeding in some women; it can also interfere with implantation of the embryo and, like uterine leiomyomas, adenomyosis can increase the risk of miscarriage or other pregnancy complications. Its presence can be suspected based on ultrasound and MRI findings, but the definitive diagnosis can only be discovered surgically. The most efficient and definitive diagnosis can only be confirmed surgically. The most efficient and definitive treatment for adenomyosis is a partial or a complete removal of the uterus, although other surgical and nonsurgical treatments such as laparoscopic myometrial electrocoagulation, uterine artery embolization, or hormonal treatments can be attempted in women that desire to preserve their fertility (Pepas, Deguara, & Davis, 2012; Wang, Liu, Fuh, Cheng, & Chao, 2009).

Uterine polyps are growths of the endometrial tissue and can be either benign or malignant. The presence of endometrial polyps, similar to other uterine pathology, can be silent or can cause abnormal uterine bleeding along with an increase in the possibility of miscarriage. A suspect diagnosis of endometrial polyps is most often based on imaging technology but a definitive diagnosis can only be done surgically. When endometrial polyps are found in women age 35 and older, there is an increased risk that the polyps could contain malignant cells and they should always be explored surgically.

Pathology of the Fallopian Tubes

The patency as well as the normal function of the fallopian tubes are a critical prerequisite for a normal fertility and pregnancy. Blockage of both the fallopian tubes prevents the oocyte from meeting the sperm; consequently, fertilization cannot occur. Any abnormal function of the fallopian tube may interfere with the normal migration of the embryo back to the uterus, increasing the risk of the embryo implanting in the fallopian tube. The resulting extrauterine (ectopic) pregnancy is potentially life threatening. Women over 40 tend to be more vulnerable to blockage of the fallopian tubes and ectopic pregnancies.

Despite the increased risk of pathology within the female reproductive tract as women age, the overall changes within the uterus and fallopian tubes have a significantly lower impact on the overall fertility when compared to the changes in the quantity and quality of the oocyte. This is evidenced by the fact that women undergoing IVF treatment in their late 40s have a success rate of less than 10 % when using their own eggs and up to 80 % or more when using an egg donor (Assisted Reproductive Technology Report, 2011; Budak et al., 2007; Navot et al., 1994; Paulson, Hatch, Lobo, & Sauer, 1997).

Cancers of the Female Reproductive System

The development of cancers in the female reproductive tract can affect fertility in different ways. Chemotherapy and radiotherapy treatments may cause irreversible destruction of the milieu of the oocyte, in addition to affecting the vascular supply to critical organs in the pelvis. Many cancers, especially those of the reproductive tract, are considered an absolute contraindication for fertility treatment and subsequent pregnancy because they both stimulate hormonal production that can aggravate the growth of any residual cancer tissue. Please see Chapter "The Impact of Reproductive Cancers on Women's Mental Health" for a more in-depth discussion about the impact of reproductive cancers on women's mental health.

Fertility Testing

Because age is such a strong contributing factor for infertility in some women, other causes for infertility and/or pregnancy loss may be overlooked. Therefore, a thorough evaluation becomes critical in determining the root cause of a woman's inability to conceive. Regardless of a woman's age, the treating physician should routinely be evaluating her for any other possible causes of infertility such as tubal disease, uterine pathology and others. For women over the age of 35, as well as women at risk of having diminish ovarian reserve such as women who have been exposed to radiation or chemotherapy, their ovarian reserve should also be tested in order to assess the quality and quantity of remaining oocytes within the ovaries and the likelihood of that particular woman responding successfully to infertility treatments.

The most commonly used tests to assess ovarian reserve are a combination of hormonal testing that includes follicular stimulating hormone (FSH) level, estradiol and anti-mullerian hormone (AMH), as well as antral follicle count that can be assessed by a pelvic sonogram.

Testing Ovarian Reserve

Day-Three FSH Level

FSH level is a hormone produced and secreted by the pituitary gland, located at the base of the brain. A high FSH level at the beginning of the menstrual cycle is one of the hallmarks of diminished ovarian reserve. The FSH travels through the bloodstream until it reaches the ovary where it stimulates the growth and development of the oocyte/follicle. At the beginning of the menstrual cycle, the secretion of FSH is inhibited by inhibin, a hormone produced by the small antral follicles. As women age and the number of follicles decreases, the secretion of inhibin also decreases, and as a result, the FSH level rises earlier during the menstrual cycle. For an appropriate use and interpretation of the FSH level, it should always be measured between the second and third day of the menstrual cycle and should routinely be interpreted in relationship to the corresponding level of estradiol, a hormone produced by the growing follicles in the ovaries.

The interpretation of the level of FSH is strictly related to the laboratory in which the test is performed since different laboratories use different cutoffs for what they consider normal range. Overall an FSH of 10 mIU/ml or higher is considered high by most fertility specialists. When a woman's FSH level is above 15 mIU/ml, she is usually considerer a poor candidate for fertility treatments. Although the FSH level tends to fluctuate from one menstrual cycle to another the measurement of one single high FSH is sufficient to diagnose diminished ovarian reserve even if a subsequent FSH is found to be normal. Previous studies have shown that the presence of an elevated FSH level during an IVF cycle correlates well with a low number of developing follicles and retrieved eggs as well as a high risk of cycle cancellation and failure to conceive (Van Rooij et al., 2003).

The FSH level should not be used as a cutoff to deny fertility treatment but should be used as a tool to diagnose possible diminished ovarian reserve and to help establish appropriate treatment as well as more realistic expectations regarding the success rate of fertility treatments. While high FSH levels may pose a contraindication for fertility treatments it does not prevent or preclude women from conceiving naturally.

Day-Three Estradiol Level

Under the stimulation of the FSH, the granulose cells that surround the oocyte produce estradiol, which is the predominant estrogen during reproductive years. Estradiol has a different mechanism of action, but its primary function is to stimulate growth in the endometrial lining of the uterus in preparation for pregnancy. Receptors to estradiol are also found in different parts of the body, such as the brain, adipose tissue, and the immune system. The secretion of estradiol is under the influence of the FSH. As women get older and the number of oocytes decreases, the FSH level begins to rise earlier in the menstrual cycle, which in turn causes early growth of the follicles and an early increase in the estradiol level. The estradiol level is influenced by other hormones, as is the FSH level, and can fluctuate significantly from one month to another.

Anti-mullerian Hormone Level

Anti – Mullerian hormone (AMH) is produced during the male fetal life where it prevents the development of the mullerian structures, which include the uterus, fallopian tubes, and upper vagina. In female fetuses, AMH is produced solely by the granulose cells that surround the oocyte, and it is not secreted until the end of the third trimester. An early secretion of AMH in the female fetus will prevent the development of the uterus, fallopian tubes, and upper vagina.

After birth, AMH is produced by the granulose cells of preantral and small antral follicles and its blood level seems to correlate well with the number of remaining oocytes in the ovaries. The role of AMH during the reproductive life is to decrease the number of follicles that are recruited each month and also to decrease their sensitivity to the action of FSH. AMH can be viewed as a stop mechanism that slows the recruitment and loss of follicles.

AMH, as opposed to FSH and estradiol, is less influenced by other hormones, and as such, it is a much more stable and reliable marker of ovarian reserve. In fact, the level of AMH when compared to FSH and estradiol rarely fluctuates from one month to another and can be tested on any day of the cycle. As women age and have fewer follicles, the AMH level tends to decrease proportionally until it reaches an almost undetectable level at menopause. AMH concentration was found to correlate well with the number of oocytes in the ovaries as well as the response to IVF.

Antral Follicle Count

Antral follicle count is one of the most efficient methods for assessing ovarian reserve. During regular menstrual cycles a number of follicles are recruited and begin to grow. As they grow, they acquire a small cavity filled with fluid and become antral. The antral follicles are also the smallest follicles that can be visualized on ultrasound where they appear as small black circles measuring between 2–10 mm in diameter. The antral follicle count is usually performed between the second and third day of the menstrual cycle. The number of follicles appears to be a good marker for ovarian reserve and correlates well with the pool of leftover follicles. In addition, it has merit in providing a more accurate assessment in regard to the potential response to the IVF treatment in conjunctions to other ovarian reserve markers. While there is no clear definition on what is considered a low number of antral follicles, when fewer than five to six of these follicles are visualized between the two ovaries at the beginning of the menstrual cycle, this usually indicates a diminished ovarian reserve.

Most fertility specialists use a combination of ovarian reserve testing in order to detect a possible aging of the reproductive system. While these tests can be helpful in diagnosing the decreased number of oocytes, none of these tests are very sensitive or specific and should be interpreted in the context of patient age and the underlying diagnosis. Most importantly, as previously stated, these tests should not be used to deny fertility treatment based on specific cutoffs, but as a tool to consult with patients appropriately and to tailor the most efficient fertility treatment for them.

The Biological Clock and Its Impact on Mood

The longing to procreate is one of the most intense and profound instincts; consequently, the inability to conceive has a profound effect on a woman's overall sense of well-being (Baldur-Felskov et al., 2013; El Kissi et al., 2013; Yael, Miri, & Ehud, 2005). When exploring any possible relationship between a woman's fertility and her mental health, evaluating any possible effects of infertility on mood as well as the potential repercussions of an existing mood disorder on infertility and pregnancy outcomes becomes essential.

Does Infertility Increase the Risk of Mood Disorder?

Numerous studies have shown that infertility and the concern about the female biological clock have deep psychological effects on women (Baldur-Felskov et al., 2013; El Kissi et al., 2013; Williams et al., 2007). A woman's inability to conceive influences her self-esteem and sense of accomplishment; it can affect her sexual function and increase her vulnerability to anxiety and depression, along with feelings of helplessness and grief with each failed treatment or when pregnancy simply cannot be achieved. Anxiety is very common in women with infertility (Baldur-Felskov et al., 2013; El Kissi et al., 2013; Yael et al., 2005) and even more so in women experiencing the ticking of their biological clock. As women begin to sense time slipping away, many often worry not only that pregnancy will never occur but also that their inability to conceive will have a dramatic impact on their relationship with their partner. Any existing anxiety is intensified by the myth that stress is the underlying cause of their infertility and that if they "just relax," pregnancy will happen. This type of friendly advice tends to create a vicious cycle, in which the anxiety and worry are now exacerbated by guilt and fear that they are the direct cause of their own infertility.

Sexual Dysfunction

Studies have shown that infertility has a significant impact on a woman's sense of sexuality (Ferraresi et al., 2013; Millheiser et al., 2010; Wischmann, 2010). Women with infertility generally report lower sex-life satisfaction along with a decrease in sexual function. Furthermore, infertility and its accompanying treatment processes often increase marital stress because of increased anxiety and pressure to conceive (Peterson, Newton, & Feingold, 2007). There is a feeling of lost intimacy when intercourse is done on demand and the intervention of the physician in a couple's sexual life and the financial burden of fertility treatments add to the stress. Along with these factors are the different coping mechanisms between female and male partners, which often create frustration and anger for both, which in turn often leads to even more of a decrease in sexual function and satisfaction, along with an escalation in marital conflict. Considering all of the above, it is highly recommended for couples that are struggling to cope with the psychological and emotional repercussions of infertility to participate in a support group or enlist the help of a therapist experienced in the issues that often surface for women and their partners (Noorbala et al., 2008; Schmidt, Tjornhoj-Thomsen, Boivin, & Nyboe Andersen, 2005).

Fertility Treatments After Age 40

When infertility is due to the age factor alone, there are different infertility treatments that are more suitable for women over the age of 40 (Pearlstone, Fournet, Gambone, Pang, & Buyalos, 1992). At this time in a woman's life, women often present clinically with a decrease in both the quantity and quality of eggs. This often results in a poorer response to fertility medications and a higher risk of failed treatment or miscarriage due to chromosome abnormalities within the oocyte.

While there are many different protocols used during treatment, the vast majority of those treatments share the same goal: increase the number of growing oocytes and facilitate the process of ovulation, fertilization, and implantation of the embryo, all of which are generally less efficient in women over 40. Some of the newer reproductive technologies attempt to decrease the miscarriage rate by transferring only those embryos that are genetically normal.

Determining through evaluation whether any underlying pathology exists, such as cancer of the female reproductive tract, becomes essential because malignancy can place a woman and/or her fetus at significant risk. Most treatments are less effective as women age; consequently, most physicians tend to be more aggressive with treatment by using higher doses of medications and, if possible, by moving more quickly into more efficient fertility treatments, such as IVF. The fertility treatments that are among the most commonly used include Clomid, gonadotropin control ovarian stimulation (COH), intrauterine insemination (IUI), and assisted reproductive technology (ART).

Clomiphene Citrate or Clomid

Clomiphene citrate or Clomid is one of the most commonly used infertility treatments. Clomid belongs to the family of selective estrogen receptor modulators (SERM). These hormones regulate the estrogen receptors by acting as either an inhibitor or a stimulator. Clomid is a pill that is taken for 5 days starting on the third, fourth, or fifth day of the menstrual cycle. Once ingested, Clomid acts by blocking the estrogen receptors in the brain. The brain senses the lack of estrogen and then triggers an increase in the secretion of FSH and LH that stimulates the growth of the follicles. The end result is the development of one or more follicles. The main indication for the use of Clomid is in women with ovulatory dysfunction due to hormonal imbalance, for example, women who may have a condition known as polycystic ovarian syndrome (PCOS). In cases such as these, Clomid has an 85 % success rate in inducing ovulation; however, in older patients, Clomid is highly inefficient and ineffective since the infertility in most of those cases is related to the decreased number and quality of the eggs (Wiser et al., 2012).

Control Ovarian Hyperstimulation (COH)

COH with the use of gonadotropins is a fertility treatment in which gonadotropin hormones, such as FSH and LH, are given as daily injections during the first days of the menstrual cycle. The gonadotropin hormones stimulate the ovaries to grow more follicles as opposed to a natural cycle in which only one oocyte develops. Once the follicles are mature enough, an injection is given in order to induce ovulation. The induction of ovulation can be combine to ether an intrauterine insemination or timed intercourse around the time of ovulation. The overall success rate of a COH cycle is approximately 25 % in the general population but less than 10 % in women over 40 simply because many of the possible limitations to infertility cannot be overcome just by increasing the number of ovulated oocytes (Wiser et al., 2012).

Intrauterine Insemination (IUI)

IUI is another commonly used fertility treatment that is generally indicated in cases where there is the presence of abnormal sperm. In addition, it is often used when there is no male partner, as in same-sex couples or a single parent, or when intercourse cannot be achieved effectively. An IUI can be performed with ether fresh or frozen sperm. In order to perform an IUI with fresh sperm, the male partner has to collect the sperm into a sterile cup. The collection of the sperm can be done in the comfort of his home and then transported to the laboratory, or it can be collected in the laboratory. Once collected, the sperm is examined and processed in preparation. There are different methods of sperm preparation. In the "simple wash " technique, the sperm are washed in a simple culture media and centrifuged. This method can be used when sperm count is low. A "swim up" or gradient centrifugation procedure allows for the selection of the most vital sperm.

Once prepared, the specimen is then aspirated into a small syringe and injected into the uterus in proximity to the ovulation time. IUI is a quick 1–2-min procedure performed in the medical office by a gynecologist or a fertility specialist. The discomfort level is minimal.

IUI can be performed during a natural cycle in which the female ovulation is detected with the use of specialized ovulation kits or a pelvic ultrasound sonogram. It can also be combined with other fertility treatments, such as the ones mentioned above.

The success rate depends on multiple factors, such as the condition of the sperm, the age of the female partner, and the underlying causes of the infertility; it ranges on average anywhere from 3 to 11 % fecundity per cycle (Merviel et al., 2010). The success rate could be higher when donor sperm is used and/or the insemination is combined with other fertility treatments, (Soria et al., 2012). For women over the age of 40, insemination alone is not as successful and is generally not recommended (De Brucker et al., 2013).

Assisted Reproductive Technology

ART includes all technologies in which the oocytes are manipulated outside of the body. The most frequently used ART procedures include:

- IVF
- Assisted hatching
- Preimplantation genetic diagnosis
- Egg freezing

In Vitro Fertilization

At the beginning of the menstrual cycle a cohort of oocyte begins to grow. From all the growing follicles, nature selects one dominant follicle which will be the only one that continues to grow and will ultimately ovulate. The remaining cohort of oocytes regresses and then dies. During the IVF process, women are given hormones to stimulate the growth of multiple oocytes. Once the oocytes mature, they are aspirated transvaginally with an ultrasound guide. The retrieved oocytes are then fertilized with the sperm, and the resulting embryos are transferred back to the uterus. IVF is considered one of the most efficient fertility treatments, and it is frequently used with women over the age of 40 (Wiser et al., 2012).

There are different IVF protocols. The choice of which IVF protocol to use depends on patient age, ovarian reserve status, and underlying diagnosis, among other factors. However, there are some IVF protocols that appear to be more suitable for women of a more advanced age, and they include short IVF protocols in which the stimulation of the ovaries is not preceded by suppression of the ovarian function. Protocols such as "flare" or "antagonist cycle" are especially suitable for women with diminished ovarian reserve and a decreased number of follicles. In natural IVF or Mini IVF, a single follicle is selected naturally or a few follicles are followed.

Natural IVF or Mini IVF

In natural IVF, and Mini IVF, single or very few follicles are selected naturally and are retrieved with a the use of a minimal dose of fertility medications or with no medications at all. The advantage of these IVF protocols is that they can be applied to all women regardless of their ovarian reserve status, as long as they still recruit follicles and ovulate. The success rate however of those IVF protocols is unusually very low, with less than 10% chance of pregnancy rate in women over 40 (Schimberni, Morgia, Colabianchi, Giallonardo, & Piscitelli, 2009).

Assisted Hatching

During a natural cycle, when the embryo reaches the uterus, it hatches from the surrounding membrane, known as zona, and begins the implantation process. During assisted hatching, a small opening is created in the zona with the use of a laser or an acidic solution prior to transferring the embryo back to the uterus. Previous studies have shown that for a selected patient's population, and especially for women of advanced maternal age, the process of assisted hatching during an IVF cycle can improve the implantation and pregnancy rate (Carney et al., 2012).

Preimplantation Genetic Diagnosis (PGS)

During preimplantation genetic diagnosis, one or more cells are removed from the embryo in order to test for genetic mutation and/or evaluate their chromosomal component. The new PGS technology is capable of evaluating all 46 chromosomes and is becoming a very attractive option for women after the age of 40 in which the majority of the embryos are chromosomally abnormal. The ability to select the "healthier "embryos and subsequently transfer them back to the uterus can potentially increase pregnancy rate and decreased the miscarriage rate especially in women after the age of 40.

Egg Freezing

As discussed earlier in this chapter, the continued loss of oocytes from the fetal stage until menopause and the rate at which women lose eggs are genetically predetermined and cannot be modified by lifestyle or medical treatments. Until recently there were no efficient treatments capable of slowing down the biological clock or stopping it from ticking. In recent years, advances in egg freezing technology have allowed for better survival and preservation of eggs for future use (Cobo & Diaz, 2011). The oocyte cryopreservation technology was originally developed for single women undergoing chemotherapy or radiation therapy, both of which can cause irreversible damage to the oocytes. This technology was ineffective for years due to poor survival rates of the oocyte during the freezing/thawing process. The first pregnancy that resulted from the use of cryopreserved oocyte was reported in 1986 (Chen, 1986). Since then, hundreds of babies have been born with the use of this technology (Noyes, Porcu, & Borini, 2009).

In recent years the development of a new freezing technology called vitrification, or fast freezing, has allowed for much better survival and is now the only recommended freezing technology to be used when freezing oocytes (Arav & Natan, 2013). The ideal conditions for successful and efficient oocyte cryopreservation cycles include women aged 35 or younger with good ovarian reserve (Rienzi et al., 2012). Because of the dramatic increase in survival and pregnancy rates as a result of this new procedure, the American Society of Reproductive Medicine (ASRM) removed the label of experimental from the procedure and it is now widely used as a fertility preservation treatment (Pfeifer et al., 2013b). Egg freezing has become an attractive option for women who anticipate a delay in childbearing or for women at risk of loss of ovarian functions due to cancer or other pathological conditions (Dondorp et al., 2012).

Oocyte Donation

The use of an egg donor in women over age 40 is a valuable option and is sometimes the only realistic one when responses to infertility treatments fail. For women aged 45 and older, egg donation is the only recommended fertility treatment (Indekeu et al., 2013). The success rate of egg donation cycles is 60–80 % compared to less than 10 % success rate in women aged 42 and older that are using their own eggs (Hourviz et al., 2009). With a donated egg, the miscarriage rate is less than 10 % in contrast to 50 % or greater miscarriage rate for women over the age of 40 who use their own eggs (Marquard, Westphal, Milki, & Lathi, 2010). The risk of conceiving a child with Down's syndrome is less than 1 in 1,450 when using an egg donor as opposed to a risk of 1 in 35 women aged 45 or older using their own eggs (Kroon, Harrison, Martin, Wong, & Yazdani, 2011; Morris, Wald, Mutton, & Alberman, 2003). An additional benefit in using an egg donor is that the amount of embryos that result from one treatment of egg donation allows for the preservation of multiple embryos for future use. The frozen embryos can be used if the fertility treatment fails or if a woman wants to have biological siblings that derive from the same donor.

Egg donors may be family members, friends, and acquaintances, or they may be anonymous donors, who are usually recruited from the local population and found through agencies or fertility clinics. Even though the majority of egg donation procedures are performed anonymously known donors can provide a higher level of comfort. Using a family member as an egg donor creates a genetic connection to the offspring that so many women believe is critical pre-requisite in their decision to go forth with this procedure. For many women, the realization that they will not be genetically connected to their child is frequently psychologically distressing. Regardless of the choice, advantages always need to be weighed against the psychological complexity of using this path towards pregnancy since it may also create interpersonal relationship issues when boundaries become this diffuse.

The ASRM endorses a number of eligibility criteria for an egg donor: age 21–34 with an excellent medical, gynecological, and genetic history (Pfeifer et al., 2013c). The issue of physical traits, i.e., hair color, eye color, or stature, becomes critically important as women try to recreate the feeling of genetic connection through outward appearance. A selected donor must undergo a medical and genetic screening as well as an in-depth psychological evaluation. Once all screening is completed and the legal contracts are ready, the fertility treatment can begin. The compensation for the donor can vary anywhere from $5,000 to more than $10,000.

Egg donation is considered the single most efficient and successful fertility treatment but also one of the most emotionally challenging considerations since it requires a woman to let go of her desire for a genetic connection. It is psychologically complicated, and the decision to use an egg donor is frequently accompanied by a deep sense of sadness and grief, leaving women more vulnerable to depression. It also raises questions in the minds of many women about their ability to love a child that is not genetically connected to them, concerns about the baby's well-being, and whether or not at some point to reveal the truth to their child. This is often accompanied by a feeling of shame and failure; however, most women who decide to move ahead with egg donation have a positive and rewarding outcome.

Gestational Carrier

A gestational carrier is a women who voluntarily agrees to carry a pregnancy for another couple or single, that are a woman who is unable to carry a pregnancy to term. In a traditional surrogacy, the gestational carrier uses her own eggs for the process. This option is rarely used today because there are potentially more legal issues, as well as risks of emotional difficulties, because a gestational carrier has a genetic connection to the child. Gestational surrogacy as opposed to "traditional surrogacy" is the most common type of surrogacy is the surrogate carries the pregnancy with the use of a donated egg; consequently, she has no genetic connection to the offspring.

Historically, the use of a gestation carrier was limited to women whose uterus was absent or severely compromised. Currently, the use of a gestational carrier has been expanded to other medical conditions that can prevent the implantation of the embryos, or increase the risk of a miscarriage, such as the presence of pathology within the uterus or cancers of the reproductive tract. In order to be considered as a gestational carrier, a the ideal candidate candidate should be 35 years of age or younger with a body mass index (BMI) of less than 25 as well as a normal obstetrical history with at least one pregnancy delivered at term. The gestational surrogate undergoes a thorough screening evaluation, similar to the screening of the egg donor. The legal contract for the surrogacy includes multiple details, such as the number of fetuses the surrogate is willing to carry and the possibility of a termination of pregnancy if needed. Once the screening process is completed the medical treatment is relatively easy. The gestational carrier undergoes preparation of the uterus for implantation of fresh or frozen embryos that can derive from an egg donor or the intended mother's own eggs.

Women that choose to become gestational carriers come from a variety of socio-economic backgrounds. Their choice to become a gestational carrier is usually a combination of altruism and financial compensation. The financial compensation to the surrogate can vary and may be anywhere from $25,000 to more than $50,000. A key element for a successful surrogacy cycle is a good match between the intended parent/parents and the gestational carrier. While this relationship may follow different patterns, given that some couples or singles may want to feel more closely connected to the gestational carrier and others may want a more distance relationship, it is paramount that the expectations and the type of relationship both parties desire are clearly defined and agreed upon prior to the initiation of the fertility treatments. With good communication and openness, the surrogacy process is usually a very positive experience.

Conclusion

Is the biological clock that has been hovering over women's lives for years really ticking? Even the idea of a fertility timekeeper has created fear and anxiety about the inevitability of the natural aging process. Its ominous presence creates an intense sense of pressure for women as they come fact to face with the limited window of their own fertility.

Although the women's movement opened the door to decisions that women make and how they take charge of their own lives, the existence of the biological clock and declining fertility feels limited, confining, and often chips away at a woman's sense that she is in control of her own destiny. We cannot ignore the existence of the biological clock, nor can we deny its effects on a female's fertility. Due to the advances in reproductive technology, a baby after the age of 40 has become a reality. With a better understanding of the underlying mechanisms that dictate the decline of fertility due to age, along with the tremendous advances in infertility treatment options, women today have significantly more reproduction choices, which brings them closer to their goal of a baby, even after age 40.

References

Angell, R. R. (1994). Aneuploidy in older women. Higher rates of aneuploidy in oocytes from older women. *Human Reproduction, 9*(7), 1199–1200.
Arav, A., & Natan, Y. (2013). Vitrification of oocytes: From basic science to clinical application. *Advances in Experimental Medicine and Biology, 761*, 69–83.

Assisted Reproductive Technology Report. (2011). Center for Disease Control. Retrieved from http://nccd.cdc.gov/DRH_ART/Apps/NationalSummaryReport.aspx

Baird, D. D., Dunson, D. B., Hill, M. C., Cousins, D., & Schectman, J. M. (2003). High cumulative incidence of uterine leiomyoma in black and white women: Ultrasound evidence. *American Journal of Obstetrics and Gynecology, 188*(1), 100–107.

Baldur-Felskov, B., Kjaer, S. K., Albieri, V., Steding-Jenssen, M., Kjaer, T., Johansen, C., ... Jensen, A. (2013). Psychiatric disorders in women with fertility problems: Results from a large Danish register-based cohort study. *Human Reproduction, 28*(3), 683–690.

Broekmans, F. J., Soules, M. R., & Fauser, B. C. (2009). Ovarian aging: Mechanisms and clinical consequences. *Endocrinological Review, 30*(5), 465–493.

Budak, E., Garrido, N., Soares, S. R., Melo, M. A., Meseguer, M., Pellicer, A., & Remohi, J. (2007). Improvements achieved in an oocyte donation program over a 10-year period: Sequential increase in implantation and pregnancy rates and decrease in high order multiple pregnancies. *Fertility and Sterility, 88*(2), 342–349.

Carney, S. K., Das, S., Blake, D., Farquhar, C., Seif, M. M., & Nelson, L. (2012). Assisted hatching on assisted conception: In vitro fertilization (IVF) and intracytoplasmic sperm injection (ICSI). *Cochrane Database Systemic Review,* (12):CD001894.

Chandra, A., Martinez, G. M., Mosher, W. D., Abma, J. C., & Jones, J. (2005). Fertility, family planning, and reproductive health of U. W. women: Data from the 2002 National Survey of Family Growth. National Center for Health Statistics. *Vital Health Statistics, 23*(25), 1–160.

Chen, C. (1986). Pregnancy after human oocyte cryopreservation. *Lancet, 327*(8486), 884–886.

Cobo, A., & Diaz, C. (2011). Clinical application of oocyte vitrification: A systematic review and meta-analysis of randomized controlled trials. *Fertility and Sterility, 96*(2), 277–285.

De Brucker, M., Tournaye, H., Haentjens, P., Verheyen, G., Collins, J., & Camus, M. (2013). Assisted reproduction counseling in women aged 40 and above: A cohort study. *Journal of Assisted Reproduction and Genetics, 30*(11), 1431–1438.

Dondorp, W., de Wert, G., Pennings, G., Shenfield, F., Devroey, P., Tarlatzis, B., ... Diedrich, K. (2012). Oocyte cryopreservation for age-related fertility loss. SHRE Task Force on Ethics and Law. *Human Reproduction, 27*(5), 1231–1237.

El Kissi, Y., Romdhane, A. B., Hidar, S., Bannour, S., Ayoubi Idrissi, K., Khairi, H., & Hadj, A. B. (2013). General psychopathology, anxiety, depression, and self-esteem couples undergoing infertility treatment: A comparative study between men and women. *European Journal of Obstetrics, Gynecology, Reproduction, & Biology, 167*(2), 185–189.

Ferraresi, S. R., Lara, L. A., De Sá, M. F., Reis, R. M., & Rosa e Silva, A. C. (2013). Current research on how infertility affects the sexuality of men and women. *Recent Patents in Endocrine Metabolic Immune Drug Discovery, 7*(3), 198–202.

Franz, M. B., & Husslein, P. W. (2010). Obstetrical management of the older gravida. *BMC Women's Health, 6*(3), 463–468.

Hamilton, B. E., Martin, J. A., & Ventura, S. J. (2012). Births: Preliminary data for 2011. National vital statistics reports, 61(5). National Center for Health Statistics. Retrieved 2012, from http://www.cdc.gov/nchs/data/nvsr/nvsr61/nvsr61_05.pdf

Hamilton, B. E., Sutton, P. D. (2013). Recent trends in births and fertility rates through December 2012. *Division of Vital Statistics.* Retrieved June 2013, from http://www.cdc.gov/nchs/data/hestat/births_fertility_december_2012/Births_Fertility_December_2012.pdf

Hourviz, A., Machtinger, R., Maman, E., Baum, M., Dor, J., & Levron, J. (2009). Assisted reproduction in women over 40 years of age: How old is too old? *Reproductive Biomedicine Online, 19*(4), 599–603.

Hull, M. G., Fleming, C. F., Hughes, A. O., & McDermott, A. (1996). The age-related decline in female fecundity: A quantitative controlled study of implanting capacity and survival of individual embryos after in vitro fertilization. *Fertility & Sterility, 65*, 783.

Indekeu, A., Dierickx, K., Schotsmans, P., Daniels, K. R., Robert, P., & Hooghe, T. (2013). Factors contributing to parental decision making in disclosing donor conception: A systematic review. *Human Reproduction Update, 19*(6), 714–733.

Kalmbach, K. H., Fontes Antunes, D. M., Dracxler, R. C., Knier, T. W., Seth-Smith, M. L., Wang, F., ... Keefe, D. L. (2013). Telomeres and human reproduction. *Fertility and Sterility, 99*(1), 23–29.

Kroon, B., Harrison, K., Martin, N., Wong, B., & Yazdani, A. (2011). Miscarriage karyotype and its relationship with maternal body mass index, age, and mode of conception. *Fertility and Sterility, 95*(5), 1827–1829.

Leridon, H. (2004). Can assisted reproduction technology compensate for the natural decline in fertility with age? A model assessment. *Human Reproduction, 19*(7), 1548.

Liu, K., & Case, A. (2011). Advanced Reproductive age and fertility. Reproductive Endocrinology and Infertility Committee: Family Physicians advisory Committee: Maternal-Fetal Medicine Committee; Executive and Council of the Society of Obstetricians. *Journal of Obstetrics and Gynecology Canada, 33*(11), 1165–1175.

Marquard, K., Westphal, L. M., Milki, A. A., & Lathi, R. B. (2010). Etiology of recurrent pregnancy loss in women over the age of 35 years. *Fertility and Sterility, 94*(4), 1473–1477.

Mathews, T. J., Hamilton, B. E. (2009). Delayed childbearing: More women are having their first child later in life. U.S. Department of Health and Human Services, Centers for Disease Control and Prevention, National Center for Health Statistics, NCHS Data Brief (21), 1–8.

Merviel, P., Heraud, M. H., Grenier, N., Lourdel, E., Sanguinet, P., & Copin, H. (2010). Predictive factors for pregnancy after intrauterine insemination (IUI): An analysis of 1038 cycles and a review of the literature. *Fertility & Sterility, 93*(1), 79–88.

Millheiser, L. S., Helmer, A. E., Quintero, R. B., Westphal, L. M., Milki, A. A., & Lathi, R. B. (2010). Is infertility a risk factor for female sexual dysfunction? A case control study. *Fertility & Sterility, 94*(6), 2022.

Montan, S. (2007). Increased risk in the elderly parturient. *Current Opinion in Obstetrics and Gynecology, 19*(2), 110–112.

Morris, J. K., Wald, N. J., Mutton, D. E., & Alberman, E. (2003). Comparison of models of maternal age specific risk for Down syndrome live births. *Prenatal Diagnosis, 23*(3), 252–258.

Munne, S. (2012). Preimplantation genetic diagnosis for aneuploidy and translocations using array comparative genomic hybridization. *Current Genomics, 13*(6), 463–470.

Navot, D., Drews, M. R., Bergh, P. A., Guzma, I., Karstaedt, A., Scott, R. T. Jr., ... Hofmann, G. E., (DATE). (1994). Age related decline in female fertility is not due to diminished capacity of the uterus to sustain embryo implantation. *Fertility & Sterility, 61*(1), 97–101.

Noorbala, A. A., Ramazanzadeh, F., Malekafzali, H., Abedinia, N., Forooshani, A. R., Shariat, M., & Jafarabadia, M. (2008). Effects of a psychological intervention on depression in infertile couples. *International Journal of Gynecology and Obstetrics, 101*(3), 248–252.

Noyes, N., Porcu, E., & Borini, A. (2009). Over 900 oocyte cryopreservation babies born with no apparent increase in congenital anomalies. *Reproductive Biomedicine Online, 18*(6), 769–776.

Paulson, R. J., Hatch, I. E., Lobo, R. A., & Sauer, M. V. (1997). Cumulative conception and live birth rates after oocyte donation: Implications regarding endometrial receptivity. *Human Reproduction, 12*(4), 835–839.

Pearlstone, A. C., Fournet, N., Gambone, J. C., Pang, S. C., & Buyalos, R. P. (1992). Ovulation induction in women age 40 and older: The importance of basal follicle-stimulating hormone level and chronological age. *Fertility & Sterility, 58*(4), 674–679.

Pepas, L., Deguara, C., & Davis, C. (2012). Update on the surgical management of adenomyosis. *Current Opinions in Obstetrics & Gynecology, 24*(4), 259–264.

Peterson, B. D., Newton, C. R., & Feingold, T. (2007). Anxiety and sexual stress in men and women undergoing infertility treatment. *Fertility & Sterility, 88*(4), 911–914.

Pfeifer, S., Goldberg, J., Lobo, R., Thomas, M., Widra, E., Licht, M., ... La Barbera, A. (2013a). Definitions of infertility and recurrent pregnancy loss: A committee of opinion. *Fertility and Sterility, 99*(1), 63.

Pfeifer, S., Goldberg, J., Lobo, R., Thomas, M., Widra, E., Licht, M., ... La Barbera, A. (2013b). Mature Oocyte cryopreservation: A guideline. *Fertility & Sterility, 99*(1), 37–43.

Pfeifer, S., Goldberg, J., Lobo, R., Thomas, M., Widra, E., Licht, M., ... La Barbera, A. (2013c). Recommendations for gamete and embryo donation: A committee opinion. *Fertility & Sterility, 99*(1), 47–62.

Qiao, J., Wang, Z. B., Feng, H. L., Miao, Y. L., Wang, Q., Yu, Y., ... Sun, Q. Y. (2013). The root of reduced fertility in aged women and possible therapeutic options: Current status and future prospects. *Molecular Aspects of Medicine, 31*(06), 399–415. S0098-2997(13)00041-1 [pii].

Rienzi, L., Cobo, A., Paffoni, A., Scarduelli, C., Capalbo, A., Vajta, G., ... Ubaldi, F. M. (2012). Consistent and predictable delivery rates after oocyte vitrification: An observational longitudinal cohort multicentric study. *Human Reproduction, 27*(6), 1606–1612.

SART. (2012). National data summary report. Retrieved from www.sartcorsonline.com

Schimberni, M., Morgia, F., Colabianchi, J., Giallonardo, A., & Piscitelli, C. (2009). Natural cycle in vitro fertilization in poor responder patients: A survey of 500 consecutive cycles. *Fertility & Sterility, 92*(4), 1297–1301.

Schmidt, L., Tjornhoj-Thomsen, T., Boivin, J., & Nyboe Andersen, A. (2005). Evaluation of a communication and stress management training programme for infertile couples. *Patient Education and Counseling 2005, 59*(3), 252–262.

Soria, M., Pradillo, G., Garcia, J., Ramon, P., Castillo, A., et al. (2012). Pregnancy predictors after intrauterine insemination: Analysis of 3012 cycles in 1201 couples. *Journal of reproduction and Infertility, 13*(3), 158–166.

The Committee on Gynecologic Practice of the American College of Obstetricians and Gynecologists and The Practice Committee of the American Society for Reproductive Medicine. (2008). Age related fertility decline: A committee opinion. *Fertility and Sterility, 90*(3), 486–487.

The Practice Committees of the American Society for Reproductive Medicine and the Society for Assisted Reproductive Technology. (2013). Mature oocyte cryopreservation: A Guideline. *Fertility & Sterility, 99*(1), 37–43.

Tietze, C. (1957). Reproductive span and rate of reproduction among Hutterite women. *Fertility & Sterility, 8*(1), 89–97.

Van Rooij, I. A. J., Bancsi, L. F. J. M. M., Broekmans, F. J. M., Looman, C. W. N., Habbema, J. D. F., & te Velde, E. R. (2003). Women older than 40 years of age and those with elevated follicle-stimulating hormone levels differ in poor response rate and embryo quality in in vitro fertilization. *Fertility & Sterility, 79*(3), 482–488.

Wang, P. H., Liu, W. M., Fuh, J. L., Cheng, M. H., & Chao, H. T. (2009). Comparison of surgery alone and combined surgical medical treatment in the management of symptomatic uterine adenomyoma. *Fertility & Sterility, 92*(3), 876.

Williams, K. E., Marsh, W. K., & Rasgon, N. L. (2007). Mood disorders and fertility in women: A critical review of the literature and implications for future research. *Human Reproduction Update, 13*(6), 607.

Wischmann, T. H. (2010). Sexual disorders in infertile couples. *Journal of Sexual Medicine, 7*(5), 1868–1876.

Wise, L. A., Palmer, J. R., Stewart, E. A., & Rosenberg, L. (2005). Age specific incidence rates for self reported uterine leiomyomata in the black women's health study. *Obstetrics and Gynecology, 105*(3), 563–568.

Wiser, A., Shalom-Paz, E., Reinblatt, S. L., Son, W. Y., Das, M., Tulandi, T., Holzer, H. (2012). Ovarian stimulation and intrauterine insemination in women aged 40 years or more. *Reproductive Biomedicine Online, 24*(2), 170–173.

Wood, M. A., & Rajkovic, A. (2013). Genomic markers of ovarian reserve. *Seminars in Reproductive Medicine, 31*(6), 399–415.

Yael, B., Miri, G., & Ehud, K. (2005). Variability in the difficulties experienced by women undergoing infertility treatments. *Fertility & Sterility, 82*(2), 275–283.

Yamada-Fukunaga, T., Yamada, M., Hamatani, T., Chikazawa N., Ogawa, S., Akutsu, H., ... Yoshimura, Y. (2013). Age associated telomere shortening in mouse oocytes. *Reproductive biology and endocrinology, 11*(1), 108.

Risk Factors for Depression During Perimenopause

Zoe Gibbs and Jayashri Kulkarni

Introduction

The relationship between transitioning into menopause and psychological disturbance has been recognised in medical literature for over 100 years (Kraepelin & Diefendorf, 1907). This transition, known as perimenopause, occurs in the majority of women between the ages of 40 and 55 years and is associated with a variety of biological and psychological changes. These include endocrine, vasomotor, cognitive, metabolic, and somatic changes, in addition to changes in mood, irritability, and hostility. Early in perimenopause, large fluctuations in estradiol, the most abundant and potent estrogen, and progesterone begin to occur. As perimenopause progresses, cycles become unpredictable and decrease, resulting in longer periods of estrogen withdrawal (Morrison, Brinton, Schmidt, & Gore, 2006). In 2001 the Stages of Reproductive Aging Workshop (STRAW) created classification guidelines for a woman's reproductive life cycle based on symptoms, menstrual cycle changes, and hormone changes (Harlow et al., 2012; Soules et al., 2001). These have now become the gold standard for assessing menopausal stage and have helped create consistency amongst researchers.

During perimenopause the rate of depression among women becomes 2–14 times higher than in the premenopausal years (Cohen, Soares, Vitonis, Otto, & Harlow, 2006; Freeman, Sammel, Lin, & Nelson, 2006; Schmidt et al., 2000). Depressive symptoms during the perimenopausal transition are also seen at an approximately 40 % greater rate than in the general population (Timur & Sahin, 2010). This has given rise to the concept of perimenopausal depression—a depressive syndrome

Z. Gibbs, Psy.D. (✉) • J. Kulkarni, MBBS
Monash Alfred Psychiatry Research Centre, Monash University, Melbourne, VIC, Australia
e-mail: zoe.gibbs@monash.edu

that is subtly different to that seen during other life stages. There are several factors that have been associated with increased rates of depressive symptoms and of major depressive disorder during perimenopause. These include biological, psychological, social, and lifestyle factors that are discussed in this chapter.

Symptomatology

Clinically, it has been suggested that the depression often seen during perimenopause is symptomatically different from depression at other stages of a woman's life (Parry, 2008; Schmidt, Roca, Bloch, & Rubinow, 1997). Perimenopausal depression is anecdotally described in the literature as feeling "blue," mildly depressed, irritable, or "grouchy," tense, or nervous (Bromberger et al., 2003). Compared to premenopausal depression, perimenopausal depression exhibits increased levels of irritability and hostility (Bromberger et al., 2003; Freeman, Sammel, Lin, Gracia, & Kapoor, 2008; Gibbs, Lee, & Kulkarni, 2013), increased mood lability (Holte & Mikkelsen, 1991), and anhedonia (Ozturk, Eraslan, Mete, & Ozsener, 2006) and is characterized by a less severely depressed presentation, rather than a major depressive episode (Dennerstein et al., 1993). In an observational study, Ozturk et al. (2006) found that premenopausal women who were depressed had higher levels of anhedonia than women with perimenopausal depression.

Prevalence

Several longitudinal studies have now shown increases in depressive symptoms during perimenopause. Freeman et al. (2006) found that participants in the Penn Study of Ovarian Aging were more than four times more likely to have high Centre for Epidemiologic Studies Depression scale (CES-D) scores (>16) compared with their scores before they entered perimenopause. Similarly, Cohen et al. (2006) found that women with no history of major depression who experienced hot flushes associated with perimenopause were significantly more likely to become depressed than women who had not entered perimenopause. Epidemiologic studies have found an increase in depressive symptoms in perimenopausal women compared with premenopausal women (Bromberger et al., 2003, 2011, 2001). Freeman, Sammel, and Liu (2004) found that women in perimenopause were up to three times more likely to report depressive symptoms than were premenopausal women. Similarly, a history of major depression has been found to increase the likelihood of developing depression in perimenopause (Harlow, Wise, Otto, Soares, & Cohen, 2003; Tam, Stucky, Hanson, & Parry, 1999). However, there is also an increased risk for first-onset depression during perimenopause (Freeman et al., 2006).

Hormonal Factors

The hormonal changes associated with perimenopause are not completely understood, mostly due to the complexity of these processes. Early changes in menstrual bleeding patterns seen during perimenopause are associated with fluctuations in reproductive hormone levels, with changes to the hormonal milieu beginning well before any somatic symptoms occur (Freeman et al., 2005; Gracia et al., 2005). Several studies have found that the perimenopausal period has distinct endocrine characteristics, with early perimenopause characteristically being a period of high gonadotropin, follicle-stimulating hormone (FSH) and luteinizing hormone (LH), levels and increased estradiol secretion, and late perimenopause is a time of high FSH levels and decreased estradiol secretion (Soules et al., 2001). In research studies, reproductive status is often confirmed by the presence of elevated plasma gonadotropin (i.e., FSH levels in the context of low plasma estradiol levels: Rubinow, Roca, & Schmidt, 2007). In the past, it has been hypothesized that declining estrogen levels during perimenopause lead to the symptoms that we associate with the transition, i.e., hot flushes and depressive symptoms. However, recent research indicates that the symptoms seen during perimenopause are related more to *fluctuations* in estradiol levels rather than a decrease in estradiol levels. This is supported by the observation that symptoms peak during mid perimenopause and begin to settle once menopause, a time of severely decreased estrogen levels, is reached (Freeman, Sammel, & Liu, 2004; Schmidt, Haq, & Rubinow, 2004).

Estrogen has widespread actions throughout the central nervous system (CNS) and modulates the transcription of many enzymes as well as the receptor proteins for several neurotransmitters and neuropeptides (Ciocca & Vargas Roig, 1995). As a result, estrogen regulates almost all the activities of the neurotransmitters serotonin and acetylcholine (Lokuge, Frey, Foster, Soares, & Steiner, 2011). For example, estrogen modulates the synthesis of serotonin (Cohen & Wise, 1988), serotonin reuptake (Fink & Summer, 1996), serotonin receptor transcription (Sumner, 1995), and response to serotonin stimulation (Matsuda, Nakano, Kanda, Iwata, & Baba, 1991). Estrogen affects widespread circuits in the human brain, including the neocortex, hypothalamus, pituitary gland, hippocampus, and brain stem. These regions are known to be responsible for maintenance of many of the functions impacted by perimenopause, including sleep, hot flushes, and fatigue, which are regulated through the hypothalamus as well as cognition and mood which are regulated through the hippocampus and neocortex. Both the central serotonergic system and the estrogenic system are prominently involved in the regulation of mood and behavioral states (Rubinow, Schmidt, & Roca, 1998). Fluctuations in estrogen levels seen in perimenopause may, therefore, directly cause all of the observed physical and psychological symptoms through altered activation of each key area of the brain.

The Relationship Between Perimenopausal Depression and Other Reproductive Event-Related Mood Disorders

There seems to be a subset of women who have extreme sensitivity to changing hormone levels associated with the menstrual cycle, and these women are most vulnerable at times of intense endocrine change, specifically premenstrually, postnatally, and perimenopausally. Community- and clinic-based studies have shown that premenstrual syndrome (PMS), premenstrual dysphoric disorder (PMDD), and postnatal depression are risk factors for subsequent perimenopausal depression (Dennerstein et al., 1993; Harlow, Cohen, Otto, Spiegelman, & Cramer, 1999; Payne, 2003; Payne et al., 2007; Payne, Teitelbaum, & Joffe, 2009; Stewart & Boydell, 1993). PMS has been identified as both an antecedent to as well as a frequent accompaniment of perimenopausal depression, leading to speculation that there is a tendency for some women to be at risk for mood destabilization during periods of reproductive endocrine change (Richards, Rubinow, Daly, & Schmidt, 2006). Studies have shown a higher-than-expected rate of PMS history in perimenopausal depressed women (Richards et al., 2006), and it has been identified as one of the strongest predictors of perimenopausal depression (Freeman, Sammel, & Liu, 2004; Freeman, Sammel, Rinaudo, & Sheng, 2004). However, in a prospective study, Schmidt, Haq, and Rubinow (2004) were unable to identify an association between either PMS or postnatal depression and perimenopausal depression.

An acknowledged problem in the literature is that many studies use retrospective self-reports of PMS, with many of the women, on closer inspection, not meeting the criteria for PMS. This unreliability of self-reporting was highlighted by Richards et al. (2006) who found that upon investigation, the actual rate of premenstrual dysphoria was not predicted by initial self-reports. However, further support for a common underlying cause comes from the nature of menstrual cycle-related mood disorders. Common symptoms that are shared by women with PMS, postpartum blues, perimenopausal transition, and menopausal depression include sleep disturbance, irritability, anxiety and panic, memory and cognitive dysfunction, and a decreased sense of well-being (Arpels, 1996). Despite inconsistencies in the research, there is compelling evidence that a past history of depression related to reproductive related events is a significant risk factor for perimenopausal depression (Freeman, Sammel, & Liu, 2004; Freeman, Sammel, Rinaudo et al., 2004).

Vasomotor and Somatic Symptoms

The most commonly associated symptoms of perimenopause are vasomotor symptoms, VMS, which refer to episodic flushing and sweating (Kronenberg, 1990). A hot flush is experienced as warmth beginning around the face and spreading to the chest, causing skin redness, diaphoresis (excessive sweating), and palpitations (Moline, Broch, Zak, & Gross, 2003). This occurs in about 75–85 % of women during perimenopause, and women experience them for up to 1 year, but as many as

25 % of women experience them for 5 years or longer (Moline et al., 2003). It has been theorized that depression during perimenopause may be secondary to the sleep disruption caused by hot flushes and night sweats, a concept known as *the Domino Theory* (Schiff, Regestein, Tulchinsky, & Ryan, 1979). This theory suggests that the ability of estrogen replacement therapies (ERT) to alleviate depressive symptoms is through alleviation of nocturnal hot flushes, resulting in an improvement in sleep (Schmidt & Rubinow, 1991).

Although not a uniform accompaniment, hot flushes are frequently associated with perimenopausal depression (Bromberger et al., 2010; Reed et al., 2009; Schmidt, Haq, & Rubinow, 2004; Seritan et al., 2010). Hot flushes have been shown to occur in over 80 % of perimenopausal women with depression, compared to only 49 % of perimenopausal women without depression (Joffe et al., 2002). The constant mild sleep deprivation that results from these VMS could explain the depression and increase in irritability and hostility that are seen during perimenopause. Sleep disruption during perimenopause is ubiquitous, with reports ranging from 44 to 61 % of perimenopausal women reporting insomnia, compared to 33–36 % of premenopausal women (Brugge, Kripke, Ancoli-Israel, & Garfinkel, 1989; Moline et al., 2003). One of the primary reasons for disturbed sleep at this time is due to nocturnal hot flushes (Moline et al., 2003).

Undermining the Domino Theory are the findings that hot flushes and perimenopause have been found to be *independent* risk factors for depression (Freeman, Sammel, & Liu, 2004; Joffe et al., 2011), thus reducing the likelihood that VMS predates all depressive symptoms. Upon further questioning of the role of VMS in depression, Bromberger et al. (2009) found that life stress and a history of psychological symptoms were more important than VMS when predicting first lifetime episodes of major depression in midlife women. In another study, Bromberger and colleagues (2011) found that VMS was not a significant predictor of first-onset major depression in midlife women. Their findings did, however, suggest that women who have a more symptomatic perimenopausal transition are at higher risk of a major depressive episode. In a longitudinal study by Hardy and Kuh (2002), it was found that VMS symptoms are strongly related to perimenopausal status, while psychological symptoms were more strongly related to current life stresses than perimenopausal status. It has also been shown that while VMS may be associated with depression, these symptoms are not able to account for the increased rate of depression (Bromberger et al., 2011). Further, it has been suggested that the experience of VMS can be influenced by concurrent depression symptoms. In an observational study assessing the relationship between climacteric symptoms and psychosocial factors, Binfa and colleagues (2004) found that vasomotor and physical symptoms of the climacteric were correlated with perimenopause, whereas psychological symptoms were more related to psychosocial factors (mainly negative life events). Based on the independent impact of VMS and perimenopause on depression rates, and the inconsistency of studies in finding a relationship between VMS and depression, it seems that the co-occurrence of VMS and depression is likely to reflect a common underlying endocrine sensitivity, rather than a causal relationship between the two. Further research to clarify this relationship is needed.

Psychosocial Factors

A relationship between stressful life events and incidence of depression has been well documented in the literature (Caspi et al., 2003; Cohen, 1987; Hecht & Mensh, 1975; Risch et al., 2009). Some studies have suggested that perimenopausal years, and midlife more generally, are associated with significantly more stressful life events than other stages of a woman's life (Schmidt, Murphy, Haq, Rubinow, & Danaceau, 2004). In 1980, Greene and Cook found that perimenopausal women reported more negative life events than younger women. This observed increase in negative life events predominantly related to events associated with interpersonal losses (e.g., children leaving the home or death of parents). This observation forms the basis of the *empty nest* construct, which refers to the grief parents feel when their children move out of home. Several studies have found that the presence of negative life events is associated with perimenopausal depression and behavior symptoms (Bromberger et al., 2010; Dennerstein, Lehert, Dudley, & Guthrie, 2001; Greene & Cooke, 1980), with an increased frequency of negative events reported by women during the early perimenopause (Cooke & Greene, 1981; Greene, 1983; Greene & Cooke, 1980). Based on these observations, it has been suggested that perimenopausal depression occurs secondary to an increase in negative life events (Freeman, 2010; Gibbs et al., 2013).

Rather than being perceived entirely negatively, however, it has been found that events associated with the empty nest construct are actually looked forward to by some groups of women (Barber, 1989; Dennerstein, Dudley, & Guthrie, 2002). It has been suggested that perimenopausal depressed women can be distinguished from non-depressed women by their greater vulnerability to the negative effect of life events on self-esteem (Greene, 1983; Veeninga & Kraaimaat, 1989). It may be that the difference between perimenopausal depressed women and non-depressed women is in the way that they perceive life events. Ballinger (1985) found that depressed perimenopausal women experienced a more negative impact of life events and more feelings of being stressed than a group of asymptomatic controls. Both the presence of negative life events as well as how negatively they are viewed may therefore be more important for predicting the risk of depression during perimenopause.

Past History of Mood Disorders

Women who develop psychiatric symptoms in midlife are more likely to have a psychiatric vulnerability (i.e., personal or family history of psychiatric disorders). In fact, over half of women with perimenopausal depression have experienced a previous depressive disorder. In a longitudinal study, Avis and colleagues (1994) found that prior depression was the most predictive index of subsequent depression in women aged 45–55 years. Depressed mood during perimenopause is particularly related to the previous experience of depressive symptoms associated with the menstrual cycle, such as PMS and postpartum depression (Dennerstein et al., 1993;

Harlow et al., 1999; Payne, 2003; Payne et al., 2007, 2009; Stewart & Boydell, 1993). In several studies conducted by Freeman et al., PMS has been found to be a predictor of perimenopausal symptoms (Freeman, Sammel, & Liu, 2004; Freeman, Sammel, Rinaudo et al., 2004). The evidence suggests that perimenopause increases susceptibility to symptoms of depression, especially in women with a lifelong vulnerability. In particular, there seems to be a subset of women who have a sensitivity to changing hormone levels associated with the menstrual cycle, and these women are most vulnerable at times of intense endocrine change, specifically at premenstrual, postnatal, and perimenopausal stages (Freeman, Sammel, & Liu, 2004; Freeman, Sammel, Rinaudo et al., 2004).

Psychosis and Perimenopause

Perimenopause is associated with a range of psychiatric pathology, not limited to depression. Most notably, there has been found to be an increase in psychosis for women in the midlife (Riecher-Rössler, 2003, 2005). Deterioration of preexisting psychosis has also been associated with women in midlife, with the course of schizophrenia in women tending to deteriorate during peri- and postmenopause (Kulkarni, Fitzgerald, & Seeman, 2012; Riecher-Rössler, 2003, 2005). Research has implicated a hormonal mechanism behind these spikes, and it is likely that a relationship exists between the midlife peak of psychotic and depressive disorders seen in women. Other periods of estrogen fluctuation have also been associated with increases in psychotic symptoms, including ante- and postnatally, after abortion, cessation of oral contraceptives, and other hormonal therapies (Mahe & Dumain, 2001; Riecher-Rössler, 2003, 2005). The vulnerability to mental health difficulties for women during and around the perimenopausal years certainly warrants further investigation given the disastrous impacts of these major mental illnesses.

Attitude Towards Perimenopause

The experience of perimenopause is influenced by cultural factors, and our perception of it is highly dependent on social learning about what to anticipate during midlife (Woods & Mitchell, 1996). The way women think about menopause and their expectations of it have been found to affect their psychological well-being during the perimenopausal period (Avis & McKinlay, 1991; Hunter, 1992; Stotland, 2002; Woods & Mitchell, 1996). In a prospective study, Avis and McKinlay (1991) found that women who have negative attitudes to menopause prior to entering the transition go on to report a more symptomatic perimenopause and were more likely to become depressed.

In the Massachusetts Women's Health Study (Avis & McKinlay, 1991), premenopausal women who reported neutral feelings or relief about the prospect of menopause developed more positive attitudes after menopause. However, women with previously negative beliefs about perimenopause were more likely to develop severe climacteric symptoms. Research has demonstrated that a person's behavior can be affected by his or her expectations, a concept known in psychological literature as "self-fulfilling prophecy" (Avis & McKinlay, 1991). Negative beliefs about menopause may act as a filter to experience, and even influence, symptoms of women's perceptions of perimenopause (Hunter, 1992). Western culture values youth and holds negative views about aging, and it is thus not surprising that women may view this marker of midlife as a negative event. Studies that have compared women across cultures, such as Asian, African, and Western, have found differences in the way menopause is viewed. Asian and African cultures have been found to view menopause more positively than Western counterparts, and women in these cultures had correspondingly more positive experiences (Aksu, Sevinçok, Kücük, Sezer, & Oğurlu, 2011; Jiménez & Pérez, 1999). These findings highlight the importance of the dialogue that exists in our culture about menopause and the need to make sure that people are receiving the right information from health providers.

Social Support

Social support has been found to be an important modulator of perimenopausal depression. Harlow et al. (1999) found that, relative to married women, women who have never been married or were divorced, widowed, or separated were at a significantly higher risk of depression during perimenopause. In a study by Schmidt and Murphy et al. (2004), depressed perimenopausal women reported significantly less satisfaction with their significant others as compared to non-depressed perimenopausal women. It is unclear as to what extent dissatisfaction in the primary partnership was preemptive of depression during perimenopause or whether the depression altered these women's perception of this relationship. In a longitudinal study, Dennerstein, Lehert, Burger, and Dudley (1999) found that risk factors for depression during midlife included interpersonal stress and that risk of depression was significantly lowered by positive feelings for their partner or by gaining a partner and decreasing stress. Ascertaining satisfaction with social support may therefore be an important indicator of potential for depression during perimenopause.

Coping Resources

The role of personality factors and coping styles in perimenopausal depression has not been adequately considered, with little research investigating this relationship (Bosworth, Bastian, Rimer, & Siegler, 2003; Gibbs, Lee, & Kulkarni, Submitted; Rostrosky & Travis, 1996). Coping refers to cognitive and behavioral strategies used by an individual in an effort to manage stressors (internal or external) that are perceived to be demanding and/or threatening (Lazarus, 1991). Adaptive coping refers to coping styles that involve efforts to remove stress and adjust the way the person thinks about stressful situations (e.g., putting things into perspective, positive reappraisal of responsibility) and efforts to effectively manage stress reactions (e.g., relaxation techniques, increased exercise). In contrast, maladaptive coping styles tend to involve withdrawal from social supports, aggression, and exaggerated use of defense mechanisms (such as avoidance) and a lack of problem-solving skills (or use of ineffective ones, such as substance use).

From the handful of studies that have looked at coping styles during menopause, there is evidence that coping style predicts both the experience and reporting of physiological symptoms (i.e., VMS) as well as depressive symptoms (Gibbs et al., 2013; Igarashi et al., 2000; Kafanelis, Kostanski, Komesaroff, & Stojanovska, 2009). In an interview-based qualitative study, Kafanelis et al. (2009) found that how well a woman copes with stressors during perimenopause seemed to be related to a perceived level of social integration, acceptance of the situation, or isolation. This is consistent with the evidence that belonging to a community or a network increases one's ability to cope and adjust to changes (Bess, Fisher, Sonn, & Bishop, 2002).

By comparison, women who were struggling to adjust were more likely to associate menopause with feelings of anger, powerlessness, and sadness over loss of youth and vitality (Kafanelis et al., 2009). Such cognitive appraisals do not encourage adaptability, help seeking, self-efficacy, or self-reflection, resulting in decreased proactive coping (Folkman, 1986, 1997; Folkman & Lazarus, 1985). Similarly, in a cross-sectional study, Gibbs et al. (2013) found that perimenopausal depression is associated with the use of self-blame and behavioral disengagement coping strategies. These findings demonstrate the importance of intrapersonal psychological factors in a woman's ability to cope with the increased vulnerability to depression during perimenopause.

Socioeconomic Status, Education, and Achievement

Socioeconomic status (SES), education, and achievement are all known to be protective against depression (Miech & Shanahan, 2000; Murrell, Himmelfarb, & Wright, 1983). The research that looks at the role of these factors for women during perimenopause is limited but suggests a protective role. In a cross-sectional study, Harlow et al. (1999) found that women who were currently employed and those living in higher SES areas were more likely to have lower depression scores. Research has also shown that higher educational achievement is associated with slightly decreased risk of depression in the perimenopausal years (Choi, Lee, Lee, Kim, & Ham, 2004; Harlow et al., 1999). There are multiple possibilities that could explain the protective nature of higher education. It may be because women who are better educated are more likely to have a better understanding of both perimenopause and depression. Also, it could be that education offers an important resource to women, better enabling them to adapt to changes during perimenopause (Choi et al., 2004). Alternatively, it may be that a higher level of education indicates a higher likelihood of a fulfilling career and that this is the factor which allows women to have a sense of purpose and meaning that goes beyond stereotypical gender roles (youthful, sexual woman, or mother) that are compromised during perimenopause (Deeks & McCabe, 2004; Raup & Myers, 1989).

Lifestyle Factors

Cigarette Smoking

Cigarette smoking has been linked to an increased risk of depression across the lifespan, with evidence that smoking specifically increases the risk of depressive symptomatology during perimenopause (Gold et al., 2000). Harlow et al. (1999) found that perimenopausal women in the highest percentile (in terms of cigarettes per day and years smoking) of cigarette smoking were significantly more likely than nonsmokers to have higher depression. This increase in depressive symptoms may be secondary to an increase in VMS associated with cigarette smoking, as cross-sectional studies have shown that cigarette smoking is associated with increased VMS (Avis, Crawford, & McKinlay, 1997; Gold et al., 2004, 2006; Whiteman, Staropoli, Benedict, Borgeest, & Flaws, 2003). It has been suggested that this increase in VMS with cigarette smoking is because cigarette smoking lowers endogenous estrogen concentrations in the body (Whiteman et al., 2003), suggesting that cigarette smoking may actually widen the window of hormonal vulnerability.

Exercise and Body Mass Index

The relationship between exercise and depression is well established within the literature (see Daley 2008 for a review), and, although a comparatively new concept, there is increasing research indicating a protective role for exercise in ameliorating perimenopausal symptoms. As part of a longitudinal study, Morse, Dudley, Guthrie, and Dennerstein (1998) found that exercise was *inversely* related to maximum numbers of perimenopausal symptoms. Similar results were found by Thurston, Joffe, Soares, and Harlow (2006), who reported that vigorous exercise in women who had a history of depression reduced the severity of severe hot flushes. This relationship between vigorous exercise and hot flushes was not, however, found in women without a history of depression. In a cross-sectional study by Lee and Kim (2008), it was found that women who were more physically active reported significantly fewer VMS, a finding supported by others (Elavsky & McAuley, 2005). However it may be dangerous to draw firm conclusions as Mirzaiinjmabadi, Anderson, and Barnes (2006) found no relationship between self-reported VMS and depression, and similar findings have been reported by others (Sternfeld, Quesenberry, & Husson,

1999; Wilbur, Dan, Hedricks, & Holm, 1990). While the relationship between VMS and exercise is unclear, exercise does seem to decrease psychological and somatic symptoms of perimenopause (Brownson et al., 2000; Gibbs et al., 2013; Mirzaiinjmabadi et al., 2006; Lee & Kim, 2008). Additionally, Harlow et al. (1999) found that increases in body mass index (BMI) produced modest increases in depression ratings, offering another potentially protective role for exercise. Because the mode in which exercise may impact perimenopausal depression is unclear, its efficacy needs to be established given its treatment potential and its associated medical benefits.

Pharmacotherapies

Estrogen therapy has been found to be an effective treatment for depressive symptoms during perimenopause (see Worsley et al., 2012 for a review). Although results have been mixed, there are currently at least two placebo-controlled trials that have found that ERT is significantly more effective than placebo in treating depressive disorders in perimenopausal women, with response rates of 68–80 % in the treatment groups compared to 20–22 % in placebo groups (Schmidt et al., 2000; Soares, Almeida, Joffe, & Cohen, 2001). They also found that treatment effect did not differ as a result of VMS, indicating that the ERT has mood-enhancing effects independent of its effects on VMS (Schmidt et al., 2000). Kornstein et al. (2010) found that perimenopausal depressed women on HRTs experience fewer physical symptoms, lower levels of melancholia, and decreased sympathetic arousal. As mentioned previously, the therapeutic effects of ERT that are seen in perimenopausal women are not seen in postmenopausal women when estrogen levels are at their lowest (Cohen et al., 2003). However, this effect has not been consistently observed, and it has been suggested that it is not the overall levels of circulating estrogen but rather fluctuations in these levels that are causing the mood disturbances (Freeman et al., 2006). In addition, it seems that the *balance* of their hormones, such as testosterone and progesterone, also has a significant effect on mood. Traditional HRT therapies are nonselective in their actions, resulting in unwanted side effects, such as endometrial and breast changes that have been associated with increased risk for breast cancer (Collaborative Group on Hormonal Factors in Breast Cancer, 1997; Writing Group for the Women's Health Initiative Investigators, 2002). This means that HRTs are not an appealing or a viable option to many women suffering from the symptoms of perimenopause. In response to these treatment limitations for standard HRT use, new trends in treatment of perimenopausal depression have emerged. To date, there has not been much research into the efficacy of SSRIs for treatment of psychological symptoms during perimenopause. However, several clinical trials have found differences in the way pre- and postmenopausal women respond to SSRIs (Kornstein et al., 2000) as well as differences between younger and older women (Cassano, Soares, & Cusin, 2005), with younger premenopausal women responding better to treatment. Comparisons between SSRI and HRT treatments have indicated similar efficacy between them (Soares et al., 2006), with some SSRI treatments showing improvement in menopausal symptoms generally (i.e., VMS) and not just in mood (Joffe et al., 2007; Soares et al., 2003).

The risks associated with traditional HRTs are of concern for some women, despite their efficacy. Tibolone is a newer and selective HRT that has a global estrogenic effect, with predominantly progestogenic effects in the endometrium (Swegle & Kelly, 2004). This particular HRT is able to alleviate menopausal VMS without stimulating the endometrium (Swegle & Kelly, 2004). Tibolone also increases circulating testosterone, which can enhance mood independently of estrogen changes (Swegle & Kelly, 2004). There are advantages to the use of this particular drug over estrogen- and/or progestogen-containing treatment options. As it does not increase mammographic density, it does not increase the risk of breast cancer whilst still having the effects on bone density and VMS seen in older HRTs (Reed & Kloosterboer, 2004). Part of the reason that tibolone is thought to be such an effective treatment is its effects as an androgen replacement. Although estrogen therapy alone has shown positive effects on mood, testosterone imbalance may contribute to lack of wellbeing (Bromberger et al., 2010; Davis, 2002). The clinical reports are supportive of the efficacy of tibolone in alleviating adverse mood symptoms experienced by postmenopausal women. To date, there is little research into the efficacy of tibolone during perimenopause. Given that a previously reported meta-analysis of estrogen therapy found a twofold increase in the effect size in perimenopausal compared to postmenopausal women (Zweifel & O'Brien, 1997), there is good reason to believe that clinical results will be positive.

Conclusion

In addition to the conflicting theories around aetiology, methodological problems have also contributed to the lack of a clear picture of perimenopausal depression. The characterization of depression has often been via self-report or has been confused with the somatic symptoms of perimenopause, and there is a lack of standardized and continuous measures of depression. Since the introduction of the STRAW criteria over 10 years ago, there have been more consensuses over perimenopausal status in research, and this seems to have resulted in more consistency in research findings.

Whereas stressful life events were initially found to be the best predictor of depression during the midlife (Woods & Mitchell, 1997), more recent research has shown that perimenopausal status, severity of VMS, hormonal fluctuation, and health and lifestyle factors are in fact better predictors of depression during the midlife than stressful life events (Cohen et al., 2006; Freeman et al., 2006; Fuh, Wang, Lee, Lu, & Juang, 2006; Woods et al., 2008). Research into pharmacological treatment of perimenopausal depression continues to make strides, with several best practice options for management now available (Parry, 2010; Worsley et al., 2012). But the anecdotally reported lack of understanding and education around perimenopause, and the subsequent distress around symptoms, is surprising given the ease with which it could be remedied. Women approaching their 40s would benefit from having discussions with health practitioners about what to expect, what their individual risk might be, and what can be done to prevent or reduce the severity of symptoms. Given that we can confidently identify many risk and protective factors, it makes sense that women at higher risk of perimenopause-related mood disorders should be identified and given preventative strategies around diet, exercise, and social supports, which could help them manage more effectively during a potentially difficult period in their reproductive lives. Further research is needed investigating how to best identify women at risk as well as what the critical period in the reproductive cycle is for early intervention.

References

Aksu, H., Sevinçok, L., Kücük, M., Sezer, S. D., & Oğurlu, N. (2011). The attitudes of menopausal women and their spouses towards menopause. *Clinical & Experimental Obstetrics & Gynecology, 38*(3), 251–255.
Arpels, J. C. (1996). The female brain hypoestrogenic continuum from the premenstrual syndrome to menopause. A hypothesis and review of supporting data. *Journal of Reproductive Medicine, 41*(9), 633–639.
Avis, N. E., Brambilla, D., McKinlay, J. B., & Vass, K. (1994). A longitudinal analysis of the association between menopause and depression: Results from the Massachusetts Women's Health Study. *Annals of Epidemiology, 4*(3), 214–220.
Avis, N. E., Crawford, S., & McKinlay, S. M. (1997). Psychosocial, behavioural, and health factors related to menopause symptomatology. *Women's Health, 3*, 103–120.
Avis, N. E., & McKinlay, S. M. (1991). A longitudinal analysis of women's attitudes toward the menopause: Results from the Massachusetts Women's Health Study. *Maturitas, 13*(1), 65–79.
Ballinger, S. (1985). Psychosocial stress and symptoms of menopause: A comparative study of menopause clinic patients and non-patients. *Maturitas, 7*, 315–327.
Barber, C. E. (1989). Transition to the empty nest. In S. J. Bahr & E. T. Peterson (Eds.), *Ageing and the family* (pp. 15–32). Lexington, MA: Health and Company.
Bess, K. D., Fisher, A. T., Sonn, C. C., & Bishop, B. J. (2002). Psychological sense of community: Theory, research and application. In A. T. Fisher, C. C. Sonn, & B. J. Bishop (Eds.), *Psychological sense of community: Research, applications, and implications* (pp. 3–24). New York, NY: Kluwer Academic/Plenum Publishers.
Binfa, L., Castelo-Branco, C., Blumel, J. E., Cancelo, M. J., Bonilla, H., Munoz, I., … Villega Rios, R. (2004). Influence of psycho-social factors on climacteric symptoms. *Maturitas, 48*, 425–431.
Bosworth, H. B., Bastian, L. A., Rimer, B. K., & Siegler, I. C. (2003). Coping styles and personality domains related to menopausal stress. *Women's Health Issues, 13*(1), 32–38.
Bromberger, J. T., Assman, S. F., Avis, N. E., Schocken, M., Kravitz, H. M., & Cordal, A. (2003). Persistent mood symptoms in a multiethnic community cohort of pre- and peri-menopausal women. *American Journal of Epidemiology, 158*, 347–356. doi:10.1093/aje/kwg155.
Bromberger, J. T., Kravitz, H. M., Chang, Y. F., Cyranowski, J. M., Brown, C., & Matthews, K. (2011). Major depression during and after the menopausal transition: Study of women's health across the nation (SWAN). *Psychological Medicine, 41*, 1879–1888. doi:10.1017/S003329171100016X.
Bromberger, J. T., Kravitz, H. M., Matthews, K., Youk, A., Brown, C., & Feng, W. (2009). Predictors of first lifetime episodes of major depression in midlife women. *Psychological Medicine, 39*, 55–64.

Bromberger, J. T., Meyer, P. M., Kravitz, H. M., Sommer, B., Cordal, A., Powell, L., ... Sutton-Tyrrell, K. (2001). Psychological distress and natural menopause: A multiethnic community study. *American Journal of Public Health, 91*(9), 1435–1442.

Bromberger, J. T., Schott, L. L., Kravitz, H. M., Sowers, M. F., Avis, N. E., Gold, E. B., ... Matthews, K. (2010). Longitudinal change in reproductive hormones and depressive symptoms across the menopausal transition. *Archives General Psychiatry, 67*(6), 598–607.

Brownson, R. C., Eyler, A. A., King, A. C., Brown, D. R., Shyu, Y. L., & Sallis, J. F. (2000). Patterns and correlates of physical activity among U.S. women 40 years and older. *American Journal of Public Health, 90*(2), 264–270.

Brugge, K. L., Kripke, D. F., Ancoli-Israel, S., & Garfinkel, L. (1989). The association of menopausal status and age with sleep disorders. *Sleep Research, 18*, 208.

Caspi, A., Sugden, K., Moffitt, T. E., Taylor, A., Craig, I. W., Harrington, H., ... Poulton, R. (2003). Influence of life stress on depression: Moderation by a polymorphism in the 5-HTT gene. *Science, 301*(5631), 386–389.

Cassano, P., Soares, C. N., & Cusin, C. (2005). Antidepressant response and well-being in pre-, peri-, and postmenopausal women with major depressive disorder treated with fluoxetine. *Psychotherapy and Psychosomatics, 74*(6), 362–365.

Choi, H., Lee, D., Lee, K., Kim, H., & Ham, E. (2004). A structural model of menopausal depression in Korean women. *Archives of Psychiatric Nursing, 18*(6), 235–242.

Ciocca, D. R., & Vargas Roig, L. M. (1995). Estrogen receptors in human nontarget tissues: Biological and clinical implications. *Endocrine Reviews, 16*, 35–62.

Cohen, S. (1987). Social factors and depressive symptoms. *Contemporary Psychology, 32*(4), 360–362. doi:10.1037/027006.

Cohen, L. S., Soares, C. N., Poitras, J. R., Prouty, J., Alexander, A. B., & Shifren, J. L. (2003). Short-term use of estradiol for depression in perimenopausal and postmenopausal women: A preliminary report. *American Journal of Psychiatry, 160*, 1519–1522.

Cohen, L. S., Soares, C. N., Vitonis, A. F., Otto, M. W., & Harlow, B. L. (2006). Risk for new onset of depression during the menopausal transition: The Harvard study of moods and cycles. *Archives of General Psychiatry, 63*(4), 385–390. doi:10.1001/archpsyc.63.4.385.

Cohen, L. S., & Wise, P. M. (1988). Effects if estradiol on the diurnal rhythm of serotonin activity in microdissected brain areas of ovariectomized rats. *Endocrinology, 122*, 2619–2625.

Collaborative Group on Hormonal Factors in Breast Cancer. (1997). Breast cancer and hormone replacement therapy: Collaborative reanalysis of data from 51 epidemiological studies of 52,705 women with breast cancer and 108,411 women without breast cancer. *The Lancet, 350*(9084), 1047–1059.

Cooke, D. J., & Greene, J. G. (1981). Types of life events in relation to symptoms at the climacterium. *Journal of Psychosomatic Research, 25*(1), 5–11. http://dx.doi.org/10.1016/0022-3999%2881%2990078-7.

Daley, A. (2008). Exercise and depression: A review of reviews. *Journal of Clinical Psychology in Medical Settings, 15*(2), 140–147. http://dx.doi.org/10.1007/s10880-008-9105-z.

Davis, S. R. (2002). The effects of tibolone on mood and libido. *Menopause, 9*(3), 162–170.

Deeks, A. A., & McCabe, M. P. (2004). Well-being and menopause: An investigation of purpose in life, self-acceptance and social role in premenopausal, perimenopausal and postmenopausal women. *Quality of Life Research, 13*, 389–398.

Dennerstein, L., Dudley, E., & Guthrie, J. (2002). Empty nest or revolving door? A prospective study of women's quality of life in midlife during the phase of children leaving and re-entering the home. *Psychological Medicine, 32*(3), 545–550. http://dx.doi.org/10.1017/S0033291701004810.

Dennerstein, L., Lehert, P., Burger, H., & Dudley, E. (1999). Mood and the menopausal transition. *Journal of Nervous and Mental Disease, 187*(11), 685–691.

Dennerstein, L., Lehert, P., Dudley, E., & Guthrie, J. (2001). Factors contributing to positive mood during the menopausal transition. *Journal of Nervous and Mental Disease, 189*(2), 84–89.

Dennerstein, L., Smith, A. M., Morse, C., Burger, H., Green, A., Hopper, J., & Ryan, M. (1993). Menopausal symptoms in Australian women. *The Medical Journal of Australia, 159*(4), 232–236.

Elavsky, S., & McAuley, E. (2005). Physical activity, symptoms, esteem, and life satisfaction during menopause. *Maturitas, 52*, 374–385.

Fink, G., & Summer, B. E. H. (1996). Oestrogen and mental state. *Nature, 383*, 306. doi:10.1038/383306a0.

Folkman, S. (1986). Dynamics of a stressful encounter: Cognitive appraisal, coping and encounter outcomes. *Journal of Personality and Social Psychology, 50*(5), 992–1003.

Folkman, S. (1997). Positive psychological states and coping with severe stress. *Social Science & Medicine, 45*, 1207–1221.

Folkman, S., & Lazarus, R. S. (1985). If it changes it must be a process: A study of emotion and coping during three stages of a college examination. *Journal of Personality and Social Psychology, 48*, 150–170.

Freeman, E. W. (2010). Associations of depression with the transition to menopause. *Menopause, 17*(4), 823–827.

Freeman, E. W., Sammel, M. D., Gracia, C. R., Kapoor, S., Lin, H., Liu, L., & Nelson, D. B. (2005). Follicular phase hormone levels and menstrual bleeding status in the approach to menopause. *Fertility and Sterility, 83*, 383–392.

Freeman, E. W., Sammel, M. D., Lin, H., Gracia, C. R., & Kapoor, S. (2008). Symptoms in the menopausal transition: Hormone and behavioural correlates. *Obstetrics and Gynecology, 111*(1), 127–136. doi:10.1097/01.AOG.0000295867.06184.b1.

Freeman, E. W., Sammel, M. D., Lin, H., & Nelson, D. B. (2006). Associations of hormones and menopausal status with depressed mood in women with no history of depression. *Archives of General Psychiatry, 63*(4), 375–382. doi:10.1001/archpsyc.63.4.375.

Freeman, E. W., Sammel, M. D., & Liu, L. (2004). Hormones and menopausal status as predictors of depression in women in transition to menopause. *Archives of General Psychiatry, 61*, 62–70.

Freeman, E. W., Sammel, M. D., Rinaudo, P. J., & Sheng, L. (2004). Premenstrual syndrome as a predictor of menopausal symptoms. *Obstetrics & Gynecology, 103*(5 pt 1), 960–966.

Fuh, J.-L., Wang, S.-J., Lee, S.-J., Lu, S.-R., & Juang, K.-D. (2006). A longitudinal study of cognition change during early menopausal transition in a rural community. *Maturitas, 53*(4), 447–453. http://dx.doi.org/10.1016/j.maturitas.2005.07.009.

Gibbs, Z., Lee, S., & Kulkarni, J. (Unpublished Manuscript). The role of coping styles in depression during perimenopause: Use of maladaptive coping styles predicts depressive symptoms in the menopausal transition.

Gibbs, Z., Lee, S., & Kulkarni, J. (2013). Factors associated with depression during the perimenopausal transition. *Women's Health Issues, 23*(5), e301–e307.

Gold, E. B., et al. (2000). Relation of demographic and lifestyle factors to symptoms in a multiracial/ethnic population of women 40–55 years of age. *American Journal of Epidemiology 152*(5), 463–473.

Gold, E. B., Block, G., Crawford, S., Lachance, L., FitzGerald, G., Miracle, H., & Sherman, S. (2004). Lifestyle and demographic factors in relation to vasomotor symptoms: Baseline results from the study of women's health across the nation. *American Journal of Epidemiology, 159*(12), 1189–1199.

Gold, E. B., Colvin, A., Avis, N., Bromberger, J., Greendale, G. A., Powell, L., … Matthews, K. (2006). Longitudinal analysis of the association between vasomotor symptoms and race/ethnicity across the menopausal transition: Study of women's health across the nation. *American Journal of Public Health, 96*(7), 1226–1235. doi: 10.2105/AJPH.2005.066936

Gracia, C. R., Sammel, M. D., Freeman, E. W., Lin, H., Langan, E., Kapoor, S., & Al, E. (2005). Defining menopausal status: Creation of a new definition to identify the early changes of the menopausal transition. *Menopause, 12*, 128–135.

Greene, J. G. (1983). Bereavement and social support at the climacteric. *Maturitas, 5*, 115–124.

Greene, J. G., & Cooke, D. J. (1980). Life Stress and symptoms at the climacterium. *British Journal of Psychiatry, 136*, 486–491.

Hardy, R., & Kuh, D. (2002). Change in psychological and vasomotor symptom reporting during the menopause. *Social Science & Medicine, 55*, 1975–1988.

Harlow, B. L., Cohen, L. S., Otto, M. W., Spiegelman, D., & Cramer, D. W. (1999). Prevalence and predictors of depressive symptoms in older perimenopausal women. *Archives of General Psychiatry, 56*, 418–424.

Harlow, S. D., Gass, M., Hall, J. E., Lobo, R., Maki, P. M., Rebar, R., ... de Villiers, T. J. (2012). Executive summary of the stages of reproductive aging workshop + 10: Addressing the unfinished agenda of staging reproductive aging. *Menopause: The Journal of the North American Menopause Society, 19*(4), 1159–1168. doi: 10.1097/gme.0b013e31824d8f40

Harlow, B. L., Wise, L. A., Otto, M. W., Soares, C. N., & Cohen, L. S. (2003). Depression and its influence on reproductive endocrine and menstrual cycle markers associated with perimenopause. *Archives of General Psychiatry, 60*, 29–36.

Hecht, E., & Mensh, I. N. (1975). Life's ups and downs may leave you down and out. *Contemporary Psychology, 20*(8), 639–640. http://dx.doi.org/10.1037/0013564.

Holte, A., & Mikkelsen, A. (1991). The menopausal syndrome: A factor analytic replication. *Maturitas, 13*(3), 193–203. http://dx.doi.org/10.1016/0378-5122(91)90194-U.

Hunter, M. (1992). The South-East England longitudinal study of the climacteric and postmenopause. *Maturitas, 14*, 117–126.

Igarashi, M., Saito, H., Morioka, Y., Oiji, A., Nadaoka, T., & Kashiwakura, M. (2000). Stress vulnerability and climacteric symptoms: Life events, coping behavior, and severity of symptoms. *Gynecologic & Obstetric Investigation, 49*(3), 170–178.

Jiménez, L. J., & Pérez, S. G. (1999). The attitude of the woman in menopause and its influence on the climacteric. *Ginecología Obstetricia de México, 67*, 319–322.

Joffe, H., Fagioli, L. P., Koukopoulos, A., Viguera, A. C., Hirschberg, A., Nonacs, R., ... Cohen, L. S. (2011). Increased estradiol and improved sleep, but not hot flashes, predict enhanced mood during the menopausal transition. *Journal of Clinical Endocrinology and Metabolism, 96*(7), 1044–1054.

Joffe, H., Hall, J. E., Soares, C. N., Hennen, J., Reilly, C. J., Carlson, K., & Cohen, L. S. (2002). Vasomotor symptoms are associated with depression in perimenopausal women seeking primary care. *Menopause, 9*, 392–398.

Joffe, H., Soares, C. N., Petrillo, L. F., Viguera, A. C., Somley, B. L., Koch, J. K., & Cohen, L. S. (2007). Treatment of depression and menopause-related symptoms with the serotonin-norepinephrine reuptake inhibitor duloxetine. *Journal of Clinical Psychiatry, 64*(6), 473–479.

Kafanelis, B. V., Kostanski, M., Komesaroff, P. A., & Stojanovska, L. (2009). Being in the script of menopause: Mapping the complexities of coping strategies. *Qualitative Health Research, 19*(1), 30–41. doi:10.1177/1049732308327352.

Kornstein, S. G., Schatzberg, A. F., Thase, M. E., Yonkers, K. A., McCullough, J. P., Keitner, G. I., ... Keller, M. B. (2000). Gender differences in treatment response to sertraline versus imipramine in chronic depression. *American Journal of Psychiatry, 157*(9), 1445–1452.

Kornstein, S. G., Young, E. A., Harvey, A. T., Wisniewski, S. R., Barkin, J. L., Thase, M. E., ... Rush, A. J. (2010). The influence of menopausal status and postmenopausal use of hormone therapy on presentation of major depression in women. *Menopause, 17*(4), 828–839. doi: 10.1097/gme.0b013e3181d770a8

Kraepelin, E., & Diefendorf, A. R. (1907). *Clinical psychiatry: A textbook for students and physicians, abstracted and adapted from the 7th German edition of Kraepelin's Lehrbuch der Psychiatrie (new ed., rev, and augmented)*. New York, NY: Macmillan.

Kronenberg, F. (1990). Hot flashes: Epidemiology and physiology. *Annals of the New York Academy of Science, 592*, 52–86.

Kulkarni, J., Fitzgerald, P., & Seeman, M. V. (2012). The clinical needs of women with schizophrenia. In D. Castle, D. Copolov, T. Wykes, & K. Mueser (Eds.), *Pharmacological and psychosocial treatments in schizophrenia* (pp. 183–201). London: Informa Healthcare.

Lazarus, R. S. (1991). Emotion and adaptation. In L. A. Pervin (Ed.), *Handbook of personality: Theory and research* (pp. 609–637). New York, NY: Guilford.

Lee, Y., & Kim, H. (2008). Relationships between menopausal symptoms, depression, and exercise in middle-aged women: A cross-sectional survey. *International Journal of Nursing Studies, 45*, 1816–1822.

Lokuge, S., Frey, B. N., Foster, J. A., Soares, C. N., & Steiner, M. (2011). Depression in women: Windows of vulnerability and new insights into the link between estrogen and serotonin. *The Journal of Clinical Psychiatry, 72*(11), e1563–e1569. doi:10.4088/JCP.11com07089.

Mahe, V., & Dumain, A. (2001). Oestrogen withdrawal associated psychoses. *Acta Psychiatrica Scandinavica, 104*, 323–331.

Matsuda, T., Nakano, Y., Kanda, T., Iwata, H., & Baba, A. (1991). Gonadal hormones affect the hypothermia induced by serotonin1A (5-HT1A) receptor activation. *Life Sciences, 48*(17), 1627–1632. http://dx.doi.org/10.1016/0024-3205(91)90122-R.

Miech, R. A., & Shanahan, M. J. (2000). Socioeconomic status and depression over the life course. *Journal of Health and Social Behavior, 41*(2), 162–176. http://dx.doi.org/10.2307/2676303.

Mirzaiinjmabadi, K., Anderson, D., & Barnes, M. (2006). The relationship between exercise, Body Mass Index and menopausal symptoms in midlife Australian women. *International Journal of Nursing Practice, 12*(1), 28–34.

Moline, M. L., Broch, L., Zak, R., & Gross, V. (2003). Sleep in women across the life cycle from adulthood through menopause. *Sleep Medicine Reviews, 7*(2), 155–177. http://dx.doi.org/10.1053/smrv.2001.0228.

Morrison, J. H., Brinton, R. D., Schmidt, P. J., & Gore, A. C. (2006). Estrogen, menopause, and the aging brain: How basic neuroscience can inform hormone therapy in women. *Journal of Neuroscience, 26*(41), 10332–10348. doi:10.1523/jneurosci.3369-06.2006.

Morse, C. A., Dudley, E., Guthrie, J., & Dennerstein, L. (1998). Relationships between premenstrual complaints and perimenopausal experiences. *Journal of Psychosomatic Obstetrics & Gynecology, 19*(4), 182–191.

Murrell, S. A., Himmelfarb, S., & Wright, K. (1983). Prevalence of depression and its correlates in older adults. *American Journal of Epidemiology, 117*(2), 173–185.

Ozturk, O., Eraslan, D., Mete, H. E., & Ozsener, S. (2006). The risk factors and symptomatology of perimenopausal depression. *Maturitas, 55*(2), 180–186. http://dx.doi.org/10.1016/j.maturitas.2006.02.001.

Parry, B. L. (2008). Perimenopausal depression. *American Journal of Psychiatry, 165*(1), 23–27. doi:10.1176/appi.ajp.2007.07071152.

Parry, B. L. (2010). Optimal management of perimenopausal depression. *International Journal of Women's Health, 2*, 143–151.

Payne, J. L. (2003). The role of estrogen in mood disorders in women. *International Review of Psychiatry, 15*, 280–290. doi:10.1080/0954026031000136893.

Payne, J. L., Roy, P. S., Murphy-Eberenz, K., Weismann, M. M., Swartz, K. L., McInnis, M. G., ... Potash, J. B. (2007). Reproductive cycle-associated mood symptoms in women with major depression and bipolar disorder. *Journal of Affective Disorders, 99*(1–3), 221–229. Retrieved from http://dx.doi.org/10.1016/j.jad.2006.08.013

Payne, J. L., Teitelbaum, P. J., & Joffe, H. (2009). A reproductive subtype of depression: Conceptualizing models and moving toward etiology. *Harvard Review of Psychiatry, 17*(2), 72–86. doi:10.1080/10673220902899706.

Raup, J. L., & Myers, J. E. (1989). The empty nest syndrome: Myth or reality? *Journal of Counseling & Development, 68*(2), 180–183.

Reed, M. J., & Kloosterboer, H. J. (2004). Tibolone: A selective tissue estrogenic activity regulator (STEAR). *Maturitas, 48*(Supplement 1), 4–6.

Reed, S. D., Ludman, E. J., Newton, K. M., Grothaus, L. C., LaCroix, A. Z., Nekhlyudov, L., ... Bush, T. (2009). Depressive symptoms and menopausal burden in the midlife. *Maturitas, 62*(3), 306–310.

Richards, M., Rubinow, D. R., Daly, R. C., & Schmidt, P. J. (2006). Premenstrual symptoms and perimenopausal depression. *American Journal of Psychiatry, 163*(1), 133–137. doi:10.1176/appi.ajp.163.1.133.

Riecher-Rössler, A. (2003). Oestrogens and schizophrenia. *Current Opinion in Psychiatry, 16*(2), 187–192.

Riecher-Rössler, A. (2005). Estrogens and schizophrenia. In N. Bergemann & A. Riecher-Rössler (Eds.), *Estrogen effects in psychiatric disorders* (pp. 31–52). Wien: Springer.

Risch, N., Herrell, R., Lehner, T., Liang, K. Y., Eaves, L., Hoh, J., ... Merikangas, K. R. (2009). Interaction between the serotonin transporter gene (5-httlpr), stressful life events, and risk of depression: A meta-analysis. *Journal of the American Medical Association, 301*(23), 2462–2471. doi: 10.1001/jama.2009.878

Rostrosky, S. S., & Travis, C. B. (1996). Menopause research and the dominance of the biomedical model 1984-1994. *Psychology of Women Quarterly, 20*, 285–312.

Rubinow, D. R., Roca, C. A., & Schmidt, P. J. (2007). Estrogens and depression in women. In R. A. Lobo (Ed.), *Treatment of the postmenopausal woman: Basic and clinical aspects*. New York, NY: Elsevier.

Rubinow, D. R., Schmidt, P. J., & Roca, C. A. (1998). Estrogen-serotonin interactions: Implications for affective regulation. *Biological Psychiatry, 44*(9), 839–850. http://dx.doi.org/10.1016/S0006-3223(98)00162-0.

Schiff, I., Regestein, Q., Tulchinsky, D., & Ryan, K. J. (1979). Effects of estrogens on sleep and psychological state of hypogonadal women. *Journal of the American Medical Association, 242*(22), 2405–2407.

Schmidt, P. J., Haq, N., & Rubinow, D. R. (2004). A longitudinal evaluation of the relationship between reproductive status and mood in perimenopausal women. *American Journal of Psychiatry, 161*(12), 2238–2244. doi:10.1176/appi.ajp.161.12.2238.

Schmidt, P. J., Murphy, J., Haq, N., Rubinow, D. R., & Danaceau, M. (2004). Stressful life events, personal losses, and perimenopause-related depression. *Archives of Women's Mental Health, 7*(1), 19–26.

Schmidt, P. J., Nieman, L., Danaceau, M. A., Tobin, M. B., Roca, C. A., Murphy, J. H., & Rubinow, D. R. (2000). Estrogen replacement in perimenopause-related depression: A preliminary report. *American Journal of Obstetrics and Gynecology, 183*(2), 414–420. Retrieved from http://dx.doi.org/10.1067/mob.2000.106004

Schmidt, P. J., Roca, C. A., Bloch, M., & Rubinow, D. R. (1997). The perimenopause and affective disorders.*Seminars in Reproductive Endocrinology, 15*(1),91–100.doi:10.1055/s-2008-1067971.

Schmidt, P. J., & Rubinow, D. R. (1991). Menopause-related affective disorders: A justification for further study. *American Journal of Psychiatry, 148*(7), 844–852.

Seritan, A. L., Iosif, A. M., Park, J. H., DeatherageHand, D., Sweet, R. L., & Gold, E. B. (2010). Self-reported anxiety, depressive, and vasomotor symptoms: A study of perimenopausal women presenting to a specialized midlife assessment center. *Menopause, 17*(2), 410–415.

Soares, C. N., Almeida, O. P., Joffe, H., & Cohen, L. S. (2001). Efficacy of estradiol for the treatment of depressive disorders in perimenopausal women: A double-blind, randomized, placebo-controlled trial. *Archives of General Psychiatry, 58*(6), 529–534.

Soares, C. N., Arsenio, H., Joffe, H., Bankier, B., Cassano, P., Petrillo, L. F., & Cohen, L. S. (2006). Escitalopram versus ethinyl estradiol and norethindrone acetate for symptomatic peri- and postmenopausal women: Impact on depression, vasomotor symptoms, sleep, and quality of life. *Menopause, 13*(5), 780–786.

Soares, C. N., Poitras, J. R., Prouty, J., Alexander, A. B., Shifren, J. L., & Cohen, L. S. (2003). Efficacy of citalopram as a monotherapy or as an adjunctive treatment to estrogen therapy for perimenopausal and postmenopausal women with depression and vasomotor symptoms. *Journal of Clinical Psychiatry, 64*(4), 473–479.

Soules, M. R., Sherman, S., Parrott, E., Rebar, R., Santoro, N., Utian, W., & Woods, N. (2001). Executive summary: Stages of reproductive aging workshop (STRAW). *Climacteric, 4*(4), 267–272.

Sternfeld, B., Quesenberry, C., & Husson, G. (1999). Habitual physical activity and menopausal symptoms. *Journal of Women's Health, 8*, 115–123.

Stewart, D. E., & Boydell, K. M. (1993). Psychologic distress during menopause: Associations across the reproductive life cycle. *International Journal of Psychiatry in Medicine, 23*, 157–162.

Stotland, N. L. (2002). Menopause: Social expectations, women's realities. *Archives of Women's Mental Health, 5*(1), 5–8. doi:10.1007/s007370200016.

Sumner, B. E. H. (1995). Estrogen increases the density of 5-hydroxytryptamine2A receptors in cerebral cortex and nucleus accumbens in the female rat. *The Journal of Steroid Biochemistry and Molecular Biology, 54*(1–2), 15. http://dx.doi.org/10.1016/0960-0760(95)00075-B.

Swegle, J. M., & Kelly, M. W. (2004). Tibolone: A unique version of hormone replacement therapy. *Annals of Pharmacotherapy, 38*(5), 874–881. doi:10.1345/aph.1D462.

Tam, L. W., Stucky, V., Hanson, R. E., & Parry, B. L. (1999). Prevalence of depression in menopause: A pilot study. *Archives of Women's Mental Health, 2*(4), 175–181.

Thurston, R., Joffe, H., Soares, C. N., & Harlow, B. L. (2006). Physical activity and risk of vasomotor symptoms in women with and without a history of depression: Results from the Harvard study of moods and cycles. *Menopause, 13*, 553–560.

Timur, S., & Sahin, N. H. (2010). The prevalence of depression symptoms and influencing factors among perimenopausal and postmenopausal women. *Menopause, 17*(3), 545–551.

Veeninga, A. T., & Kraaimaat, F. W. (1989). Life stress and symptoms in menopause clinic patients and non-patients. *Journal of Psychosomatic Obstetrics & Gynecology, 10*(3), 269–277. doi:10.3109/01674828909016700.

Whiteman, M. K., Staropoli, C. A., Benedict, J. C., Borgeest, C., & Flaws, J. A. (2003). Risk factors for hot flashes in midlife women. *Journal of Women's Health, 12*, 459–472.

Wilbur, J., Dan, A., Hedricks, C., & Holm, K. (1990). The relationship among menopausal status, menopausal symptoms, and physical activity in midlife women. *Family and Community Health, 13*, 67–78.

Woods, N. F., & Mitchell, E. S. (1996). Patterns of depressed mood in midlife women: Observations from the Seattle midlife women's health study. *Research in Nursing and Health, 19*, 111–123.

Woods, N. F., & Mitchell, E. S. (1997). Pathways to depressed mood for midlife women: Observations from the Seattle midlife women's health study. *Research in Nursing and Health, 20*, 119–129.

Woods, N. F., Smith-DiJulio, K., Percival, D. B., Tao, E. Y., Mariella, A., & Mitchell, E. S. (2008). Depressed mood during the menopausal transition and early postmenopause: Observations from the Seattle midlife women's health study. *Menopause: The Journal of The North American Menopause Society, 15*(3), 223–232.

Worsley, R., Davis, S. R., Gavrilidis, E., Gibbs, Z., Lee, S., Burger, H., & Kulkarni, J. (2012). Hormonal therapies for new onset and relapsed depression during perimenopause. *Maturitas, 73*(2), 127–133. doi: 10.1016/j.maturitas.2012.06.011

Writing Group for the Women's Health Initiative Investigators. (2002). Risks and benefits of estrogen plus progestin in healthy postmenopausal women: Principal results from the women's health initiative randomized controlled trial. *Journal of the American Medical Association, 288*(3), 321–333. doi:10.1001/jama.288.3.321.

Zweifel, J. E., & O'Brien, W. H. (1997). A meta-analysis of the effect of hormone replacement therapy upon depressed mood. *Psychoneuroendocrinology, 22*(3), 189–212.

Part IV
Across the Lifespan

Eating Disorders Across the Life-Span: From Menstruation to Menopause

Stephanie Zerwas and Elizabeth Claydon

Introduction

In this chapter we review key issues for reproductive mental health in women with anorexia nervosa, bulimia nervosa, binge eating disorder (BED), and purging disorder. We take a developmental lens and cover four main periods across the female life-span that can impact the onset, course, and maintenance of eating disorders. First, we define eating disorders. Second, we address prenatal issues associated with eating disorders in adolescence and young adulthood including the role of estradiol for eating disorder risk, endocrine dysfunction, amenorrhea and oligomenorrhea that accompany the illness, and fertility concerns for women with eating disorders. Third, we cover perinatal issues associated with eating disorders during pregnancy including course of illness during pregnancy, pregnancy outcomes, birth outcomes, and perinatal mental health. Fourth, we discuss the postpartum issues associated with eating disorders including weight retention concerns, postpartum mood disorders, and early child feeding. Finally, we discuss midlife issues for eating disorder onset and relapse. By examining eating disorder behaviors across the life-span, we can explicate the dynamic interplay between women's physical development, eating disorder symptoms, and overall mental health.

S. Zerwas, Ph.D. (✉)
Department of Psychiatry, School of Medicine at the University of North Carolina, Chapel Hill, NC, USA
e-mail: stephanie_zerwas@med.unc.edu

E. Claydon, M.P.H.
Department of Chronic Disease Epidemiology,
Yale University School of Public Health, New Haven, CT, USA

Eating Disorders

Although eating disorders have distinct features, they share common symptoms including the overevaluation of weight for self-worth, dysregulation in eating behavior, and obsessive ruminative thoughts about food, weight, and body shape. In particular, anorexia nervosa (AN) is marked by extremely low body weight of less than 85 % of an ideal body weight for height and age, cognitive distortions related to body shape and weight perception, and severe food restriction. Bulimia nervosa (BN) is marked by periods of binge eating in which a large amount of food is consumed with a perceived sense of loss of control over eating. Binge eating is followed by inappropriate behavior to compensate for the amount of food consumed including purging, excessive exercise, and fasting (American Psychiatric Association, 2013).

The most recent version of the *Diagnostic and Statistical Manual* (DSM-5) also witnessed the addition of a new eating disorder diagnosis: BED. BED is marked by repeated binge eating episodes combined with loss of control but no inappropriate compensatory behavior in response. In addition, although it is not recognized in DSM-5, many researchers also consider purging disorder (PD) to be a possible diagnostic category worthy of further study. PD is marked by purging episodes, but unlike purging in BN, purging does not follow binge eating episodes with a loss of control but instead accompanies average-size meals or snacks (Keel, Haedt, & Edler, 2005). In the best epidemiological studies of eating disorder prevalence, approximately 1 % of women will suffer from AN, 1.5 % will suffer from BN, and 1 % will suffer from PD over their life. BED is by far the most prevalent eating disorder with a lifetime prevalence of 3.5 % for women (Hudson, Hiripi, Pope, & Kessler, 2007).

The medical and psychological consequences of AN, BN, BED, and PD can be both debilitating and life threatening. AN, in particular, has the highest mortality of any psychiatric illness (Berkman, Lohr, & Bulik, 2007; Birmingham, Su, Hlynsky, Goldner, & Gao, 2005; Harris & Barraclough, 1998; Millar et al., 2005; Papadopoulos, Ekbom, Brandt, & Ekselius, 2009; Sullivan, 1995). The psychiatric correlates of eating disorders include depression, anxiety, social withdrawal, and heightened self-consciousness (Birmingham et al., 2005; Fernandez-Aranda et al., 2007; Godart, Flament, Perdereau, & Jeammet, 2002; Halmi et al., 1991; Javaras et al., 2008; Kaplan, 1993; Katzman, 2005; Kaye et al., 2004; Keel, Mitchell, Miller, Davis, & Crow, 1999; Millar et al., 2005; Mitchell, Specker, & de Zwaan, 1991; Papadopoulos et al., 2009; Reichborn-Kjennerud, Bulik, Sullivan, Tambs, & Harris, 2004; Sharp & Freeman, 1993; Sullivan, 1995; Zipfel, Lowe, Reas, Deter, & Herzog, 2000). The medical sequelae include electrolyte imbalances, cardiac arrhythmias, osteoporosis and osteopenia, tooth decay, gastroesophageal reflux disease, and gastric rupture (Brown & Mehler, 2013; Brownell & Fairburn, 1995; Bulik & Reichborn-Kjennerud, 2003; Katzman, 2005). Medical complications such as osteoporosis can persist throughout life even after weight restoration and recovery (Rigotti, Neer, Skates, Herzog, & Nussbaum, 1991). Most notably for reproductive mental health, eating disorders are also associated with significant disruptions to the neuroendocrine system (Abraham, Pettigrew, Boyd, Russell, & Taylor, 2005; Andersen & Ryan, 2009;

Pinheiro et al., 2007; Watson & Andersen, 2003). The impact of malnutrition associated with eating disorders on reproductive hormones is discussed throughout the chapter with a focus on the unique impact at each life stage.

Etiology

For many years eating disorders were conceptualized primarily from a sociocultural model, with much of the blame unfairly directed towards families and parenting as being the primary causal factor for the development of eating disorders. However, over the past 30 years, an enhanced understanding of the biology of eating disorders has resulted in the identification of genetic, neurological, and environmental risk factors (Bulik et al., 2006; Strober, Freeman, Lampert, Diamond, & Kaye, 2000). Thus, the current view maintains a biopsychosocial model of eating disorder etiology in which the development of eating psychopathology is due to biological, psychological, and social factors (Keel, Leon, & Fulkerson, 2001; Rutter, Moffitt, & Caspi, 2006).

Eating disorders run in families due to genetic factors rather than due to parenting behaviors explained by shared environment. Heritability estimates range from 33 to 84 % for AN, 28 to 83 % for BN, and 41 to 57 % for BED, with the remaining variance typically attributable to unique environment factors (Bulik & Tozzi, 2004; Javaras et al., 2008; Thornton, Mazzeo, & Bulik, 2011). No studies have yet been published on the heritability of PD, although self-induced vomiting is highly heritable (72 %; Sullivan, Bulik, & Kendler, 1998). In addition, research on the neurocircuitry of eating disorders has demonstrated that eating disorders are accompanied by altered reward mechanisms including possible anterior ventral striatal pathway dysfunction and altered gustatory processing in the anterior insula (Kaye, Wagner, Fudge, & Paulus, 2011).

Although they can occur throughout the life-span, these disorders primarily begin in mid to late adolescence with an average age of onset between 15 and 22 years of age (Hudson et al., 2007). Puberty and its associated neuroendocrine changes, in particular, may trigger the expression of an eating disorder for those with a genetic predisposition. Cross-sectional and longitudinal studies comparing early-adolescent to middle- and late-adolescent twins have demonstrated a negligible heritability of disordered eating behaviors and weight and shape concerns in younger twins, but higher heritability with the onset of puberty (Baker et al., 2009; Klump et al., 2010; Klump, Keel, Sisk, & Burt, 2010). Although the biological mechanisms that lead to the increase of heritability in puberty are unknown, twin studies have suggested a potential role for estradiol (Klump, Burt et al., 2010; Klump, Keel et al., 2010). However, in some animal models ovarian hormones were not found to contribute to binge eating behavior (Klump, Suisman, Culbert, Kashy, & Sisk, 2011).

Social and psychological risk factors for the development of eating disorders include life trauma (Bulik, Prescott, & Kendler, 2001; Kendler et al., 2000), childhood anxiety (Raney et al., 2008), harm avoidance and perfectionism (Fassino, Amianto, Gramaglia, Facchini, & Abbate Daga, 2004), difficulties with set shifting (Steinglass, Walsh, & Stern, 2006; Tchanturia et al., 2004), impulsivity

(Racine, Culbert, Larson, & Klump, 2009; Wonderlich, Connolly, & Stice, 2004), and problems with emotion regulation (Harrison, Tchanturia, & Treasure, 2010; Heatherton & Baumeister, 1991). However, all biological, psychological, social risk, and protective factors for eating disorders are best conceptualized as probabilistic rather than deterministic (Rutter et al., 2006).

Of special interest for reproductive mental health, environmental risk factors experienced at birth such as preterm birth or neonatal immaturity may also place children and adults at risk for later eating disorders. Research on "fetal programming" posits that environmental influences on the fetal environment could lead to long-term, and perhaps permanent, effects on the structure and functioning of organs leading to risk for the long-term physical and mental health of offspring (Barker, 2004; Gluckman & Hanson, 2004; Schlotz & Phillips, 2009).

Bulik and colleagues have hypothesized that maternal eating disorders during pregnancy lead to a cycle of risk for eating disorder development in subsequent generations (Bulik, Reba, Siega-Riz, & Reichborn-Kjennerud, 2005). In addition to genetic risk factors, maternal eating disorders during pregnancy could lead to fetal undernutrition, overexposure to stress hormones, labor and delivery complications, and low birth weight (Micali & Treasure, 2009). These experiences during the sensitive fetal period could, in turn, place the children of mothers with eating disorders at increased risk for diminished cognitive function, behavioral problems, stress reactivity, and psychopathology throughout their life-span (Schlotz & Phillips, 2009). In fact, with data from large medical birth registries, research has demonstrated that pregnancy and obstetric complications such as gestational diabetes, maternal anemia, and placental infarction are significant risk factors for the development of eating disorders (Favaro, Tenconi, & Santonastaso, 2006). Thus, the combination of genetic risk for eating disorders and increased risk of perinatal malnutrition and birth complications associated with maternal eating disorders may lead to a cycle of long-term and trans-generational risk.

Antenatal Eating Disorders

Prior to conception, there are many ways in which eating disorders can, and do, affect a woman's reproductive viability, her attitude towards pregnancy, and ultimately the outcome of a potential pregnancy. This section addresses some of the antenatal changes and consequences that can result as a consequence of eating disorder behaviors and symptoms.

Amenorrhea/Oligomenorrhea

Although commonly associated with the restrictive subtype of anorexia, amenorrhea or the absence of regular menstrual cycles can also be present in individuals with BN and BED (Abraham et al., 2005; Andersen & Ryan, 2009; Ehrmann, 2005; Naessén &

Hirschberg, 2011; Pinheiro et al., 2007; Watson & Andersen, 2003). Oligomenorrhea, or the presence of menstrual periods that are infrequent or exceptionally light, can also be a consequence of most eating disorders. A survey of 241 inpatients with eating disorders illustrated the prevalence of amenorrhea/oligomenorrhea across diagnosis with 24 % of patients presenting with eating disorder not otherwise specified (EDNOS) and 18 % of patients with BN experiencing menstrual disturbance (Abraham et al., 2005). However, the cause of amenorrhea and oligomenorrhea may emanate from different origins and they have diverging trajectories for each diagnosis.

In anorexia, amenorrhea typically results from low body fat due to restricted caloric and nutrient intake (Pinheiro et al., 2007). With lower body fat content there also comes a decrease in naturally occurring levels of leptin and ghrelin, two important hormones that influence energy balance and menstruation (Andersen & Ryan, 2009; Pinelli & Tagliabue, 2007). As part of the hypothalamic-pituitary-ovarian axis, these changes influence the body's ability to meet the energy requirements needed for menstruation. Even in diagnoses of EDNOS that have AN-like symptoms, there is evidence that women struggle with amenorrhea and oligomenorrhea despite being above the 85th percentile in weight (Watson & Andersen, 2003). Therefore, factors other than weight can play a role in the advent and continuation of amenorrhea or irregular menses, including excessive exercise (Pinheiro et al., 2007).

Polycystic ovarian syndrome (PCOS) has also routinely been found to be associated with eating disorders, especially BN and BED. PCOS modifies both sex hormones and menstrual cycles significantly and has also been correlated with craving sweets and binge eating due to the disrupted hormones (Hirschberg, Naessen, Stridsberg, Bystrom, & Holtet, 2004). High androgen levels as a result of PCOS may also lead to bulimic behavior through increased cravings and diminished impulse control (Resch, Szendei, & Haasz, 2004a, 2004b). Binge eating is actually cited as a more common occurrence among individuals with oligomenorrhea, secondary to their eating disorder (Pinheiro et al., 2007).

Prenatal and Perinatal Eating Disorders

Sexual Functioning

Pregnancy in women with AN was long thought to be rare due to the psychological and psychosocial features of the disorder coupled with the endocrinological disturbances and amenorrhea associated with malnutrition. In general, women with eating disorders report higher levels of sexual dysfunction. A significant percentage of women with AN, BN, and PD report a loss of libido (75 %, 39 %, and 45.4 %, respectively), and overall women with active eating disorders report decreased sexual desire (66.9 %) and increased sexual anxiety (59.2 %; Pinheiro et al., 2010). In particular, a lower body mass index (BMI) predicts a greater loss of libido, more sexual anxiety, and fewer sexual relationships.

From a biological perspective, low body weight affects the physiological functioning of sexual organs, and changes in BMI have been directly associated with fluctuations in sexual interest (Beumont, Abraham, & Simson, 1981; Hsu, 1980; Morgan, Lacey, & Reid, 1999). From a psychological perspective, women who attain a lower BMI body may also feel more dissatisfaction with body weight and body shape and experience more distortion of body size. Thus, they may also experience more discomfort with physical contact and physical exposure, which contributes to a loss of libido and an increase in sexual anxiety. With weight restoration and recovery, women with eating disorders commonly report an increase in sexual drive, likely due to both biological and psychosocial factors (Morgan, Lacey, & Reid, 1999). Changes in sexual functioning are likely to be multifactorial in patients with eating disorders and represent a convergence of physiological and psychological factors.

Fertility

Clinically, worries about current or future fertility represent one of the most reported motivators for treatment and weight restoration in women. However, studies on fertility outcomes in women with eating disorders have been equivocal. Some have not found differences in fertility between women with histories of AN or BN when compared with controls, demonstrating that despite high levels of amenorrhea and oligomenorrhea, women with AN can become pregnant (Brinch, Isager, & Tolstrup, 1988; Bulik et al., 1999). However, others have found that women with AN have children at one-third the rate of women without an eating disorder history (Brinch et al., 1988). Moreover, there is an especially high prevalence (16–20 %) of women meeting eating disorder criteria within a fertility specialist clinic setting in comparison to the lifetime prevalence of eating disorders in women within the general population (~5–6 %; Bulik et al., 1999; Freizinger, Franko, Dacey, Okun, & Domar, 2010; Hudson et al., 2007). In a large population-based longitudinal study, women with AN were more likely to have seen a doctor for fertility concerns, taken longer than 6 months to conceive, and needed fertility treatment in order to conceive (Easter, Treasure, & Micali, 2011). Thus, at an individual clinical level, assessing whether lifetime eating disorder status will have a long-term effect on fertility is difficult, and there are no clear predictive algorithms to determine fertility during the eating disorder or after recovery.

Attitudes Towards Pregnancy

Upon becoming pregnant, many women with eating disorders and eating disorder histories struggle in adapting to this significant life transition. Women with eating disorders are more likely to report that they experienced negative feelings upon discovering that they were pregnant (Easter et al., 2011). However, by 18 weeks of gestation, there is no significant difference in their attitudes when compared to women without eating disorders. Pregnant women with eating disorders have also been found to be two times more likely than referent women to endorse that motherhood meant giving up something important and were more likely to view motherhood as a personal sacrifice (Easter et al., 2011).

Again, the difficulty that women with eating disorders face during the transition to motherhood may be due to a combination of factors, both physical and psychological. First, women with AN have been found significantly more likely to be younger than the referent group at their first pregnancy and are perhaps not as prepared emotionally and developmentally for the challenges associated with pregnancy and parenting (Bulik et al., 2009; Micali, Treasure, & Simonoff, 2007). Second, the likelihood of an unplanned pregnancy is markedly higher for women with AN and BN than for women without eating disorders. There is a twofold increase in the risk of unplanned pregnancy for women with AN and a 30-fold increase of unplanned pregnancy for women with BN (Bulik et al., 2010; Morgan, Lacey, & Chung, 2006). Women with AN are also significantly more likely to have terminated a pregnancy at some point in their lives than women without an eating disorder (24.2 % vs. 14.6 %; Bulik et al., 2010). Although the reasons for a higher likelihood of an unplanned and terminated pregnancy are unclear, researchers speculate that it may be due to patients' belief that amenorrhea or oligomenorrhea conveys a lack of fertility and thus they do not arrange for adequate contraception under the mistaken belief that they cannot become pregnant (Bulik et al., 2010). An unplanned pregnancy may reduce the likelihood that women with eating disorders can arrange for the critical nutritional and emotional support needed to manage the demands of pregnancy and motherhood, especially early in their pregnancy.

Finally, the demands of pregnancy and motherhood represent an immense challenge for women already struggling to recover both medically and psychologically from an eating disorder (Easter et al., 2011). Pregnancy requires a radical transformation in weight, size, and shape. In general, women with eating disorders report that they worry about gestational weight gain more than women without eating disorders. Specifically, 62.9 % of those with AN, 61.5 % of those with BN, 50 % of those with PD, and 24 % of those with BED endorse being "very worried" about gestational weight gain in comparison to 6.9 % of those without eating disorders (Swann et al., 2009). They may perceive the loss of the pre-pregnancy body that accompanies motherhood as a "sacrifice" (Easter et al., 2011). Pregnant women with eating disorders may feel additional stress as they struggle to adapt to "eating for the baby" while also managing the negative emotions and cognitions that accompany an increase in gestational weight and radical changes to their shape.

Eating Disorder Course

Fortunately, despite the anticipatory worry that many women report at the beginning of their pregnancies, large population-based prospective studies have found that the most common course of eating disorders during pregnancy is remission. For full remission, rates are 78 % for PD and 34 % for BN with an additional 29 % of women with BN attaining partial remission during pregnancy (Bulik et al., 2007).

However, estimates of remission from AN are extremely difficult to obtain because there are no clear criteria to establish maternal underweight during pregnancy (Bulik et al., 2007). Cohort studies have also found that weight and shape concerns decrease during pregnancy in women with active eating disorders (Fairburn, Stein, & Jones, 1992; Micali et al., 2007). Some women with eating disorders also report believing that pregnancy could be a means to recover from their disorder because they view gestational weight gain and a larger body size as more acceptable during pregnancy than under other circumstances (Lemberg & Phillips, 1989).

Although eating disorder diagnoses most often remit during pregnancy, women with eating disorders report greater continued use of laxatives, self-induced vomiting, and higher levels of vigorous exercise (defined as greater than 1 h of moderate–vigorous activity daily) during pregnancy than women without eating disorders (Micali et al., 2007). Women with AN are also more likely to smoke during pregnancy (37.1 % compared to 9.2 % in women without eating disorders), possibly due to concerns about weight and appetite control (Bulik et al., 2009).

Notably, women with BED are most likely to continue their eating disorder behaviors during pregnancy. In a large population-based Norwegian sample (the Mother and Baby Cohort Study—MoBa), a full 61 % of women with BED continued to have binge eating episodes with a loss of control while pregnant. Moreover, incident cases of BED are more common than any other eating disorder. In MoBa, 2 % of the ~42,000 mothers in the sample developed a new diagnosis of BED with repeated binge eating episodes and loss of control over eating. Thus, pregnancy may be a window of vulnerability for binge eating (Bulik et al., 2007).

From a biological perspective, a cascade of adaptive neuroendocrine changes occur during pregnancy that can affect brain functioning, metabolism, appetite, and mood (Russell, Douglas, & Ingram, 2001). Also, from a nutritional perspective, binge eating episodes often immediately follow a period of food restriction (Hagan et al., 2002). Women who attempt to eat with the same frequency and amount as prior to their pregnancy may unwittingly set themselves up for periods of intense hunger and as a result trigger a dysregulated eating pattern (Bulik et al., 2007).

From a psychological perspective, the emotional, financial, and social stress of pregnancy and anticipated motherhood may also trigger binge eating episodes. In the MoBa cohort, the mothers at greatest risk for incident BED were also more likely to have fewer years of education, more previous pregnancies, and lower income (Bulik et al., 2007).

New onset of AN, BN, and PD during pregnancy is extremely rare. However, in AN, there is also evidence that of those who had experienced a recovery from AN before becoming pregnant, approximately a third (33 %) relapsed in their eating disorder behavior during pregnancy (Koubaa, Hallstrom, Lindholm, & Hirschberg, 2005). In addition, some women with a history of eating disorders reported that they experienced an increase in overall weight and shape concerns during pregnancy (Micali et al., 2007). Thus, for women with histories of AN and BN, pregnancy can also be a sensitive period for the reemergence of symptoms.

Hyperemesis Gravidarum

Some have questioned whether self-induced vomiting prior to pregnancy could be a risk factor for hyperemesis gravidarum during pregnancy. Indeed, women with purging-type eating disorders are more likely to report both nausea and vomiting during pregnancy than those without an eating disorder (Torgersen et al., 2008), and some have also found an increased risk of hyperemesis gravidarum (Koubaa et al., 2005). Underweight pregnant women are more likely to use antiemetic drugs during their pregnancy and are also more likely to be hospitalized for the weight loss and electrolyte dysfunction associated with hyperemesis (Cedergren, Brynhildsen, Josefsson, Sydsjo, & Sydsjo, 2008). However, the mechanism predisposing women with pre-pregnancy vomiting and underweight to hyperemesis is unclear. Some women with pre-pregnancy eating disorders may attempt to hide their ongoing struggle with purging behaviors under the guise of hyperemesis (Lingam & McCluskey, 1996). However, neurobiological mechanisms and/or automatic learned behaviors could also contribute to the risk of both hyperemesis and continued self-induced vomiting. Self-induced vomiting is highly heritable which may suggest a biological pathway, although the neurobiology of hyperemesis is unclear (Goodwin, 2002; Sullivan et al., 1998).

Women with repeated experiences of self-induced purging may also have lower thresholds for vomiting in response to pregnancy-associated nausea than women without a history of purging. Nevertheless, women with a history of intentional purging behaviors should be counseled that intentional purging during pregnancy can have a significant impact on fetal nutrition and development, despite the fact that pregnancy-related vomiting is commonplace. Qualitatively, women with eating disorders report that they are also able to distinguish between pregnancy-related vomiting and intentional compensatory purging, a distinction, which could be leveraged in clinical care (Lacey & Smith, 1987).

Untreated Eating Disorders During Pregnancy

One of the primary challenges in knowing how to help a patient suffering with an eating disorder during pregnancy is that the physicians must know that their patient either has an eating disorder or has a history of one. Many obstetricians do not inquire into eating disorder histories and statuses, and expectant mothers do not always volunteer this information. Due to the heightened risk for caesarian sections and a trifold likelihood of postpartum depression among women with active eating disorders when compared to the general population, women with eating disorders should be considered to be in high-risk pregnancies and monitored closely by physicians both during and after pregnancy (Franko et al., 2001).

Postpartum Eating Disorders

The complications that ensue due to the presence of a maternal eating disorder do not end at delivery. Women with a lifetime or a recent history of an eating disorder are at greater risk for postpartum depression than the general population, and the risk of relapse and problems with breastfeeding are considerable concerns.

Postpartum Depression and Relapse

Multiple researchers have found that among pregnant women with active eating disorders, the likelihood of postpartum depression or postpartum distress is considerably higher than the general population (Abraham, Taylor, & Conti, 2001; Franko et al., 2001). BED and BN have the strongest correlation with postpartum depression with a two- to threefold increased risk, but there is still a trend seen in AN, which is in need of greater study (Mazzeo et al., 2006). Regardless, one of the hallmark traits of AN, perfectionism, seems to play a role in determining the severity of postpartum depression (Mazzeo, Slof-Op't Landt et al., 2006). Mothers with eating disorders also appear to struggle more with adjusting to lives with their newborns. Among women who were suffering from eating disorders (specifically AN or BN) prior to pregnancy, 92 % reported problems adjusting compared to only 13 % in the control group ($p<0.001$; Koubaa, Hallstrom, & Hirschberg, 2008).

Women with eating disorders may have a similar or a greater risk of developing perinatal and postpartum depression compared to women with a history of major depressive disorder and no eating disorder (Gavin et al., 2005; Mazzeo, Mitchell, Gerke, & Bulik, 2006). Active BN during pregnancy is a strong predictor of postpartum depression, inferring almost a threefold risk compared with women with quiescent BN during pregnancy (Morgan et al., 2006; Morgan, Lacey, & Sedgwick, 1999). Moreover, women with eating disorders are over-represented in women seeking postpartum depression treatment. In one study, 37 % of women seeking treatment for perinatal depression reported a lifetime diagnosis of an eating disorder, a three- to fourfold higher lifetime prevalence than in national general population samples (Meltzer-Brody et al., 2011). In addition, women with lifetime eating disorders, particularly those with a history of BN and PD, have also reported more severe perinatal depression (as measured by the Edinburgh Depression Inventory) than women with no eating disorder history (Meltzer-Brody et al., 2011).

Women with a higher residual postpartum weight—due to the likelihood of greater weight gain among women with eating disorders—may have a stronger desire to lose weight, thus falling back on some maladaptive weight-loss strategies they used in the past and some perhaps relapsing during this fragile time (Bulik et al., 2009). The presence of postpartum depression magnifies the risk of recurrence of a previous eating disorder or even crossover to a new diagnosis. Remission is the most typical course in pregnant women, but it is essential to understand that pregnancy does not offer a lasting protective effect for everyone (Bulik et al., 2009).

In a large-scale population-based study of postpartum eating disorders, only 59 % of women with AN, 30 % with BN, 57 % with PD, and 42 % with BED prior to pregnancy were in remission 3 years postpartum (Knoph et al., 2013). Both social support and psychological factors were associated with continuation of eating disorder symptoms. Women who reported less relationship satisfaction and greater psychological distress during the postpartum period were more likely to experience a continuation of eating disorder symptoms (in particular, BED symptoms; Knoph et al., 2013). These results highlight the need to provide women with eating disorders adequate social support and treatment for postpartum mood in order to preserve the symptom remission often seen during pregnancy.

Postpartum Dieting, Nutrition, and Body Image

Weight gain during pregnancy can be a source of stress for many women, and most women attempt to lose residual gestational weight in the weeks and months following delivery. In general, concerns about weight and weight loss attempts are normative with 75 % of women concerned about their weight in the first few weeks postpartum (Hiser, 1987; Stein & Fairburn, 1996) and an additional 70 % of women worried about their "flabby figure" (Hiser, 1987; Stein & Fairburn, 1996).

Perhaps because of this heightened awareness of weight and shape concerns among the majority of postpartum women, it is not surprising that almost three-quarters are still trying to lose weight at 4 months postpartum (Baker, Carter, Cohen, & Brownell, 1999; Stein & Fairburn, 1996). Therefore, this pattern of weight concerns and desire for weight loss postpartum are not solely restricted to women with histories of eating disorders. However, among individuals with eating disorders, especially anorexia, these feelings are exponentially heightened due to the preexisting hyper-focus on body weight and shape that defines the disease. There is also evidence that women with AN, BN, PD, and BED gain more gestational weight than women without eating disorders (Bulik et al., 2009). Therefore, it is not surprising that among women with eating disorders, Eating Disorder Examination Questionnaire (EDE-Q) scores are higher at postpartum than among women without an eating disorder diagnosis (Stein & Fairburn, 1996). Consequently, although weight concerns and weight loss are a prevalent concern among new mothers, the presence of an eating disorder exacerbates and exponentially heightens the distress around weight and the compulsion to lose gestational weight.

Breastfeeding and Infant Feeding

There is significant evidence that breastfeeding is the optimal practice for both maternal and child health due to immunological benefits for the child and a reduced risk of maternal breast and ovarian cancer, hypertension, and type 2 diabetes

(Galson, 2008; Schwarz et al., 2010; Stuebe et al., 2010, 2011). The American Academy of Pediatrics recommends exclusive breastfeeding for the first 6 months with continuation through the first year or longer to ensure optimal benefit (AAP, 2012). However, breastfeeding is still not utilized as the primary source of feeding for many mothers; among mothers with a history of an eating disorder, breastfeeding is often more truncated due to multiple concerns.

While one study found that women with lifetime histories of AN and BN are more likely to initiate breastfeeding and breastfeed just as long as or longer than women in the general population (Micali, Simonoff, & Treasure, 2009), others have found that those women with prenatal AN or EDNOS (including PD) are approximately two times more likely to stop breastfeeding early when compared to women without eating disorders (Blais et al., 2000; Larsson & Andersson-Ellstrom, 2003; Torgersen et al., 2010). This premature cessation of breastfeeding in mothers with a history of eating disorders begins soon after delivery. In a Scandinavian sample of women who self-reported histories of eating disorders, by the time their child was 3 months old, 19 % had ceased breastfeeding compared to only 7 % of mothers without a history of an eating disorder (Larsson & Andersson-Ellstrom, 2003).

As partial explanation for their shortened duration of breastfeeding, women with eating disorders often find the act of breastfeeding embarrassing and worry that this could alter their appearance (Stein & Fairburn, 1989; Waugh & Bulik, 1999). Some mothers with eating disorders do not even initiate breastfeeding due to these concerns (Waugh & Bulik, 1999). Mothers with eating disorders also endorse worrying that their breast milk will be insufficient for their infant's needs and that their infant may be allergic to their breast milk and are more likely to rigidly adhere to a prescribed feeding schedule, experiencing anxiety when their infant signals hunger cues outside of the prescribed feeding window (Evans & le Grange, 1995).

These differences also continue to rise in infant feeding. Women with a history of an eating disorder or a current episode during pregnancy are more likely to have infants with feeding difficulties, primarily due to the presence of maternal distress (Micali, Simonoff, Stahl, & Treasure, 2011). Maternal distress from perinatal depression and anxiety also partially mediates the relationship between eating disorder status and early infant feeding difficulties (Micali et al., 2011). Maternal emotional dysregulation, specifically in response to food or weight concerns, impairs the mother's ability to feed her newborn without a certain level of anxiety, which potentially could be conveyed to the infant. Women with eating disorders are also more likely to rate their infants as having a more difficult and fussy temperament, which may also contribute to feeding difficulties (Zerwas et al., 2012).

Midlife Eating Disorders

Typically eating disorders have been conceptualized as diseases that are bracketed within the teenage and young adult years. However, there is increasing evidence to suggest that the landscape for eating disorders has considerably changed to include an older age range than previously thought. Midlife eating disorders also comprise a more heterogeneous mix than eating disorders earlier in life (Bulik, 2013). For many, eating disorders in midlife could be the progression of a chronic eating disorder that began many years earlier in adolescence or early adulthood. For a smaller minority, it could represent a new diagnosis in a formerly healthy individual or a relapse from recovery (Bulik, 2013). Consequently, recognizing and treating these varied presentations and establishing effective treatments for chronic, recurrent, and new-onset eating disorders in midlife women are crucial.

Although there is little epidemiological data documenting increased eating disorders in midlife clinically, treatment centers report that they are witnessing greater numbers of women in midlife than seen previously. Among women over age 50, the greatest predictors for eating disorder symptoms, concerns, and behaviors are a younger age and a higher BMI (Gagne et al., 2012). Therefore it seems that the fear of aging and weight may be more pronounced in middle age and then decrease in the elderly population (Lewis & Cachelin, 2001).

This may be due to a cohort effect. Because an older generation of women did not have as much exposure to fat talk, "old talk," and unrealistic representations of beauty that dominate the current media landscape, they may have experienced less environmental pressure towards developing eating disorder symptoms (Becker, Diedrichs, Jankowski, & Werchan, 2013). This fear of aging has been directly tied to disordered eating and can emanate from both a personal source, but also in response to media focus on defying the effects of age, as well as "old talk" by friends and family members (Becker et al., 2013; Lewis & Cachelin, 2001). "Old talk" is defined as a parallel but distinct form of "fat talk" that specifically addresses nonconformance with the thin young ideal of female beauty (Becker et al., 2013; Lewis & Cachelin, 2001). Having this type of talk perpetuates body- and age-related anxiety and increases body image disturbances as well as eating disorder pathology among women most exposed to it (Becker et al., 2013). It also suggests that when women are young, the most salient feature of beauty is weight, whereas youth becomes a much more significant and salient concern as women age.

The hyper-focus on eating disorders in youth can be problematic for older individuals dealing with eating disorders for multiple reasons. Stigma and embarrassment about experiencing these problems in midlife could keep women suffering with eating disorders from seeking help. Because of the focus on youth eating disorders and eating disorder risk, they may feel ignored both by public attitudes on eating disorders and by treatment providers. Additionally, the majority of evidence-based treatments for eating disorders are targeted towards and based on findings from a younger population.

Menopause

In relation to understanding eating disorders in an older age range of women than previously studied, it is important to acknowledge one of the major life changes women face that may be associated with eating pathology. Menopause marks the cessation of menstruation and also changing hormone levels that affect metabolism and weight in women, thus contributing to factors that could increase the risk for disordered eating.

This is a relatively new area of study, and therefore the research concerning menopause and eating disorders is still rather limited; however, *anorexia tardive* was a term established in the 1980s to describe late onset of anorexia, occurring anytime after a woman's marriage and containing diagnoses that happened at or after menopause (Dally, 1984). This loss of weight was, at the time, seen as a desire to die, rather than expressing marital crises (Dally, 1984). A more recent conception of eating disorders around menopause suggests that the biological changes to the body and its deviation from both the thin and young ideal could cause women experiencing these changes to adopt maladaptive strategies to control their weight and slow the aging process (Becker et al., 2013).

Recently, a large-scale survey about shape and weight concerns was conducted in an older population of women, aged 50 and older. More than 70 % said that they were currently trying to lose weight, and 41 % said that they scrutinized their body at least once a day (Gagne et al., 2012). Additionally, several responses to an open-ended question reflected frustration with menopause-related weight gain (Gagne et al., 2012). Therefore, there is evidence to suggest that menopausal women are at risk for disordered eating and body image disturbances as well as possible eating disorders. Thus far, only one study has examined eating disorders, body image, and menopausal status in women at midlife (Mangweth-Matzek et al., 2006).

Perimenopausal women were significantly more likely to report eating disorder symptoms when compared to a referent group of premenopausal women (Mangweth-Matzek et al., 2006). Moreover, they were significantly more likely to report body image concerns including "feeling fat" and dissatisfaction with their weight (Mangweth-Matzek et al., 2006). Women with menopause due to hysterectomies also reported significantly higher eating and body image concerns (Mangweth-Matzek et al., 2006). Clearly, however, more research is needed to clarify the specific triggers and prognosis for eating disorders during the menopausal transition, and examining eating disorders in midlife could be a rich area of future study.

Clinical Implications

Fostering a greater understanding and screening of eating disorders across the lifespan are essential for women's physical and mental health and for the health of future generations. Clinicians in primary care and gynecology are an untapped resource to detect and treat women who are struggling with eating disorders (Mitchell-Gieleghem, Mittelstaedt, & Bulik, 2002; Sim et al., 2010). However, all too often, large-scale surveys have demonstrated that clinicians do not ask about eating disorder symptoms, and patients frequently do not discuss their struggle with eating disorders. For example, among patients who presented for treatment to an infertility clinic with oligomenorrhea or amenorrhea, 58–76.4 % of women met clinical indicators for eating disorders, but none had disclosed symptoms to their providers (Freizinger et al., 2010; Stewart, Robinson, Goldbloom, & Wright, 1990). Furthermore, 64 % of pregnant women did not report their eating disorder status to their obstetrician-gynecologists (OB-GYN), and of those who discussed their eating disorders with their OB-GYNs, only half found this to be helpful (Lemberg & Phillips, 1989).

Obstetrician-gynecologists also report that they are not confident in making an eating disorder diagnosis. Only 20 % report confidence in their ability to diagnose eating disorders, and only 54 % of gynecologists report that eating disorder assessment and screening fell within their scope of practice. However, 90.8 % reported that eating disorders could have a negative impact on pregnancy and birth outcomes (Leddy, Jones, Morgan, & Schulkin, 2009; Morgan, 1999). Much of the reluctance to screen for eating disorders may be due to lack of education, with an overwhelming majority reporting (88.5–96.2 %) that their training in diagnosing and treating eating disorders was barely adequate (Leddy et al., 2009).

Paradoxically, although primary care providers surveyed express reluctance to screen for eating disorders, the perinatal period could be viewed as a unique window of opportunity for recovery. Routine perinatal care gives OB-GYN providers the chance to screen for mental health issues and engage their patients in repeated monthly or even weekly visits (Borri et al., 2008; Hawkins & Gottlieb, 2013; Reck et al., 2008). In addition, women with eating disorders express motivation to eat and avoid inappropriate compensatory measures "for the baby" during their pregnancies and view weight gain during this period as more "socially acceptable." Moreover, postpartum women will report disordered eating symptoms when directly asked by providers (Broussard, 2012). Treatment and support may also be especially acute in the postpartum period, as the pressure to lose gestational weight and stress accompanying the demands of caring for a newborn often leads to the reemergence of symptoms (Knoph et al., 2013; Lacey & Smith, 1987; Morgan, Lacey, & Sedgwick, 1999).

Given the increased risk of perinatal depression and anxiety in women with eating disorders, additional screening for symptoms of depression and anxiety is critical. Although the awareness and assessment of perinatal and postpartum depression within the OB-GYN community have dramatically improved (Yonkers et al., 2009), raising awareness and screening of eating disorder symptoms during pregnancy are still desperately needed in order to capitalize on this unique window for eating disorder remission and recovery (Franko et al., 2001; Franko & Spurrell, 2000). Currently, screening for domestic violence and depression in pregnant and postpartum women is routine, but screening for eating disorders has only been recommended in women with a documented history (Agency for Healthcare Research and Policy, 2013). Given the fact that many providers do not ask about eating disorder histories and many patients do not tell, limiting screening to a documented history could fail to capture many women who are struggling during this important juncture.

Clinicians in primary care should also be educated about the risk of eating disorder emergence or reemergence during the perimenopausal period. Creating a safe environment for disclosure of symptoms also means identifying and addressing clinician biases about who can and cannot be affected by eating disorders. Although the highest risk of eating disorder onset is in mid-adolescence to early adulthood, increasingly women have been presenting with eating disorder symptoms in midlife (Hudson et al., 2007). Educating providers about the role of the menopausal transition for eating psychopathology may be necessary in order to ensure that providers do not assume that eating disorders are restricted only to young women.

Screening

Routine uniform screening for eating disorders across all levels of primary care and in OB-GYN offices would be the best way to improve their detection and treatment (Harris, 2010). The SCOFF questions (Luck et al., 2002; Morgan, Reid, & Lacey, 1999) have universally been identified as an excellent measure to assist providers when screening for eating disorders (Harris, 2010; Hawkins & Gottlieb, 2013; Hoffman, Zerwas, & Bulik, 2011; Sim et al., 2010). The SCOFF includes five short yes/no questions about possible eating disorder symptoms, and the acronym originates from the words used in the questions:

- S—Do you make yourself *sick/vomit* because you are uncomfortably full?
- C—Do you worry about loss of *control* over your eating?
- O—Have you recently lost *one* stone (14 lb) in 3 months?
- F—Do you believe you are *fat* although others say that you are thin?
- F—Would you say *food* predominates your life? (Morgan, Reid, & Lacey, 1999)

A positive screen (answering yes to two or more questions) suggests a referral to an eating disorder specialist and nutrition providers is necessary in order to ensure continued assessment and care.

Future Directions

The director of the National Institute of Mental Health, Dr. Thomas Insel, cites the mathematician and physicist Freeman Dyson to describe how innovations in technology have disrupted the past 10 years of mental health research, "New directions in science are launched by new tools much more often than by new concepts (Dyson, 1997)." Because of new tools, we have witnessed the launch of a new era of inquiry into the biological bases of mental health and a dramatic change in our understanding of genetic and epigenetic mechanisms for the transmission of psychiatric illness. The combination of the publication of the human genome sequence by the international Human Genome Project (HGP) in the spring of 2001 and the rapidly accelerating pace of computing power paved the way for genome-wide association studies (GWAS), a new form of genetic case–control association studies. In turn, results from GWAS have pointed towards new biological pathways that confer the risk for mental illness and possible new treatments (Kim, Zerwas, Trace, & Sullivan, 2011; Lander et al., 2001).

In eating disorder research, two GWAS are under way. In one GWAS, funded by the International Wellcome Trust Case Control Consortium (WTCCC3), a consortium of investigators from 17 countries is combining 3,000 blood samples from women with AN (Bulik, Collier, & Sullivan, 2011). In the second, the Anorexia Nervosa Genetics Initiative (ANGI), a second consortium of investigators from four countries is currently collecting 8,000 blood samples with AN (Bulik & Baker, 2013). Understanding the genes that predispose individuals to eating disorders will be a powerful tool for understanding the biology of eating psychopathology and ultimately elucidate how genetic risk markers are expressed over the life-span from menses to menopause.

Particularly relevant for reproductive mental health and eating disorders are the new tools to understand epigenetic modulation of the genome. Epigenetic modulation or epigenetics refers to any factor that affects gene expression such as DNA methylation, histone modification, and small interfering RNA (Campbell, Mill, Uher, & Schmidt, 2011). In particular, reduced representation bisulfite sequencing allows researchers to analyze DNA methylation on a genome-wide basis (Fouse, Nagarajan, & Costello, 2010). The prenatal period is considered a critical window for modulation of the epigenome because prenatal nutrition, particularly deficiencies in micronutrients, can alter gene expression of offspring through methylation (Davis et al., 2007; Entringer, Kumsta, Hellhammer, Wadhwa, & Wust, 2009; Lemberg & Phillips, 1989; Micali & Treasure, 2009; O'Connor et al., 2005; Seckl, 2008). When micronutrients are deficient during pregnancy, children are more likely to have impairments in their development (Chmurzynska, 2010). For example, when mothers experienced the Dutch Famine early in their pregnancies, their children had less DNA methylation of the imprinted insulin-like growth factor 2 (IGF2) gene as adults, even though the children's weight was within the normal range at birth (Heijmans et al., 2008). Moreover, since epigenetic marks may be heritable, these effects may not be limited just to immediate offspring but could be passed on to grandchildren (Champagne, 2008; Lim & Ferguson-Smith, 2010; Richards, 2006).

Although this research has not been extended to eating disorders during pregnancy, women struggling with restrictive eating disorders during pregnancy may be more likely to have micronutrient deficiencies. Unplanned pregnancies may be more common in women with AN and prenatal vitamin consumption prior to conception or in early pregnancy unlikely (Bulik et al., 2010; Dellava et al., 2011). Moreover, there is some evidence to suggest that women with eating disorders have systematic differences in their DNA methylation. Global DNA hypermethylation of the *DRD2* promoter, associated with dopamine regulation, has been found in AN and BN, and hypermethylation of the atrial natriuretic peptide (ANP) gene promoter region which regulates corticotropin and cortisol has been found in BN (Frieling et al., 2008, 2010; Groleau et al., 2013). Understanding how methylation is programmed in utero and varies across development constitutes a new biological pathway for understanding the interaction between genetic risk for eating disorders and environmental influences on gene expression. New technologies in genetics and epigenetics combined with prospective longitudinal studies measuring these biomarkers across multiple time points will pave the way towards a new understanding of the interaction between reproductive hormones and genetics as risk and resilience factors for the development of eating disorders.

In sum, eating disorder prevention and treatment can have a tremendous impact on public health. Preconception, antenatal, postpartum, and perimenopausal care should include screening in order to reduce the medical and financial burden these devastating disorders place on individuals, families, and communities. Leveraging disruptive new technologies to understand how genetics and epigenetics interact in development will create new ways of understanding the biological bases of eating disorders across the life-span.

References

AAP. (2012). Breastfeeding and the use of human milk. *Pediatrics, 129*(3), e827–e841.

Abraham, S. F., Pettigrew, B., Boyd, C., Russell, J., & Taylor, A. (2005). Usefulness of amenorrhoea in the diagnoses of eating disorder patients. *Journal of Psychosomatic Obsetrics and Gynecology, 26*(3), 211–215.

Abraham, S. F., Taylor, A., & Conti, J. (2001). Postnatal depression, eating, exercise, and vomiting before and during pregnancy. *International Journal of Eating Disorders, 29*(4), 482–487.

Agency for Healthcare Research and Policy. (2013). Eating disorders during pregnancy and postpartum. Retrieved July 17, 2013, from http://www.guidelines.gov/content.aspx?id=25631

American Psychiatric Association. (2013). *Diagnostic and statistical manual of mental disorders. Fifth edition text revision*. Washington, DC: American Psychiatric Press.

Andersen, A. E., & Ryan, G. L. (2009). Eating disorders in the obstetric and gynecologic patient population. *Obstetrics and Gynecology, 114*(6), 1353–1367.

Baker, C. W., Carter, A. S., Cohen, L. R., & Brownell, K. D. (1999). Eating attitudes and behaviors in pregnancy and postpartum: Global stability versus specific transitions. *Annals of Behavioral Medicine, 21*(2), 143–148.

Baker, J. H., Maes, H. H., Lissner, L., Aggen, S. H., Lichtenstein, P., & Kendler, K. S. (2009). Genetic risk factors for disordered eating in adolescent males and females. *Journal of Abnormal Psychology, 118*(3), 576–586.

Barker, D. J. (2004). The developmental origins of well-being. *Philosophical Transactions of the Royal Society Biological Sciences, 359*(1449), 1359–1366.

Becker, C. B., Diedrichs, P. C., Jankowski, G., & Werchan, C. (2013). I'm not just fat, I'm old: Has the study of body image overlooked "old talk"? *International Journal of Eating Disorders, 1*(6), 1–12.

Berkman, N. D., Lohr, K. N., & Bulik, C. M. (2007). Outcomes of eating disorders: A systematic review of the literature. *International Journal of Eating Disorders, 40*, 293–309.

Beumont, P. J. V., Abraham, S. F., & Simson, K. G. (1981). The psychosexual histories of adolescent girls and young women with anorexia nervosa. *Psychological Medicine, 11*, 131–140.

Birmingham, C. L., Su, J., Hlynsky, J. A., Goldner, E. M., & Gao, M. (2005). The mortality rate from anorexia nervosa. *International Journal of Eating Disorders, 38*, 143–146.

Blais, M. A., Becker, A. E., Burwell, R. A., Flores, A. T., Nussbaum, K. M., Greenwood, D. N., … Herzog, D. B. (2000). Pregnancy: Outcome and impact on symptomatology in a cohort of eating-disordered women. *International Journal of Eating Disorders, 27*(2), 140–149.

Borri, C., Mauri, M., Oppo, A., Banti, S., Rambelli, C., Ramacciotti, D., … Cassano, G. B. (2008). Axis I psychopathology and functional impairment at the third month of pregnancy: Results from the Perinatal Depression-Research and Screening Unit (PND-ReScU) study. *Journal of Clinical Psychiatry, 69*(10), 1617–1624.

Brinch, M., Isager, T., & Tolstrup, K. (1988). Anorexia nervosa and motherhood: Reproduction pattern and mothering behavior of 50 women. *Acta Psychiatrica Scandinavica, 77*, 611–617.

Broussard, B. (2012). Psychological and behavioral traits associated with eating disorders and pregnancy: A pilot study. *Journal of Midwifery and Women's Health, 57*(1), 61–66.

Brown, C. A., & Mehler, P. S. (2013). Medical complications of self-induced vomiting. *Eating Disorders, 21*(4), 287–294.

Brownell, K. D., & Fairburn, C. G. (1995). *Eating disorders and obesity: A comprehensive handbook.* New York, NY: Guilford Press.

Bulik, C. M. (2013). *Midlife eating disorders: Your journey to recovery.* New York, NY: Walker Publishing Company.

Bulik, C. M., Baker, J. H. (2013). ANGI-anorexia nervosa genetics initiative. Retrieved from http://www.med.unc.edu/psych/eatingdisorders/our-research/angi

Bulik, C. M., Collier, D., & Sullivan, P. (2011). *WTCCC3 and GCAN: A genome-wide scan for anorexia nervosa.* Paper presented at the International Conference on Eating disorders, Miami, FL, 2011.

Bulik, C. M., Hoffman, E. R., Von Holle, A., Torgersen, L., Stoltenberg, C., & Reichborn-Kjennerud, T. (2010). Unplanned pregnancy in women with anorexia nervosa. *Obstetrics and Gynecology, 116*(5), 1136–1140.

Bulik, C. M., Prescott, C. A., & Kendler, K. S. (2001). Features of childhood sexual abuse and the development of psychiatric and substance use disorders. *British Journal of Psychiatry, 179*, 444–449.

Bulik, C. M., Reba, L., Siega-Riz, A. M., & Reichborn-Kjennerud, T. (2005). Anorexia nervosa: Definition, epidemiology, and cycle of risk. *International Journal of Eating Disorders, 37*(Suppl), S2–S9. discussion S20–21.

Bulik, C. M., & Reichborn-Kjennerud, T. (2003). Medical morbidity in binge eating disorder. *International Journal of Eating Disorders, 34*(Suppl), S39–S46.

Bulik, C. M., Sullivan, P. F., Fear, J., Pickering, A., Dawn, A., & McCullin, M. (1999). Fertility and reproduction in women with a history of anorexia nervosa: A controlled study. *Journal of Clinical Psychiatry, 60*, 130–135.

Bulik, C. M., Sullivan, P. F., Tozzi, F., Furberg, H., Lichtenstein, P., & Pedersen, N. L. (2006). Prevalence, heritability, and prospective risk factors for anorexia nervosa. *Archives of General Psychiatry, 63*(3), 305–312.

Bulik, C. M., & Tozzi, F. (2004). Genetics in eating disorders: State of the science. *CNS Spectrums, 9*, 511–515.

Bulik, C. M., Von Holle, A., Hamer, R., Knoph Berg, C., Torgersen, L., Magnus, P., … Reichborn-Kjennerud, T. (2007). Patterns of remission, continuation and incidence of broadly defined eating disorders during early pregnancy in the Norwegian Mother and Child Cohort Study (MoBa). *Psychological Medicine, 37*(8), 1109–1118.

Bulik, C. M., Von Holle, A., Siega-Riz, A. M., Torgersen, L., Lie, K. K., Hamer, R. M., … Reichborn-Kjennerud, T. (2009). Birth outcomes in women with eating disorders in the Norwegian Mother and Child cohort study (MoBa). *International Journal of Eating Disorders, 42*(1), 9–18.

Campbell, I. C., Mill, J., Uher, R., & Schmidt, U. (2011). Eating disorders, gene-environment interactions and epigenetics. *Neuroscience and Biobehavioral Reviews, 35*(3), 784–793. doi:10.1016/j.neubiorev.2010.09.012.

Cedergren, M., Brynhildsen, J., Josefsson, A., Sydsjo, A., & Sydsjo, G. (2008). Hyperemesis gravidarum that requires hospitalization and the use of antiemetic drugs in relation to maternal body composition. *American Journal of Obstetrics and Gynecology, 198*(4), 412.e1–412.e5. doi:10.1016/j.ajog.2007.09.029.

Champagne, F. A. (2008). Epigenetic mechanisms and the transgenerational effects of maternal care. *Frontiers in Neuroendocrinology, 29*(3), 386–397. doi:10.1016/j.yfrne.2008.03.003.

Chmurzynska, A. (2010). Fetal programming: Link between early nutrition, DNA methylation, and complex diseases. *Nutrition Reviews, 68*(2), 87–98. doi:10.1111/j.1753-4887.2009.00265.x.

Dally, P. (1984). Anorexia tardive: Late onset marital anorexia nervosa. *Journal of Psychosomatic Research, 28*(5), 423–428.

Davis, E. P., Glynn, L. M., Schetter, C. D., Hobel, C., Chicz-Demet, A., & Sandman, C. A. (2007). Prenatal exposure to maternal depression and cortisol influences infant temperament. *Journal of the American Academy of Child & Adolescent Psychiatry, 46*(6), 737–746.

Dellava, J. E., Von Holle, A., Torgersen, L., Reichborn-Kjennerud, T., Haugen, M., Meltzer, H. M., & Bulik, C. M. (2011). Dietary supplement use immediately before and during pregnancy in Norwegian women with eating disorders. *International Journal of Eating Disorders, 44*(4), 325–332. doi: 10.1002/eat.20831

Dyson, F. (1997). *Imagined worlds*. Cambridge, MA: Harvard University Press.

Easter, A., Treasure, J., & Micali, N. (2011). Fertility and prenatal attitudes towards pregnancy in women with eating disorders: Results from the Avon Longitudinal Study of Parents and Children. *BJOG: An International Journal of Obstetrics and Gynaecology, 118*(12), 1491–1498.

Ehrmann, D. A. (2005). Polycystic ovary syndrome. *New England Journal of Medicine, 352*(12), 1223–1236.

Entringer, S., Kumsta, R., Hellhammer, D. H., Wadhwa, P. D., & Wust, S. (2009). Prenatal exposure to maternal psychosocial stress and HPA axis regulation in young adults. *Hormones and Behavior, 55*(2), 292–298.

Evans, J., & le Grange, D. (1995). Body size and parenting in eating disorders: A comparative study of the attitudes of mothers toward their children. *International Journal of Eating Disorders, 18*, 39–48.

Fairburn, C. G., Stein, A., & Jones, R. (1992). Eating habits and eating disorders during pregnancy. *Psychosomatic Medicine, 54*(6), 665–672.

Fassino, S., Amianto, F., Gramaglia, C., Facchini, F., & Abbate Daga, G. (2004). Temperament and character in eating disorders: Ten years of studies. *Eating and Weight Disorders, 9*, 81–90.

Favaro, A., Tenconi, E., & Santonastaso, P. (2006). Perinatal factors and the risk of developing anorexia nervosa and bulimia nervosa. *Archives of General Psychiatry, 63*, 82–88.

Fernandez-Aranda, F., Pinheiro, A. P., Tozzi, F., Thornton, L. M., Fichter, M. M., Halmi, K. A., … Bulik, C. M. (2007). Symptom profile of major depressive disorder in women with eating disorders. *Australian and New Zealand Journal of Psychiatry, 41*(1), 24–31.

Fouse, S. D., Nagarajan, R. O., & Costello, J. F. (2010). Genome-scale DNA methylation analysis. *Epigenomics, 2*(1), 105–117. doi:10.2217/epi.09.35.

Franko, D. L., Blais, M. A., Becker, A. E., Delinsky, S. S., Greenwood, D. M., Flores, A. T., … Herzog, D. B. (2001). Pregnancy complications and neonatal outcomes in women with eating disorders. *American Journal of Psychiatry, 158*, 1461–1466.

Franko, D. L., & Spurrell, E. B. (2000). Detection and management of eating disorders during pregnancy. *Obstetrics and Gynecology, 95*, 942–946.

Freizinger, M., Franko, D. L., Dacey, M., Okun, B., & Domar, A. D. (2010). The prevalence of eating disorders in infertile women. *Fertility and Sterility, 93*(1), 72–78. doi:10.1016/j.fertnstert.2008.09.055.

Frieling, H., Bleich, S., Otten, J., Romer, K. D., Kornhuber, J., de Zwaan, M., … Hillemacher, T. (2008). Epigenetic downregulation of atrial natriuretic peptide but not vasopressin mRNA expression in females with eating disorders is related to impulsivity. *Neuropsychopharmacology, 33*(11), 2605–2609.

Frieling, H., Romer, K. D., Scholz, S., Mittelbach, F., Wilhelm, J., De Zwaan, M., … Bleich, S. (2010). Epigenetic dysregulation of dopaminergic genes in eating disorders. *International Journal of Eating Disorders, 43*(7), 577–583. doi: 10.1002/eat.20745

Gagne, D. A., Von Holle, A., Brownley, K. A., Runfola, C. D., Hofmeier, S., Branch, K. E., & Bulik, C. M. (2012). Eating disorder symptoms and weight and shape concerns in a large web-based convenience sample of women ages 50 and above: Results of the gender and body image (GABI) study. *International Journal of Eating Disorders, 45*(7), 832–844.

Galson, S. K. (2008). Mothers and children benefit from breastfeeding. *Journal of the American Dietetic Association, 108*(7), 1106–1107.

Gavin, N. I., Gaynes, B. N., Lohr, K. N., Meltzer-Brody, S., Gartlehner, G., & Swinson, T. (2005). Perinatal depression: A systematic review of prevalence and incidence. *Obstetrics and Gynecology, 106*(5 Pt 1), 1071–1083.

Gluckman, P. D., & Hanson, M. A. (2004). Developmental origins of disease paradigm: A mechanistic and evolutionary perspective. *Pediatric Research, 56*(3), 311–317. doi:10.1203/01.PDR.0000135998.08025.FB.

Godart, N. T., Flament, M. F., Perdereau, F., & Jeammet, P. (2002). Comorbidity between eating disorders and anxiety disorders: A review. *International Journal of Eating Disorders, 32*, 253–270.

Goodwin, T. M. (2002). Nausea and vomiting of pregnancy: An obstetric syndrome. *American Journal of Obstetrics and Gynecology, 186*(5 Suppl Understanding), S184–S189.

Groleau, P., Joober, R., Israel, M., Zeramdini, N., Deguzman, R., & Steiger, H. (2013). Methylation of the dopamine D2 receptor (DRD2) gene promoter in women with a bulimia-spectrum disorder: Associations with borderline personality disorder and exposure to childhood abuse. *Journal of Psychiatric Research, 48*(1), 121–127. doi:10.1016/j.jpsychires.2013.10.003.

Hagan, M. M., Wauford, P. K., Chandler, P. C., Jarrett, L. A., Rybak, R. J., & Blackburn, K. (2002). A new animal model of binge eating: Key synergistic role of past caloric restriction and stress. *Physiology & Behavior, 77*(1), 45–54.

Halmi, K. A., Eckert, E., Marchi, P., Sampugnaro, V., Apple, R., & Cohen, J. (1991). Comorbidity of psychiatric diagnoses in anorexia nervosa. *Archives of General Psychiatry, 48*, 712–718.

Harris, A. A. (2010). Practical advice for caring for women with eating disorders during the perinatal period. *Journal of Midwifery and Women's Health, 55*(6), 579–586.

Harris, E. C., & Barraclough, B. (1998). Excess mortality of mental disorder. *British Journal of Psychiatry, 173*, 11–53.

Harrison, A., Tchanturia, K., & Treasure, J. (2010). Attentional bias, emotion recognition, and emotion regulation in anorexia: State or trait? *Biological Psychiatry, 68*(8), 755–761.

Hawkins, L. K., & Gottlieb, B. R. (2013). Screening for eating disorders in pregnancy: How uniform screening during a high-risk period could minimize under-recognition. *Journal of Women's Health (Larchmt), 22*(4), 390–392. doi:10.1089/jwh.2013.4313.

Heatherton, T. F., & Baumeister, R. F. (1991). Binge eating as escape from self-awareness. *Psychological Bulletin, 110*, 86–108.

Heijmans, B. T., Tobi, E. W., Stein, A. D., Putter, H., Blauw, G. J., Susser, E. S., … Lumey, L. H. (2008). Persistent epigenetic differences associated with prenatal exposure to famine in humans. *Proceedings of the National Academy of Sciences of the United States of America, 105*(44), 17046–17049. doi: 10.1073/pnas.0806560105

Hirschberg, A. L., Naessen, S., Stridsberg, M., Bystrom, B., & Holtet, J. (2004). Impaired cholecystokinin secretion and disturbed appetite regulation in women with polycystic ovary syndrome. *Gynecological Endocrinology, 19*(2), 79–87.

Hiser, P. L. (1987). Concerns of multiparas during the second postpartum week. *Journal of Obstetric, Gynecologic, & Neonatal Nursing, 16*(3), 195–203. doi:10.1111/j.1552-6909.1987.tb01457.x.

Hoffman, E. R., Zerwas, S. C., & Bulik, C. M. (2011). Reproductive issues in anorexia nervosa. *Expert Review of Obstetrics and Gynecology, 6*(4), 403–414. doi:10.1586/eog.11.31.

Hsu, L. K. G. (1980). Outcome of anorexia nervosa: A review of the literature (1954-1978). *Archives of General Psychiatry, 37*, 1041–1046.

Hudson, J. I., Hiripi, E., Pope, H. G., Jr., & Kessler, R. C. (2007). The prevalence and correlates of eating disorders in the National Comorbidity Survey Replication. *Biological Psychiatry, 61*, 348–358.

Javaras, K. N., Laird, N. M., Reichborn-Kjennerud, T., Bulik, C. M., Pope, H. G., Jr., & Hudson, J. I. (2008). Familiality and heritability of binge eating disorder: Results of a case-control family study and a twin study. *International Journal of Eating Disorders, 41*(2), 174–179.

Kaplan, A. S. (1993). Medical aspects of anorexia nervosa and bulimia nervosa. In S. H. Kennedy (Ed.), *Handbook of eating disorders* (pp. 22–29). Toronto, ON: University of Toronto.

Katzman, D. K. (2005). Medical complications in adolescents with anorexia nervosa: A review of the literature. *International Journal of Eating Disorders, 37*(Suppl), S52–S59. discussion S87–S89.

Kaye, W. H., Bulik, C. M., Thornton, L., Barbarich, B. S., Masters, K., & Group, Price Foundation Collaborative. (2004). Comorbidity of anxiety disorders with anorexia and bulimia nervosa. *American Journal of Psychiatry, 161*, 2215–2221.

Kaye, W. H., Wagner, A., Fudge, J. L., & Paulus, M. (2011). Neurocircuitry of eating disorders. *Current Topics in Behavioral Neuroscience, 6*, 37–57.

Keel, P. K., Haedt, A., & Edler, C. (2005). Purging disorder: An ominous variant of bulimia nervosa? *International Journal of Eating Disorders, 38*(3), 191–199.

Keel, P. K., Leon, G. R., & Fulkerson, J. A. (2001). Vulnerability to eating disorders in childhood and adolescence. In R. E. Ingram & J. M. Price (Eds.), *Vulnerability to psychopathology: Risk across the lifespan*. New York, NY: Guilford Press.

Keel, P. K., Mitchell, J. E., Miller, K. B., Davis, T. L., & Crow, S. J. (1999). Long-term outcome of bulimia nervosa. *Archives of General Psychiatry, 56*(1), 63–69.

Kendler, K. S., Bulik, C. M., Silberg, J., Hettema, J. M., Myers, J., & Prescott, C. A. (2000). Childhood sexual abuse and adult psychiatric and substance use disorders in women: An epidemiological and cotwin control analysis. *Archives of General Psychiatry, 57*(10), 953–959.

Kim, Y., Zerwas, S., Trace, S. E., & Sullivan, P. F. (2011). Schizophrenia genetics: Where next? *Schizophrenia Bulletin, 37*(3), 456–463. doi:10.1093/schbul/sbr031.

Klump, K. L., Burt, S. A., Spanos, A., McGue, M., Iacono, W. G., & Wade, T. D. (2010). Age differences in genetic and environmental influences on weight and shape concerns. *International Journal of Eating Disorders, 43*(8), 679–688.

Klump, K. L., Keel, P. K., Sisk, C., & Burt, S. A. (2010). Preliminary evidence that estradiol moderates genetic influences on disordered eating attitudes and behaviors during puberty. *Psychological Medicine, 40*(10), 1745–1753.

Klump, K. L., Suisman, J. L., Culbert, K. M., Kashy, D. A., & Sisk, C. L. (2011). Binge eating proneness emerges during puberty in female rats: A longitudinal study. *Journal of Abnormal Psychology, 120*(4), 948–955.

Knoph, C., Von Holle, A., Zerwas, S., Torgersen, L., Tambs, K., Stoltenberg, C., … Reichborn-Kjennerud, T. (2013). Course and predictors of maternal eating disorders in the postpartum period. *International Journal of Eating Disorders, 46*(4), 355–368.

Koubaa, S., Hallstrom, T., & Hirschberg, A. L. (2008). Early maternal adjustment in women with eating disorders. *International Journal of Eating Disorders, 41*(5), 405–410.

Koubaa, S., Hallstrom, T., Lindholm, C., & Hirschberg, A. L. (2005). Pregnancy and neonatal outcomes in women with eating disorders. *Obstetrics and Gynecology, 105*(2), 255–260.

Lacey, J. H., & Smith, G. (1987). Bulimia nervosa: The impact of pregnancy on mother and baby. *British Journal of Psychiatry, 150*, 777–781.

Lander, E. S., Linton, L. M., Birren, B., Nusbaum, C., Zody, M. C., Baldwin, J., … Chen, Y. J. (2001). Initial sequencing and analysis of the human genome. *Nature, 409*(6822), 860–921.

Larsson, G., & Andersson-Ellstrom, A. (2003). Experiences of pregnancy-related body shape changes and of breast-feeding in women with a history of eating disorders. *European Eating Disorders Review, 11*(2), 116–124.

Leddy, M. A., Jones, C., Morgan, M. A., & Schulkin, J. (2009). Eating disorders and obstetric-gynecologic care. *Journal of Women's Health (Larchmt), 18*(9), 1395–1401.

Lemberg, R., & Phillips, J. (1989). The impact of pregnancy on anorexia nervosa and bulimia. *International Journal of Eating Disorders, 8*, 285–295.

Lewis, D. M., & Cachelin, F. M. (2001). Body image, body dissatisfaction, and eating attitudes in midlife and elderly women. *Eating Disorders, 9*(1), 29–39.

Lim, A. L., & Ferguson-Smith, A. C. (2010). Genomic imprinting effects in a compromised in utero environment: Implications for a healthy pregnancy. *Seminars in Cell and Developmental Biology, 21*(2), 201–208. doi:10.1016/j.semcdb.2009.10.008.

Lingam, R., & McCluskey, S. (1996). Eating disorders associated with hyperemesis gravidarum. *Journal of Psychosomatic Research, 40*(3), 231–234.

Luck, A. J., Morgan, J. F., Reid, F., O'Brien, A, Brunton, J., Price, C., … Lacey, J. H. (2002). The SCOFF questionnaire and clinical interview for eating disorders in general practice: Comparative study. *British Medical Journal, 325*, 755–756.

Mangweth-Matzek, B., Rupp, C. I., Hausmann, A., Assmayr, K., Mariacher, E., Kemmler, G., ... Biebl, W. (2006). Never too old for eating disorders or body dissatisfaction: A community study of elderly women. *International Journal of Eating Disorders, 39*(7), 583–586.

Mazzeo, S. E., Mitchell, K. S., Gerke, C. K., & Bulik, C. M. (2006). Parental influences on children's eating behavior. *Current Nutrition and Food Science, 2*, 275–295.

Mazzeo, S. E., Slof-Op't Landt, M. C., Jones, I., Mitchell, K., Kendler, K. S., Neale, M. C., ... Bulik, C. M. (2006). Associations among postpartum depression, eating disorders, and perfectionism in a population-based sample of adult women. *International Journal of Eating Disorders, 39*(3), 202–211.

Meltzer-Brody, S., Zerwas, S., Leserman, J., Holle, A. V., Regis, T., & Bulik, C. (2011). Eating disorders and trauma history in women with perinatal depression. *Journal of Women's Health (Larchmt), 20*(6), 863–870.

Micali, N., Simonoff, E., Stahl, D., & Treasure, J. (2011). Maternal eating disorders and infant feeding difficulties: Maternal and child mediators in a longitudinal general population study. *Journal of Child Psychology and Psychiatry, 52*(7), 800–807.

Micali, N., Simonoff, E., & Treasure, J. (2009). Infant feeding and weight in the first year of life in babies of women with eating disorders. *Journal of Pediatrics, 154*(1), 55–60.e1.

Micali, N., & Treasure, J. (2009). Biological effects of a maternal ED on pregnancy and foetal development: A review. *European Eating Disorders Review, 17*(6), 448–454.

Micali, N., Treasure, J., & Simonoff, E. (2007). Eating disorders symptoms in pregnancy: A longitudinal study of women with recent and past eating disorders and obesity. *Journal of Psychosomatic Research, 63*(3), 297–303.

Millar, H. R., Wardell, F., Vyvyan, J. P., Naji, S. A., Prescott, G. J., & Eagles, J. M. (2005). Anorexia nervosa mortality in Northeast Scotland, 1965-1999. *American Journal of Psychiatry, 162*(4), 753–757.

Mitchell, J. E., Specker, S. M., & de Zwaan, M. (1991). Comorbidity and medical complications of bulimia nervosa. *Journal of Clinical Psychiatry, 52*(Suppl), 13–20.

Mitchell-Gieleghem, A., Mittelstaedt, M. E., & Bulik, C. M. (2002). Eating disorders and childbearing: Concealment and consequences. *Birth, 29*(3), 182–191.

Morgan, J. F. (1999). Eating disorders and gynecology: Knowledge and attitudes among clinicians. *Acta Obstetricia and Gynecologica Scandinavica, 78*(3), 233–239.

Morgan, J. F., Lacey, J. H., & Chung, E. (2006). Risk of postnatal depression, miscarriage, and preterm birth in bulimia nervosa: Retrospective controlled study. *Psychosomatic Medicine, 68*(3), 487–492.

Morgan, J. F., Lacey, J. H., & Reid, F. (1999). Anorexia nervosa: Changes in sexuality during weight restoration. *Psychosomatic Medicine, 61*(4), 541–545.

Morgan, J. F., Lacey, J. H., & Sedgwick, P. M. (1999). Impact of pregnancy on bulimia nervosa. *British Journal of Psychiatry, 174*, 135–140.

Morgan, J. F., Reid, F., & Lacey, J. H. (1999). The SCOFF questionnaire: Assessment of a new screening tool for eating disorders. *BMJ, 319*, 1467–1468.

Naessén, S., & Hirschberg, A. (2011). Sex hormones and appetite in women: A focus on bulimia nervosa. In V. R. Preedy, R. R. Watson, & C. R. Martin (Eds.), *Handbook of behavior, Food and Nutrition* (pp. 1759–1767). New York, NY: Springer.

O'Connor, T. G., Ben-Shlomo, Y., Heron, J., Golding, J., Adams, D., & Glover, V. (2005). Prenatal anxiety predicts individual differences in cortisol in pre-adolescent children. *Biological Psychiatry, 58*(3), 211–217.

Papadopoulos, F. C., Ekbom, A., Brandt, L., & Ekselius, L. (2009). Excess mortality, causes of death and prognostic factors in anorexia nervosa. *British Journal of Psychiatry, 194*(1), 10–17.

Pinelli, G., & Tagliabue, A. (2007). Nutrition and fertility. *Minerva Gastroenterologica Dietol, 53*(4), 375–382.

Pinheiro, A. P., Raney, T. J., Thornton, L. M., Fichter, M. M., Berrettini, W. H., Goldman, D., ... Bulik, C. M. (2010). Sexual functioning in women with eating disorders. *International Journal of Eating Disorders, 43*(2), 123–129.

Pinheiro, A. P., Thornton, L. M., Plotonicov, K. H., Tozzi, F., Klump, K. L., Berrettini, W. H., ... Bulik, C. M. (2007). Patterns of menstrual disturbance in eating disorders. *International Journal of Eating Disorders, 40*(5), 424–434.

Racine, S. E., Culbert, K. M., Larson, C. L., & Klump, K. L. (2009). The possible influence of impulsivity and dietary restraint on associations between serotonin genes and binge eating. *Journal of Psychiatric Research, 43*(16), 1278–1286.

Raney, T. J., Thornton, L. M., Berrettini, W., Brandt, H., Crawford, S., Fichter, M. M., ... Bulik, C. M. (2008). Influence of overanxious disorder of childhood on the expression of anorexia nervosa. *International Journal of Eating Disorders, 41*(4), 326–332.

Reck, C., Struben, K., Backenstrass, M., Stefenelli, U., Reinig, K., Fuchs, T., ... Mundt, C. (2008). Prevalence, onset and comorbidity of postpartum anxiety and depressive disorders. *Acta Psychiatrica Scandinavica, 118*(6), 459–468.

Reichborn-Kjennerud, T., Bulik, C. M., Sullivan, P. F., Tambs, K., & Harris, J. R. (2004). Psychiatric and medical symptoms in binge eating in the absence of compensatory behaviors. *Obesity Research, 12*, 1445–1454.

Resch, M., Szendei, G., & Haasz, P. (2004a). Bulimia from a gynecological view: Hormonal changes. *Journal of Obstetrics and Gynaecology, 24*(8), 907–910.

Resch, M., Szendei, G., & Haasz, P. (2004b). Eating disorders from a gynecologic and endocrinologic view: Hormonal changes. *Fertility and Sterility, 81*(4), 1151–1153.

Richards, E. J. (2006). Inherited epigenetic variation – Revisiting soft inheritance. *Nature Reviews Genetics, 7*(5), 395–401. doi:10.1038/nrg1834.

Rigotti, N. A., Neer, R. M., Skates, S. J., Herzog, D. B., & Nussbaum, S. R. (1991). The clinical course of osteoporosis in anorexia nervosa: A longitudinal study of cortical bone mass. *Journal of the American Medical Association, 265*(9), 1133–1137.

Russell, J. A., Douglas, A. J., & Ingram, C. D. (2001). Brain preparations for maternity: Adaptive changes in behavioral and neuroendocrine systems during pregnancy and lactation. An overview. *Progress in Brain Research, 133*, 1–38.

Rutter, M., Moffitt, T. E., & Caspi, A. (2006). Gene-environment interplay and psychopathology: Multiple varieties but real effects. *Journal of Child Psychology and Psychiatry, 47*(3–4), 226–261.

Schlotz, W., & Phillips, D. I. (2009). Fetal origins of mental health: Evidence and mechanisms. *Brain, Behavior, and Immunity, 23*(7), 905–916.

Schwarz, E. B., Brown, J. S., Creasman, J. M., Stuebe, A., McClure, C. K., Van Den Eeden, S. K., & Thom, D. (2010). Lactation and maternal risk of type 2 diabetes: A population-based study. *American Journal of Medicine, 123*(9), 863.e1–863.e6.

Seckl, J. R. (2008). Glucocorticoids, developmental 'programming' and the risk of affective dysfunction. *Progress in Brain Research, 167*, 17–34.

Sharp, C. W., & Freeman, C. P. L. (1993). The medical complications of anorexia nervosa. *British Journal of Psychiatry, 162*, 452–462.

Sim, L. A., McAlpine, D. E., Grothe, K. B., Himes, S. M., Cockerill, R. G., & Clark, M. M. (2010). Identification and treatment of eating disorders in the primary care setting. *Mayo Clinical Proceedings, 85*(8), 746–751.

Stein, A., & Fairburn, C. G. (1989). Children of mothers with bulimia nervosa. *British Medical Journal, 299*(6702), 777–778.

Stein, A., & Fairburn, C. G. (1996). Eating habits and attitudes in the postpartum period. *Psychosomatic Medicine, 58*, 321–325.

Steinglass, J. E., Walsh, B. T., & Stern, Y. (2006). Set shifting deficit in anorexia nervosa. *Journal of the International Neuropsychological Society, 12*, 431–435.

Stewart, D. E., Robinson, G. E., Goldbloom, D. S., & Wright, C. (1990). Infertility and eating disorders. *American Journal of Obstetrics and Gynecology, 163*, 1196–1199.

Strober, M., Freeman, R., Lampert, C., Diamond, J., & Kaye, W. (2000). Controlled family study of anorexia nervosa and bulimia nervosa: Evidence of shared liability and transmission of partial syndromes. *American Journal of Psychiatry, 157*(3), 393–401.

Stuebe, A. M., Kleinman, K., Gillman, M. W., Rifas-Shiman, S. L., Gunderson, E. P., & Rich-Edwards, J. (2010). Duration of lactation and maternal metabolism at three years postpartum. *Journal of Women's Health (Larchmt), 19*(5), 941–950.

Stuebe, A. M., Schwarz, E. B., Grewen, K., Rich-Edwards, J. W., Michels, K. B., Foster, E. M., ... Forman, J. (2011). Duration of lactation and incidence of maternal hypertension: A longitudinal cohort study. *American Journal of Epidemiology, 174*(10), 1147–1158.

Sullivan, P. F. (1995). Mortality in anorexia nervosa. *American Journal of Psychiatry, 152*(7), 1073–1074.

Sullivan, P. F., Bulik, C. M., & Kendler, K. S. (1998). The genetic epidemiology of binging and vomiting. *British Journal of Psychiatry, 173*, 75–79.

Swann, R. A., Von Holle, A., Torgersen, L., Gendall, K., Reichborn-Kjennerud, T., & Bulik, C. M. (2009). Attitudes toward weight gain during pregnancy: Results from the Norwegian mother and child cohort study (MoBa). *International Journal of Eating Disorders, 42*(5), 394–401.

Tchanturia, K., Morris, R. G., Anderluh, M. B., Collier, D. A., Nikolaou, V., & Treasure, J. (2004). Set shifting in anorexia nervosa: An examination before and after weight gain, in full recovery and relationship to childhood and adult OCPD traits. *Journal of Psychiatric Research, 38*(5), 545–552.

Thornton, L. M., Mazzeo, S. E., & Bulik, C. M. (2011). The heritability of eating disorders: Methods and current findings. *Current Topics in Behavioral Neuroscience, 6*, 141–156. doi:10.1007/7854_2010_91.

Torgersen, L., Von Holle, A., Reichborn-Kjennerud, T., Berg, C. K., Hamer, R., Sullivan, P., & Bulik, C. M. (2008). Nausea and vomiting of pregnancy in women with bulimia nervosa and eating disorders not otherwise specified. *International Journal of Eating Disorders, 41*(8), 722–727.

Torgersen, L., Ystrom, E., Haugen, M., Meltzer, H. M., Von Holle, A., Berg, C. K., ... Bulik, C. M. (2010). Breastfeeding practice in mothers with eating disorders. *Maternal & Child Nutrition, 6*(3), 243–252.

Watson, T. L., & Andersen, A. E. (2003). A critical examination of the amenorrhea and weight criteria for diagnosing anorexia nervosa. *Acta Psychiatrica Scandinavica, 108*, 175–182.

Waugh, E., & Bulik, C. M. (1999). Offspring of women with eating disorders. *International Journal of Eating Disorders, 25*(2), 123–133.

Wonderlich, S. A., Connolly, K. M., & Stice, E. (2004). Impulsivity as a risk factor for eating disorder behavior: Assessment implications with adolescents. *International Journal of Eating Disorders, 36*(2), 172–182.

Yonkers, K. A., Wisner, K. L., Stewart, D. E., Oberlander, T. F., Dell, D. L., Stotland, N., ... Lockwood, C. (2009). The management of depression during pregnancy: A report from the American Psychiatric Association and the American College of Obstetricians and Gynecologists. *Obstetrics and Gynecology, 114*(3), 703–713.

Zerwas, S., Von Holle, A., Torgersen, L., Reichborn-Kjennerud, T., Stoltenberg, C., & Bulik, C. M. (2012). Maternal eating disorders and infant temperament: Findings from the Norwegian mother and child cohort study. *International Journal of Eating Disorders, 45*(4), 546–555.

Zipfel, S., Lowe, B., Reas, D. L., Deter, H. C., & Herzog, W. (2000). Long-term prognosis in anorexia nervosa: Lessons from a 21-year follow-up study. *Lancet, 355*(9205), 721–722.

The Use of Hormonal Contraception and Its Impact on Women's Moods

Lauren Schiff

Introduction

It is commonly believed that hormonal contraception can have significant effects on a woman's mood, including worsening of depression, bipolar disorder, postpartum depression, anxiety disorders, and post-traumatic stress disorders as well as improving symptoms of premenstrual syndrome. However this belief has not been well substantiated and the literature is replete with conflicting data. Inconsistent research findings echo the frequent clinical observation that patients experience disparate reactions to hormonal contraception, making it challenging to recommend an ideal contraceptive technique to a given patient. The relationship between exogenous hormones and mood disorders has not been studied in sufficient depth to provide a definitive answer to the question of whether these hormones have a direct effect on clinical psychiatric outcomes.

In recent years, scientific research addressing the effects of hormones on mood has increased significantly and although much of this research is promising, clinical application in women is mostly theoretical. Further clinical research is needed to understand how these hormones interact with neuromodulators to impact mood and anxiety disorders. The female hormonal milieu is based in the hypothalamic–pituitary–ovarian–adrenal axis: the system of endocrine glands that self-regulates to secrete the sex hormones, estrogen, and progesterone, regulating the menstrual cycle. It is also known that cortisol, prolactin, and oxytocin and the neurotransmitters dopamine, serotonin, and norepinephrine are part of an intricate web of neurochemical signaling that affect cognitive, behavioral, and emotional functioning. While obstetricians and gynecologists focus on the somatic effects of estrogen and

L. Schiff, M.D. (✉)
University of North Carolina at Chapel Hill, Chapel Hill, North Carolina, USA
e-mail: schiff.lauren@gmail.com

progesterone and their dysregulation (producing disease states such as menorrhagia or amenorrhea), psychiatrists focus on the mood-altering effects of serotonin, norepinephrine, and dopamine. The lingering question is do these hormones, when dysregulated, interact to directly alter mood and functional effects? Currently there is no means to predict, recognize, and treat dysregulations in a way that produces reliable clinical outcomes. In other words, all perimenopausal women with a history of major depression and menorrhagia will not react predictably similarly to Lupron (a GnRH agonist used for ovarian suppression to inhibit bleeding); some may have no effect, while others may experience a resurgence of depression. Similarly, although most women with a history of dysthymia who receive depot medroxyprogesterone acetate, DMPA, for postpartum contraception will not develop postpartum depression, some will. Clinical studies have not been able to identify a model for predicting who, amongst women sharing similar medical and psychiatric histories, will experience psychiatric sequelae from exogenous hormones.

Without clear causal, dose–effect relationships between hormonal contraception and mood outcomes being demonstrated in the literature, clinicians generally conclude that there is no substantial effect. The World Health Organization (WHO) produces the most relied upon clinical guide to contraceptive use for women with medical comorbidities and recommends without reservation all contraceptive techniques to women with "depressive disorders" (WHO, 2010). However, the most recent literature reviews of the effects of hormonal contraception (exogenous gonadal steroids) on women's mental health acknowledges a large gap in our understanding of this relationship and calls for further rigorous study in the field. The conclusion in the psychiatric and neurochemistry fields is that a true relationship exists that we have not yet clearly defined.

This chapter guides clinicians towards making the best contraceptive choices for their patients who have, or are at risk for developing, mood and anxiety disorders. The first section offers a brief review of the current biological basis for mood outcomes and its relationship to the endocrine axis that controls the menstrual cycle. The second section outlines the current contraceptive options available in the USA and highlights the indications, risks, and common side effects of these contraceptives. The third section presents common case scenarios and offers recommendations based on the available literature and ultimately demonstrates that identifying the ideal contraceptive method for a given patient must be a patient-centered, individualized, process.

Neurobiochemistry of Mood and the HPOA Axis

The hypothalamus is the neuroendocrine gland within the brain that is the central "processor" of the neuroendocrine system and controls the hypothalamic–pituitary–adrenal (HPA) axis and the hypothalamic–pituitary–ovarian (HPO) axis. Because these endocrine axes are interdependent, they are often referred to together as the HPOA axis.

The regulatory hormones of the HPOA axis do not have a singular purpose; they intricately interact to suppress and stimulate one another's receptors (Fritz & Speroff, 2011, pp. 157–163). Specifically estrogen and progesterone have been shown to have neuroregulatory effects outside of their reproductive function, including mood and cognition (Meltzer-Brody, 2011). The extent of the physiologic, cognitive, and affective outcomes produced by interactions between these hormones is not well understood. Mapping of neuropeptide interaction is a focus of basic scientists, which promises to further our understanding of how exogenous hormones alter this balance.

The role of the HPOA axis in the development of mood disorders is being defined in emerging literature. Marked variations in estrogen and progesterone levels have been described in depressed postpartum women when compared to their non-depressed counterparts (Bloch, Daly, & Rubinow, 2003). Estrogen has been shown to increase serotonin and to have anxiolytic effects, while depletion of estrogen levels has been seen in depressed women (Ryan & Ancelin, 2012). Additionally, the HPA axis is hyperactive and suppresses the HPO axis in the setting of depression (Swaab, Boa, & Lucassen, 2005). This relationship between the HPA axis and the HPO axis in depression has led researchers to believe that sex steroids interact with the HPA axis in a way that can regulate mood outcomes. For example, cortisol has been a focus in the study of mood disorders and is now well accepted to play an important role in the development of major depressive disorder and postpartum depression (Meltzer-Brody, 2011). Cortisol is essential for the regulation of stress response. During pregnancy, cortisol levels are particularly high; however, these levels fall precipitously following delivery of the placenta. Unlike their euthymic counterparts, depressed patients in the postpartum period do not re-regulate cortisol for a prolonged period (Magiakou et al., 1996; Taylor, Glover, Marks, & Kammerer, 2009). This persistent depletion of cortisol in women with postpartum depression is intimately tied to the major fluctuation of gonadal steroids that occurs in the postpartum period. During pregnancy, the gonadal steroids, estrogen and progesterone, are at multifold higher levels than normal. Immediately following delivery, they both drop precipitously, a rapid fluctuation, which although is a normal physiologic event in childbearing, has been suggested to produce negative mood outcomes in a subset of susceptible women (Bloch et al., 2005).

It is likely that there is also a subset of women predisposed to the emergence of mood disorders when HPOA dysregulation or alteration occurs outside of the postpartum period, such as in the administration of exogenous hormones. While neurochemical studies have repeatedly demonstrated a link between altered HPOA axis hormones and mood disorders, clinical studies have been unable to reproduce this effect of gonadal hormones on mood outcomes in a causal fashion.

The missing link in the study of neurohormones to mood disorders is the less quantifiable contribution of life events, personality traits, and genetics. Animal models have shown that distinct neurochemical changes occur in response to stressful life events, such as maternal separation and isolation, and result in behavioral outcomes akin to human mood disorders. For example, in studies of oxytocin knockout mice, lack of oxytocin (the neurohormone responsible for labor, milk let-down, and infant bonding) was associated with anhedonic or poor maternal care behaviors and increased anxiety behaviors (Pedersen, Vadlamudi, Boccia, & Amico, 2006). Evidence from human models also demonstrates a likely role of oxytocin in depression (Purba, Hoogendijk, Hofman, & Swaab, 1996) with depressed women being more likely than their non-depressed counterparts to display a dysregulated pattern of peripheral oxytocin release (Cyranowski et al., 2008). The field of behavioral epigenetics is further defining how life events, genetics, and neurochemical regulation produce mood and behavioral outcomes. The expression or the suppression of genes may be altered from exposure to stressful early life events and subsequently alter future behavior. An elegant study by Champagne and colleagues (Champagne et al., 2006) demonstrates that socialization directly affects genetic expression: rodent offspring of mothers who displayed strong maternal behavior showed high estrogen receptor expression compared to poorly nurtured offspring. When the offspring of highly nurturing and poorly nurturing mothers were cross fostered, however, the estrogen receptor expression reversed, thus demonstrating an epigenetic effect on estrogen receptor expression. Similarly, gene expression of the glucocorticoid receptor has been shown to be affected by stressful life events resulting in an increased stress response (Weaver et al., 2004). These studies suggest that HPOA regulation and its downstream effects can be directly altered by life events and may be at the heart of why certain women are more vulnerable than others to gonadal steroid alterations. This may be why clinicians have such difficulty predicting the mood and behavior effects of hormonal contraception in women. Not only do life events affect changes in DNA expression, but also these changes are carried to the next generation of animal offspring suggesting that the susceptibility to steroid alterations incurred by life events in one generation may predispose the subsequent generations to similar susceptibilities (Franklin et al., 2010).

In epidemiologic terms, the ability to power a study to identify a difference between two groups of women with a homogeneous enough genetically predetermined susceptibility to hormonal contraception may prove impossible. Neuroendocrinologic and genetic research supports the fact that some women are vulnerable to experience mood and behavioral effects from hormonal contraception; we must take the experiences of our patients, including family histories of mood disorders along with the available clinical data, to make our recommendations for their use of hormonal contraception.

Contraceptive Options and Their Indications

Contraceptive options have significantly expanded over the past 20–30 years allowing physicians to tailor the contraceptive approach to each individual patient's lifestyle, family planning goals, medical comorbidities, and comfort level. Contraceptive options are generally divided between hormonal methods, barrier methods, and surgical methods (i.e., sterilization). Aside from permanent sterilization, hormonal contraceptive methods are the most commonly used in the USA with the best efficacy profile (WHO, 2010). They exist in many forms, the main differences lying in the type and dosage of hormones used, the schedule of use, and the level of user maintenance required. In this section, we briefly review each class of hormonal contraceptive available on the US market, their indications, and their risk/benefit profile.

Oral Contraceptive Pills

Oral contraceptive pills (OCPs) are the most commonly used form of hormonal contraceptive. These include both combined estrogen–progestin pills and progestin-only pills (POP or "mini-pill"). The mini-pill is not considered to be a reliable contraceptive method due to the potential for breakthrough ovulation if the pill is taken more than 24 h apart. It is most commonly prescribed in the postpartum period to avoid potential side effects of estrogen during this time, including venous thromboembolism (VTE) and theoretical decrease in milk supply. The mini-pill should not be relied upon as a long-term contraceptive solution. Breakthrough bleeding is the most common benign side effect of this method. The combined oral contraceptive, COC, pill comes in varying estrogen and progestin doses, types of progestins, and prescribed schedules. Older COCs, no longer commonly used in the USA, contained higher levels of estrogen (50 mcg estradiol); however, they were thought to be related to higher thrombosis risk. Estradiol at 20–30 mcg is sufficient in most women to suppress ovulation without increasing side effects. COCs require a high level of user reliability: they must be taken every day and at approximately the same time. Most commonly reported side effects include weight gain or loss, nausea, mood changes, breast soreness, and changes in libido. Continuous OCPs can be used to induce ovulation suppression without increasing side effects such as bone loss or VTE risk; however, breakthrough bleeding may occur. An abbreviated list of conditions in which COCs are contraindicated include those with ischemic cardiovascular disease or its risk equivalents, risk for or personal history of thrombosis or stroke, heavy smokers over the age of 35, and migraine headache with aura (WHO, 2010). Please reference the WHO medical eligibility for contraceptive use for complete risk profile.

Combined Hormonal Patch and Ring

The combined contraceptive patch and ring have the same mechanism of action as COCs: to inhibit follicular maturation, ovulation, fallopian tube mobility, cervical mucous passage, and endometrial receptivity. Women who benefit from estrogen-containing hormonal contraception (for dysmenorrhea, bleeding control, acne relief, etc.) and are unable to reliably take a daily pill may desire to use the contraceptive patch. The patch must be changed weekly for optimal use. The contraceptive ring offers a similar risk/benefit profile to other combined hormonal methods. Once inserted, the ring is left in place for 3 weeks at a time, with removal prior to the fourth week to allow for a withdrawal bleed. If vaginal application is tolerable to the user, it provides the benefit of a less rigorous schedule. Due to the local action of the ring, plasma estradiol levels are significantly lower than those with COC or the patch (Timmer & Mulders, 2000). Common side effects that differ in the ring from other combined methods are increased local vaginal effects including vaginitis, discharge, and potential coital discomfort requiring transient removal.

Injectables

The most common form of hormonal contraception is depot medroxy progesterone-acetate, DMPA, a slow-release progestin-only method. Newer combined hormonal injectables have been developed and show great promise with decreased hormonal concentrations and potentially decreased side effects. These are not readily available in the USA, although ongoing research is encouraging (WHO, 2010). DMPA is an injection administered every 3 months and is ideal for patients who desire a low maintenance method. There is no extended efficacy beyond 3 months; therefore, careful follow-up with repeat injections or initiation of a new method must be observed for successful contraception. DMPA has been shown to have efficacy in reducing dysfunctional uterine bleeding and reducing pain associated with endometriosis. Return to fertility is delayed and unpredictable and can last for up to 2 years. Women desiring fertility within 2 years of use should be counseled towards another method if appropriate. Weight gain is a commonly reported side effect and has been suggested in the literature (Lopez et al., 2013). Bone mass density decreases do occur; however, return to baseline occurs with discontinuation of the method and risk for reduced peak bone mass or increased fracture risk later in the life in women with average risk of osteoporosis is unlikely (Nappi, Bifulco, Tommaselli, Gargano, & Di Carlo, 2012).

Long-Acting Reversible Contraception

Long-acting reversible contraception (LARC) refers to contraceptive methods that are inserted intrauterinally or are implanted subdermally with duration of efficacy ranging from 3 to 10 years depending on the method. These methods are ideal for women not planning pregnancy for 3 or more years, and cost-effectiveness has been demonstrated even if the method is discontinued after 2 years of use (Trussell et al., 2009). Once inserted, these methods require no user maintenance, until replacement is indicated or discontinuation is desired. The intrauterine device, IUD, exists in two types: progestin-eluding, levonorgestrel-IUD, LNG-IUD, and the non-hormone-eluding copper IUD (Cu-IUD), the brand names in the USA being Mirena and ParaGard, respectively. The most commonly used subdermal implants used in the USA are the single-rod progestin, etonogestrel-releasing implants (brand names Implanon and Nexplanon). A similar two-rod device eluding levonorgestrel (brand name Jadelle) is commonly available outside the USA.

In addition to having a superior efficacy rate (99.8 %), the LNG-IUD has FDA-approved medical applications as well as off-label uses that are ideal for addressing both contraceptive and medical concerns simultaneously. By releasing progestin to the endometrium, it can be used to control menorrhagia, dysmenorrhea, and reverse simple endometrial hyperplasia and treat atypical endometrial hyperplasia in non-surgical candidates (Scarselli et al., 2011). Additionally, studies have shown that the LNG-IUD may be effective in controlling pelvic pain associated with endometriosis and adenomyosis (Abou-Setta, Houston, Al-Inany, & Farquhar, 2013; Sheng, Zhang, Zhang, & Lu, 2009). It also may be placed immediately postpartum (within 10 min of placental delivery) with relatively low expulsion rates and is considered to be safe when breastfeeding. The most commonly reported side effect of the LNG-IUD is irregular bleeding. Absolute contraindications are few and include initiation at the time of active pelvic inflammatory disease and anatomical uterine abnormalities incompatible with placement (WHO, 2010).

The Cu-IUD is an efficacious long-term contraceptive, ideal for those who cannot, or decline to, use a hormonal method. Its efficacy is slightly inferior to the LNG-IUD (99.2 %). Advantages include that it lasts for up to 10 years and can be used as a successful emergency contraceptive method with the benefit of providing ongoing contraception (Cheng, Che, & Gülmezoglu, 2012). The Cu-IUD may increase the amount of menstrual bleeding, duration, and dysmenorrhea and should not be recommended to women with menorrhagia or dysmenorrhea. It should be avoided in women with distortion of the endometrial cavity (septum, fibroid, etc.) as correct placement within the cavity is necessary for efficacy.

Sterilization (Hysteroscopic/Tubal Ligation)

Two main methods are currently used in the USA for female permanent sterilization: the hysteroscopic sterilization with the Essure® device and tubal ligation either immediately postpartum or at a 6-week interval via the laparoscopic approach. According to WHO, female sterilization is slightly less efficacious than both the LNG-IUD and etonogestrel single-rod implant (99.5 % efficacy vs. 99.8 % vs. 99.95 % efficacy, respectively) (WHO, 2010). In clinical practice, these methods are considered of equal efficacy and should be recommended based on the family planning needs and the health risks of the individual patient. Surgical risks of sterilization via hysteroscopic or abdominal/laparoscopic methods are minimal and related to general surgical and anesthetic risks. Permanent sterilization can be associated with the feeling of regret, which is reported to be highest (20.3 %) in women under the age of 30 (Peterson, 2008).

Hormonal Contraception and Mood Disorders in Context

Clinical Scenarios

When choosing a contraceptive method for an individual patient, four questions should be answered:

1. What are the family planning goals of this patient?
2. What are the comorbid gynecologic conditions that may be addressed by contraception?
3. What are the medical comorbidities and/or factors that may limit contraceptive choices?
4. What are the psychiatric comorbidities and/or risk factors to consider in choosing a contraceptive method?

Answering these four questions will invariably point to the optimal choice, or range of choices, of contraceptive techniques for each patient. It is important to note before further discussion regarding the relationship of mood and hormonal contraception that the fourth question outlined above is controversial. Despite frequent patient subjective reports, anecdotal evidence, and formal neurobiochemical studies, no definitive data has been presented to date that demonstrates unequivocally that hormonal contraception directly produces effects on mood.

Each of the common case scenarios below in which hormonal contraception is prescribed is followed by a review of the most up-to-date literature and recommendations for treatment options. This review demonstrates that each patient must be considered on an individual basis and that recommendations be made on the best medical evidence in combination with the patient's mood and behavioral history.

No Prior Mood Disorder

> Case: A 28-year-old, otherwise healthy, nulli-gravid woman presents seeking contraception. She desires to maintain her fertility; however, does not plan to become pregnant in the next five years. She reports no gynecologic, medical, or psychiatric history.

For a patient without any history of mood disorder and no medical concerns and who has never been pregnant before, there is no special consideration that needs to be given to contraceptive choices; however, this does not ensure that an individual starting hormonal contraception may not return to the office complaining of effects such as mood swings, tearfulness, or irritability. While hormonal shifts that occur through the menstrual cycle may increase vulnerability for worsening depression, specifically premenstrually (Almagor & Ben-Porath, 1991; Endicott, 1993), no directional relationship between hormonal changes during the menstrual cycle and mood outcome has been shown. Additionally, while older studies suggest potential negative mood effects from exogenous hormones (Oinonen & Mazmanian, 2002), more recent studies have refuted this claim and suggest that hormonal contraception is not associated with negative influence on mental health (Toffol, Heikinheimo, Koponen, Luoto, & Partonen, 2012).

Recommendations

If a patient reports the onset of new mood symptoms after the initiation of hormonal contraception, it is important to not dismiss this occurrence and to investigate the extent and severity of these symptoms. Development of such symptoms may suggest that the patient has an underlying psychiatric disorder, as women who report COC-induced adverse mood are more likely to have a diagnosed mood disorder (Segebladh, Borgström, Odlind, Bixo, & Sundström-Poromaa, 2009). A thorough depression inventory and history, menstrual-mood relationship history, and family history for mood disorders should be taken.

When mood symptoms occur with initiation of combined oral contraceptives, the type and dose of contraceptive should be examined. Monophasic pills, lower dose pills (Oinonen & Mazmanian, 2002), and drospirenone containing OCP are associated with reducing premenstrual symptoms, PMS, or stabilizing moods (Lopez, Kaptein, & Helmerhorst, 2012). These may be used as an alternative on a trial basis. If it is not medically contraindicated and the patient is amenable to LNG-IUD or progestin implant, these tend to have decreased reported mood side effects compared to the oral contraceptive and vaginal ring options. Cu-IUD will eliminate all potential for mood-altering effects and may remain as an option for a patient who does not tolerate other hormonal contraceptive options.

Premenstrual Mood Symptoms/Premenstrual Mood Disorder

Case: A 34-year-old gravida two para two presents desiring birth control without specific plans for her future fertility. She reports a 28-day menstrual cycle with heavy flow, worsening premenstrual bloating, cramping, moodiness, and irritability since the birth of her last child. She denies medical problems.

In this case, caution must be taken to understand whether the patient meets diagnostic criteria for premenstrual dysphoric disorder, PMDD, as opposed to PMS given that greater than 90 % of women report at least one PMS per cycle, whereas only 2–3 % of women actually meet diagnostic criteria for PMDD (Nevatte et al., 2013). Please see chapter "Menstruation and Premenstrual Dysphoric Disorder: Its Impact on Mood" for a detailed review of PMDD.

Recommendations

Oral contraception, and particularly continuous COC (with or without drospirenone), may be ideal in a patient seeking contraception with a history of PMDD as the data suggests a possible mood-stabilizing effect (Nevatte et al., 2013; Borenstein, Yu, Wade, Chiou & Rapkin, 2003; Yonkers et al., 2005; Lopez et al., 2012; Freeman et al., 2012). Those with PMS without a true diagnosis of PMDD may benefit from COC and are unlikely to experience worsening symptoms from COC. Mood deterioration with COC use has also been reported, although not consistently (Nevatte et al., 2013); patients may experience negative mood effects, which remains a clinical challenge. Deterioration of mood with COC use may more likely occur in women with a history of true depression (Joffe, Lee, & Harlow, 2003), as compared to PMS or PMDD. Such mood deterioration should prompt the provider to more closely evaluate the patient for other mood disorders. Notably, the prevalence of major depression in women with PMDD may be as high as 24.6 % (Forrester-Knauss, Zemp Stutz, Weiss, & Tschudin, 2011).

Perimenopausal women with PMDD may benefit from GnRH agonists with estradiol/progesterone add back, limited to every 3 months to minimize recurrence of symptoms (Pincus, Alam, Rubinow, Bhuvaneswar, & Schmidt, 2011; Schmidt, Nieman, Danaceau, Adams, & Rubinow, 1998). Alternate methods of contraception in patients with PMDD have not been studied and should be used as indicated for medical or regimen adherence reasons. The transdermal patch and vaginal ring have not been studied in relation to PMDD. It is conceivable that patients may experience relief of PMDD symptoms with either of these methods due to their shared mechanism of action. Uninterrupted use may be hypothesized to help in a similar way. In patients for whom combined hormonal contraception is not ideal due to medical risks or regimen adherence concerns, implantables (Implanon/Nexplanon), LNG-IUD or DMPA, may be an ideal contraceptive technique. While no data exists evaluating their effect on PMDD, mood deterioration, in the setting of their use, may indicate an underlying mood disorder and prompt the use of alternate methods of contraception.

Major Depression

> Case: A 21-year-old G1P0010 presents for her routine gynecologic exam. She reports being sexually active, has used oral contraceptive pills in the past, but is not using them currently, and denies medical problems. She is having increased difficulty concentrating at school, finds herself feeling angry, frequently tearful, and feeling hopeless. She reports these symptoms have occurred in the past pre-menstrually, but have become more consistent lately. She was treated for depression at age 17 following her parents' divorce.

While having a history of major depression has been identified as a risk factor for developing COC-related mood deterioration in the premenstrual period (Joffe et al., 2003), the estradiol component of COCs has been suggested to lessen the severity of depressive symptoms due to its serotonin-activating effects (Young et al., 2007). It has also shown to be successful in patients with major depression who experience worsening of symptoms premenstrually (Joffe et al., 2007).

An alternate explanation for the observed overall emotional well-being improvement seen with COCs is offered by Huber and colleagues who suggest that progesterone metabolites induce the GABA A receptor to cause anxiolytic effects (Huber, Heskamp, & Schramm, 2008). Their theory is in contrast to the frequently referenced depressogenic effects of progesterone, which were originally reported in the 1960s and 1970s and have led providers to avoid progesterone-only methods in depressed patients. Few recent studies exist that specifically study progestin-only methods. Westhoff and colleagues (Westhoff et al., 1998) studied changes in depressive symptoms with the use of DMPA and Norplant and found that those who continued the contraceptive therapy for 12 months and 2 years in the DMPA and Norplant groups, respectively, had overall improvement from baseline in their depression symptom scores. Their findings are confounded by a large dropout and loss to follow-up rate making it challenging to assess whether depressive symptoms led to discontinuation. Their findings do suggest that while a subgroup of depressed patients may not tolerate DMPA or Norplant, most may improve or may not be affected.

Recommendations

The available data cannot advise against the use of any particular kind of hormonal contraception in major depression with any certainty and may recommend an estrogen-containing method in these patients. Women with major depression may see an improvement in depression with estrogen-containing hormonal contraception and will likely tolerate progestin-only methods without deleterious mood-related side effects. Progestin therapies should be used once a thorough history has been taken of response to similar therapies in the past. No specific studies examining LNG-IUD and major depression have been undertaken, and it may be assumed that this will be equally well tolerated. Anecdotal clinical reports suggest potential worsening in the setting of progestin therapy in patients with a history of depression with psychotic features; however, no current data exists to guide this choice. Risk–benefit analysis with the patient should be undertaken to balance both medical goals and potential psychiatric risks.

For the patient case presented at the start of this section, reasons for the patient's discontinuation of her use of COC before should be identified. Additionally, the patient should be referred to psychiatry for evaluation of the reported mood symptoms. The key to determining the best method for each patient again hinges on the patient's past experience with exogenous hormones. Close post-initiation follow-up of mood symptoms is advised, especially with progestin-only methods where the data remains murky.

Postpartum Depression

> Case: a 35-year-old G2P1 with a history of "postpartum blues" after her first delivery, delivers a healthy baby girl at full term. Prior to discharge from the hospital she discusses her birth control plan and reports that she would like to return to taking DMPA but is concerned about whether that will cause post-partum depression to recur.

The postpartum period is the period of greatest risk for women to develop major depression or postpartum depression (Brummelte & Galea, 2010), and the effect of exogenous hormones on women with a predisposition to postpartum depression remains unknown. In a double-blind, placebo-controlled trial, Bloch et al. (2000) demonstrated that acute withdrawal of gonadal steroids after supra-physiological gonadal steroid injection induced depression relapse in subjects with a history of postpartum depression, while it had no effect on those with no such history. This added support to the theory that gonadal steroid fluctuations produce deleterious outcomes in those predisposed to depression, although they had no effect on those with no vulnerability. The question that remains to be answered is how to risk stratify our postpartum patients based on their history to identify vulnerability in order to predict mood outcomes from gonadal steroid administration.

It is general practice amongst obstetricians to prescribe a birth control method at the time of discharge from the hospital; however, methods containing estrogen are avoided for three to six weeks postpartum due to increased VTE risk during this period (WHO, 2010). For this reason, patients amenable to hormonal contraception frequently have an immediate postpartum LNG-IUD placed after placental delivery, are prescribed the progestin-only mini-pill, receive the first injection of DMPA, or have an implantable progestin-only device (Implanon/Nexplanon) inserted prior to discharge.

Some psychiatrists will warn against the use of progestin-only methods, such as DMPA, in postpartum patients with a history of depression. This was supported by a 1998 study (Lawrie et al., 1998) demonstrating that those who received an injection of a synthetic progestin postpartum had an almost two times risk of displaying depressive symptoms by 6 weeks postpartum. This finding was contested by a 2010 retrospective chart review (Tsai & Schaffir, 2010) comparing women who did and did not receive DMPA immediately postpartum, and the results showed no difference in depression scores between the two groups at postpartum week 6.

Recommendations

The available studies do suggest that DMPA is an acceptable method in overall healthy postpartum women and should not be withheld due to concern for development of de novo depression. The effects on those with a history of depression, bipolar disorder, or a history of postpartum depression in prior pregnancies cannot be determined based on the available data. Use of progestin-only methods postpartum in a high-risk group should be undertaken with close follow-up. Progestin-only pills have not been studied in the postpartum setting; however, they may be posited to have a similar effect as DMPA. If concern is raised for DMPA postpartum contraception, the LNG-IUD may be ideal given that serum hormone levels eluded from the LNG-IUD are significantly lower than DMPA. Unlike DMPA, whose effects last for 3 months, the IUD can be removed readily in the setting of worsening depressive symptoms. The progestin-only implantables (Implanon/Nexplanon) may also be ideal as detectable plasma hormone levels are also lower than DMPA; however, removal may be slightly more challenging depending on the skills of the provider. If menstrual or medical history does not preclude the use of the Cu-IUD, this remains a viable option for those with significant concern for postpartum hormonal intervention.

Transition to an estrogen-containing method at 6 weeks postpartum, after which increased coagulability due to pregnancy has abated, may help some with depressive symptoms (Galea, Wide, & Barr, 2001; Gregoire, Kumar, Everitt, Henderson, & Studd, 1996; Sichel, Cohen, Robertson, Ruttenberg, & Rosenbaum, 1995). Recent studies have continued to demonstrate a relationship between abrupt estrogen withdrawal and onset of depressive symptoms (Ben Dor et al., 2013; Schiller, O'Hara, Rubinow, & Johnson, 2013), supporting further study into estrogen treatment for postpartum depression. However, clinical data does not definitively support this method (Karuppaswamy & Vlies, 2003). While estradiol treatment in patients with severe postpartum depression has been reported with good outcomes (Dennis, Ross, & Herxheimer, 2008), caution must be taken when administering estrogen in the postpartum period due to thrombosis risk. Estrogen use within three weeks postpartum is contraindicated by the WHO with additional precautions advised for longer periods depending on personal risk factors.

The most important element in postpartum contraceptive choice is the follow-up to assess potential side effects given our ability to predict that the outcome is poor and the outcomes of untreated postpartum depression can be devastating. Concurrent use of the appropriate psychotropic regimen should be considered as first-line 3 to treatment.

Bipolar Disorder

Case: A 17-year-old G0 with a history of treatment resistant bipolar II disorder presents to her gynecologist due to irregular menstrual cycles and desires oral contraceptives for regulation. She reports having taken COC before and feeling "crazy" when she took them, but cannot clearly relate the timing of her COC to her periods of worsening psychiatric symptomatology.

Women with bipolar disorder have been reported to experience worsening symptoms associated with menstrual, postpartum, and menopausal transition periods (Blehar et al., 1998). The relationship between bipolar disorder and physiologic hormonal fluctuations has prompted research into the effects of exogenous hormones on this disorder. While some studies observed significant mood alterations during the menstrual cycle in bipolar patients (Rasgon, Bauer, Glenn, Elman, & Whybrow, 2003), others have suggested that no discernible pattern of mood changes occur (Shivakumar et al., 2008; Sit, Seltman, & Wisner, 2011).

There is very limited data on the specific effect of exogenous hormones on bipolar disorder. Most studies have included very small number of participants and have been observational in nature (Berenson, Asem, Tan, & Wilkinson, 2011; Rasgon et al., 2003). It is important to recognize that increased sexual promiscuity (as may be seen in this population) or history of prior pelvic inflammatory disease is not a contraindication to IUD placement (ACOG, 2011).

If choosing to use a combined hormonal method in patients on mood stabilizers for bipolar disorder, review of medication interactions is essential. Certain mood stabilizers, also known as antiepileptic drugs (AEDs), can decrease the efficacy of both the oral contraceptive pill and the AED. Specifically COCs lower the effectiveness of valproate and lamotrigine, while COC effectiveness is reduced by phenobarbital, phenytoin, carbamazepine, felbamate, oxcarbazepine, and topiramate (Seeman & Ross, 2011). This is not the case with DMPA, LNG-IUD, progestin-only implantables, or Cu-IUD, and these methods can be used without reservation. The interaction of these drugs with progestin-only pills has not been confirmed, and its use is not recommended (WHO, 2010).

Recommendations

In summary, COC use is not contraindicated in bipolar disorder and may offer mood-stabilizing effects. A patient reporting symptom worsening in the setting of COC, as does the patient in the case scenario at the start of this section, warrants careful review of symptom profiling in relation to her menstrual cycle and exogenous hormone use. There is no evidence that DMPA causes deleterious effects on bipolar disorder, and it may be suited to patients who cannot remember to take a daily pill, keeping in mind, however, that its discontinuation rates are high. The LNG-IUD appears to be the most suitable method of choice in these patients based on the limited data available. As there is no definitive evidence to support the use or non-use of hormonal contraception in bipolar disorder, in the setting of negative mood side effects or poor adherence, transition to an alternate method employing a different hormonal regimen or system of delivery (i.e., LNG-IUD, implantable, vaginal ring) may be tried to assess the improvement of adherence and mood response.

Schizophrenia

Case: A 41-year-old G3P3 is brought to the gynecology clinic by her home health aid for a routine check-up. The patient has a history of schizophrenia and lives independently, although she does require daily assistance from her health aid to manage her medications. The patient reports being sexually active with more than one partner, occasionally uses condoms, and does not recall whether she has had a sexually transmitted infection.

Women with schizophrenia tend to undergo gynecologic examination, discuss family planning with their doctors, and correctly use contraception less frequently than their unaffected counterparts (Seeman & Ross, 2011). This is believed to be due to inadequate counseling, inability to adhere to the regimen due to deficits in daily functioning, or reduction in efficacy from co-prescribed medications (Seeman & Ross, 2011).

Use of combined oral contraceptives may be challenging in the schizophrenia population due to the need for daily regimen adherence and monitoring for drug interactions with mood-stabilizing medications (AEDs) (see review in section "Bipolar Disorder" above). Additionally, oral contraceptives reduce clearance of the antipsychotic medications clozapine and chlorpromazine, commonly prescribed in schizophrenia, potentially leading to toxic levels. The corollary is also true; cessation of oral contraceptives will reduce the plasma levels of these antipsychotic medications and necessitate up-titration to maintain effectiveness. Therefore if a patient abruptly discontinues her COC without discussing this with her psychiatrist, relapse may occur. Notably the antipsychotic medication, ziprasidone, has not been shown to interact as robustly with COCs, and dose adjustments with concurrent use of this medication are not required (Muirhead, Harness, Holt, Oliver, & Anziano, 2000).

Low estrogenic states, immediately postpartum, premenstrual, and menopause, are times of increased schizophrenia relapse (Riecher-Rössler, 2002), and estrogen replacement has been noted to have potential therapeutic effects by decreasing psychotic symptoms (Kulkarni et al., 2008). Use of estrogen treatment is limited by the cardiovascular/thrombotic estrogen risks, which may be more common in patients with schizophrenia due to the weight gain side effects of antipsychotic medications. Despite this risk, however, estrogen-containing contraceptives are likely a benefit rather than a risk to the severity of schizophrenia symptoms and thus should be used without reservation in those patients for whom all other COC-associated concerns are immaterial.

DMPA may be an appropriate method for a patient requiring a less demanding regimen; however, there is no data to support the use or the non-use in this population. Continuation rates would be expected to be equivalently low in this compared to the general population, and the potential for weight gain with DMPA (Steenland, Zapata, Brahmi, Marchbanks, & Curtis, 2013) in patients taking obesity-inducing antipsychotics may advise against its use.

LARC, such as implantables and IUDs, are ideal for these patients when pregnancy is not intended within at least 2 years. There are no contraindications in terms of the common comorbid medical disorders in women with schizophrenia, and there is no interaction with AEDs or antipsychotic medications due to lack of first pass metabolism in the liver. The LARC affords the patient the highest contraceptive efficacy with the lowest requirements of the individual for maintenance.

Recommendations

In summary, a combined hormonal contraceptive method (COC, the vaginal ring, the transdermal patch) may be beneficial to women with schizophrenia by providing estrogen-associated decrease in symptom relapse, with use being limited to women without significant medical comorbidities. DMPA is untested in this group and is limited only by its high rate of discontinuation. LARC technologies are considered as the ideal contraception in this population with no reported deleterious mood outcomes, low-risk profile, low user maintenance, and prolonged efficacy.

Conclusion

The available evidence supports the ongoing use of hormonal contraception in women with mood disorders. There is no conclusive evidence that hormonal contraception causes deleterious effects on mood, and in fact, estrogen may improve or stabilize moods in most mood disorders. The role of progestins remains less clear with contradictory evidence suggesting no effect, improvement, or worsening in different settings. We can say with confidence that the neuroendocrine systems directing the menstrual cycle are linked to mood, cognition, and behavior; however, a dose–response relationship has not yet been defined. There are clearly populations of women who display vulnerability to mood effects from both physiologic dysregulation of endogenous hormones as well as administration of exogenous hormones. This susceptibility is multifactorial, and we are thus far unable to definitively identify those women or predict who amongst them will experience these effects.

It is always essential to individualize care when recommending hormonal contraception to patients. Reactions to hormonal contraception reported by patients should be carefully sought and clearly documented. Close collaboration between psychiatrists and contraception prescribers is vital to successful outcomes. While there is no method of hormonal contraception that is absolutely contraindicated in patients with mood disorders, careful attention to an individual's menstrual-mood history and past experience with hormonal contraception will help us provide the contraceptive plan that best meets each patient's needs.

References

Abou-Setta, A. M., Houston, B., Al-Inany, H. G., & Farquhar, C. (2013). Levonorgestrel-releasing intrauterine device (LNG-IUD) for symptomatic endometriosis following surgery. *The Cochrane Database of Systematic Reviews, 31*(1), CD005072.

Almagor, M., & Ben-Porath, Y. S. (1991). Mood changes during the menstrual cycle and their relation to the use of oral contraceptive. *Journal of Psychosomatic Research, 35*(6), 721–728.

American College of Obstetricians and Gynecologists. (2011). ACOG Practice Bulletin No. 121: Long-acting reversible contraception: Implants and Intrauterine Devices. *Obstetrics and Gynecology, 105*, 223–232.

Ben Dor, R., Harsh, V. L., Fortinsky, P., Koziol, D. E., Rubinow, D. R., & Schmidt, P. J. (2013). Effects of pharmacologically induced hypogonadism on mood and behavior in healthy young women. *American Journal of Psychiatry, 170*(4), 426–433.

Berenson, A. B., Asem, H., Tan, A., & Wilkinson, G. (2011). Continuation rates and complications of intrauterine contraception in women diagnosed with bipolar disorder. *Obstetrics and Gynecology, 118*(6), 1331–1336.

Blehar, M. C., Depaulo, J. R., Gershon, E. S., Reich, T., Simpson, S. G., & Nurnberger, J. I. (1998). Women with bipolar disorder: Findings from the NIMH genetics initiative sample. *Psychopharmacology Bulletin, 34*, 239–243.

Bloch, M., Daly, R. C., & Rubinow, D. R. (2003). Endocrine factors in the etiology of postpartum depression. *Comprehensive Psychiatry, 44*(3), 234–246.

Bloch, M., Rubinow, D. R., Schmidt, P. J., Lotsikas, A., Chrousos, G. P., & Cizza, G. (2005). Cortisol responses to ovine corticotropin-resealing hormone in a model of pregnancy and parturition in euthymic women with and without a history of postpartum depression. *Journal of Clinical Endocrinology and Metabolism, 90*, 924–930.

Bloch, M., Schmidt, P. J., Danaceau, M., Murphy, J., Nieman, L., & Rubinow, D. R. (2000). Effects of gonadal steroids in women with a history of postpartum depression. *American Journal of Psychiatry, 157*(6), 924–930.

Borenstein, J., Yu, H. T., Wade, S., Chiou, C. F., & Rapkin, A. (2003). Effect of an oral contraceptive containing ethinyl estradiol and drospirenone on premenstrual symptomatology and health-related quality of life. *The Journal of Reproductive Medicine, 48*(2), 79–85.

Brummelte, S., & Galea, L. A. (2010). Depression during pregnancy and postpartum: Contribution of stress and ovarian hormones. *Progress in Neuro-Psychopharmacology and Biological Psychiatry, 34*(5), 766–776.

Champagne, F. A., Weaver, I. C., Dioro, J., Dymov, S., Szyf, M., & Meaney, M. J. (2006). Maternal care associated with methylation of the estrogen receptor-alpha1b promoter and estrogen receptor-alpha expression in the medial preoptic area of female offspring. *Endocrinology, 147*, 2909–2915.

Cheng, L., Che, Y., & Gülmezoglu, A. M. (2012). Interventions for emergency contraception. *The Cochrane Database of Systematic Reviews, 15*(8), CD001324.

Cyranowski, J. M., Hofkens, T. L., Frank, E., Seltman, H., Cai, H. M., & Amico, J. A. (2008). Evidence of dysregulated peripheral oxytocin release among depressed women. *Psychosomatic Medicine, 70*(9), 967–975.

Dennis, C. L., Ross, L. E., & Herxheimer, A. (2008). Oestrogens and progestins for preventing and treating postpartum depression. *The Cochrane Database of Systematic Reviews.* (4), CD001690.

Endicott, J. (1993). The menstrual cycle and mood disorders. *Journal of Affective Disorders, 29*(2–3), 193–200.

Forrester-Knauss, C., Zemp Stutz, E., Weiss, C., & Tschudin, S. (2011). The interrelation between premenstrual syndrome and major depression: Results from a population-based sample. *BMC Public Health, 11*, 795.

Franklin, T. B., Russig, H., Weiss, I. C., Gräff, J., Linder, N., Michalon, A., ... Mansuy, I. M. (2010). Epigenetic transmission of the impact of early stress across generations. *Biological Psychiatry. 68*, 408–415.

Freeman, E. W., Halbreich, U., Grubb, G. S., Rapkin, A. J., Skouby, S. O., Smith, L., ... Constantine, G. D. (2012). An overview of four studies of a continuous oral contraceptive (levonorgestrel 90 mcg/ethinyl estradiol 20mcg) on premenstrual dysphoric disorder and premenstrual syndrome. *Contraception, 85*(5), 437–45.

Fritz, M. A., & Speroff, L. (2011). *Clinical gynecologic endocrinology and infertility* (8th ed., pp. 157–163). Philadelphia, PA: Lippincott Williams & Wilkins.

Galea, L. A., Wide, J. K., & Barr, A. M. (2001). Estradiol alleviates depressive-like symptoms in a novel animal model of post-partum depression. *Behavioural Brain Research, 122*(1), 1–9.

Gregoire, A. J., Kumar, R., Everitt, B., Henderson, A. F., & Studd, J. W. (1996). Transdermal oestrogen for the treatment of severe postnatal depression. *Lancet, 347*(9006), 930–933.

Huber, J. C., Heskamp, M. L., & Schramm, G. A. (2008). Effect of an oral contraceptive with chlormadinone acetate on depressive mood: analysis of data from four observational studies. *Clinical Drug Investigation, 28*(12), 783–791.

Joffe, H., Lee, C., & Harlow, B. (2003). Impact of oral contraceptive pill use on premenstrual mood. Predictors of improvement and deterioration. *American Journal of Obstetrics and Gynecology, 189*(6), 1523–1530.

Joffe, H., Petrillo, L. F., Viguera, A. C., Gottshcall, H., Soares, C. N., Hall, J. E., & Cohen, L. S. (2007). Treatment of premenstrual worsening of depression with adjunctive oral contraceptive pills: a preliminary report. *Journal of Clinical Psychiatry, 68*(12), 1954–1962.

Karuppaswamy, J., & Vlies, R. (2003). The benefit of oestrogens and progestogens in postnatal depression. *Journal of Obstetrics and Gynaecology, 23*(4), 341–346.

Kulkarni, J., de Castella, A., Fitzgerald, P. B., Gurvich, C. T., Bailey, M., Bartholomeusz, C., & Burger, H. (2008). Estrogen in severe mental illness: A potential new treatment approach. *Archives of General Psychiatry, 65*, 955–960.

Lawrie, T. A., Hofmeyr, G. J., de Jager, M., Berk, M., Paiker, J., & Viljoen, E. (1998). A double-blind randomised placebo controlled trial of postnatal norethisterone enanthate: The effect on postnatal depression and serum hormones. *British Journal of Obstetrics and Gynaecology, 105*, 1082–1090.

Lopez, L. M., Edelman, A., Chen, M., Otterness, C., Trussell, J., & Helmerhorst, F. M. (2013). Progestin-only contraceptives: Effects on weight. *The Cochrane Database of Systematic Reviews, 2*(7), CD008815.

Lopez, L. M., Kaptein, A. A., & Helmerhorst, F. M. (2012). Oral contraceptives containing drospirenone for premenstrual syndrome (Review). *The Cochrane Database of Systematic Reviews, 15*(2), CD006586.

Magiakou, M. A., Mastorakos, G., Rabin, D., Dubbert, B., Gold, P. W., & Chrousos, G. P. (1996). Hypothalamic corticotropin-releasing hormone suppression during the postpartum period: Implications for the increase in psychiatric manifestations at this time. *Journal of Clinical Endocrinology and Metabolism, 81*(5), 1912–1917.

Meltzer-Brody, S. (2011). New insights into perinatal depression: Pathogenesis and treatment during pregnancy and postpartum. *Dialogues in Clinical Neuroscience, 13*(1), 89–100.

Muirhead, G. J., Harness, J., Holt, P. R., Oliver, S., & Anziano, R. J. (2000). Ziprasidone and the pharmacokinetics of a combined oral contraceptive. *British Journal of Clinical Pharmacology, 49*(Suppl. 1), 49S–56S.

Nappi, C., Bifulco, G., Tommaselli, G. A., Gargano, V., & Di Carlo, C. (2012). Hormonal contraception and bone metabolism: A systematic review. *Contraception, 86*(6), 606–621.

Nevatte, T., O'Brien, P. M., Bäckström, T., Brown, C., Dennerstein, L., Endicott, J., … Consensus Group of the International Society for Premenstrual Disorders. (2013). ISPMD consensus on the management of premenstrual disorders. *Archives of Women's Mental Health, 16*(4), 279–291.

Oinonen, K. A., & Mazmanian, D. (2002). To what extent do oral contraceptives influence mood and affect? *Journal of Affective Disorders, 70*(3), 229–240.

Pedersen, C., Vadlamudi, S., Boccia, M., & Amico, J. A. (2006). Maternal behavior deficits in nulliparous oxytocin knockout mice. *Genes, Brain and Behavior, 5*, 274–281.

Peterson, H. (2008). Sterilization. *Obstetrics and Gynecology, 111*(1), 189–203.

Pincus, S., Alam, S., Rubinow, D. R., Bhuvaneswar, C. G., & Schmidt, P. J. (2011). Predicting response to leuprolide of women with premenstrual dysphoric disorder by daily mood rating dynamics. *Journal of Psychiatric Research, 45*(3), 386–394.

Purba, J., Hoogendijk, W., Hofman, M., & Swaab, D. F. (1996). Increased number of vasopressin- and oxytocin-expressing neurons in the paraventricular nucleus of the hypothalamus in depression. *Archives of General Psychiatry, 52*, 137–143.

Rasgon, N., Bauer, M., Glenn, T., Elman, S., & Whybrow, P. C. (2003). Menstrual cycle related mood changes in women with bipolar disorder. *Bipolar Disorder, 5*(1), 48–52.

Riecher-Rössler, A. (2002). Oestrogen effects in schizophrenia and their potential therapeutic implications—review. *Archives of Women's Mental Health, 5*, 111–118.

Ryan, J., & Ancelin, M. L. (2012). Polymorphisms of estrogen receptors and risk of depression: Therapeutic implications. *Drugs, 72*(13), 1725–1738.

Scarselli, G., Bargelli, G., Taddei, G. L., Marchionni, M., Peruzzi, E., Pieralli, A., … Fambrini, M. (2011). Levonorgestrel-releasing intrauterine system (LNG-IUS) as an effective treatment option for endometrial hyperplasia: A 15-year follow-up study. *Fertility and Sterility, 95*, 420.

Schiller, C. E., O'Hara, M. W., Rubinow, D. R., & Johnson, A. K. (2013). Estradiol modulates anhedonia and behavioral despair in rats and negative affect in a subgroup of women at high risk for postpartum depression. *Physiology and Behavior, 119*, 137–144.

Schmidt, P. J., Nieman, L. K., Danaceau, M. A., Adams, L. F., & Rubinow, D. R. (1998). Differential behavioral effects of gonadal steroids in women with and in those without premenstrual syndrome. *New England Journal of Medicine, 338*, 209–216.

Seeman, M., & Ross, R. (2011). Prescribing contraceptives for women with schizophrenia. *Journal of Psychiatric Practice, 17*(4), 258–269.

Segebladh, B., Borgström, A., Odlind, V., Bixo, M., & Sundström-Poromaa, I. (2009). Prevalence of psychiatric disorders and premenstrual dysphoric symptoms in patients with experience of adverse mood during treatment with combined oral contraceptives. *Contraception, 79*(1), 50–55.

Sheng, J., Zhang, W. Y., Zhang, J. P., & Lu, D. (2009). The LNG-IUS study on adenomyosis: a three-year follow-up study on the efficacy and side effects of the use of levonorgestrel intrauterine system for the treatment of dysmenorrhea associated with adenomyosis. *Contraception, 79*(3), 189–193.

Shivakumar, G., Bernstein, I. H., Suppes, T., Stanley Foundation Bipolar Network., Keck, P. E., McElroy, S. L., ... Post, R. M. (2008). Are bipolar mood symptoms affected by the phase of the menstrual cycle? *Journal Women's Health, 17*(3), 473–478.

Sichel, D. A., Cohen, L. S., Robertson, L. M., Ruttenberg, A., & Rosenbaum, J. F. (1995). Prophylactic estrogen in recurrent postpartum affective disorder. *Biological Psychiatry, 38*(12), 814–818.

Sit, D., Seltman, H., & Wisner, K. L. (2011). Menstrual effects on mood symptoms in treated women with bipolar disorders. *Bipolar Disorder, 13*(3), 310–317.

Steenland, M. W., Zapata, L. B., Brahmi, D., Marchbanks, P. A., & Curtis, K. M. (2013). Appropriate follow up to detect potential adverse events after initiation of select contraceptive methods: A systematic review. *Contraception, 87*(5), 611–624.

Swaab, D. F., Boa, A. M., & Lucassen, P. J. (2005). The stress system in the human brain in depression and neurodegeneration. *Ageing Research Reviews, 4*(2), 141–194.

Taylor, A., Glover, V., Marks, M., & Kammerer, M. (2009). Diurnal pattern of cortisol output in postnatal depression. *Psychoneuroendocrinology, 34*, 1184–1188.

Timmer, C. J., & Mulders, T. M. (2000). Pharmacokinetics of etonogestrel and ethinylestradiol released from a combined contraceptive vaginal ring. *Clinical Pharmacokinetics, 39*, 233.

Toffol, E., Heikinheimo, O., Koponen, P., Luoto, R., & Partonen, T. (2012). Further evidence for lack of negative associations between hormonal contraception and mental health. *Contraception, 86*(5), 470–480.

Trussell, J., Lalla, A. M., Doan, Q. V., Reyes, E., Pinto, L., & Gricar, J. (2009). Cost effectiveness of contraceptives in the United States. *Contraception, 79*, 5.

Tsai, R., & Schaffir, J. (2010). Effect of depot medroxyprogesterone acetate on postpartum depression. *Contraception, 82*(2), 174–177.

Weaver, I. C., Cervoni, N., Champagne, F. A., D'Alessio, A. C., Sharma, S., Seckl, J. R., ... Meaney, M. J. (2004) Epigenetic programming by maternal behavior. *Nature Neuroscience. 7*(8), 847–854.

Westhoff, C., Truman, C., Kalmuss, D., Cushman, L., Davidson, A., Rulin, M., & Heartwell, S. (1998). Depressive symptoms and Depo-Provera. *Contraception, 57*(4), 237–240.

World Health Organization. (2010). *Medical eligibility criteria for contraceptive use: A WHO family planning cornerstone* (4th ed.). Geneva: Switzerland.

Yonkers, K., Brown, C., Pearlstein, T. B., Foegh, M., Sampson-Landers, C., & Rapkin, A. (2005). Efficacy of a new low-dose oral contraceptive with drospirenone in premenstrual dysphoric disorder. *Obstetrics and Gynecology, 106*(3), 492–501.

Young, E. A., Kornstein, S. G., Harvey, A. T., Wisniewski, S. R., Barkin, J., Fava, M., ... Rush, A. J. (2007). Influences of hormone-based contraception on depressive symptoms in premenopausal women with major depression. *Psychoneuroendocrinology, 32*(7), 843–853.

The Impact of Reproductive Cancers on Women's Mental Health

Doreen L. Wiggins, Carmen Monzon, and Beth R. Hott

Introduction

It is estimated that in 2014 there will be 14 million cancer survivors in the USA (de Moor et al., 2013). Today, women with breast (22 %) and gynecologic (8 %) cancers account for 30 % of all survivors (Siegel et al., 2012). Improvements in screening and treatment continue to increase the number of individuals living 5 years beyond their cancer diagnosis, and it is projected that long-term survival will continue to increase over the next decade (Howlader et al. 2009).

Cancer is quickly becoming viewed as a chronic illness associated with long-term side effects of treatment, including decreased functional capacity, pain, fatigue, decreased fertility and sexual function, anxiety, and depression (Carr et al., 2002). The psychological impact of a cancer diagnosis varies with disease origin, age of diagnosis, physiologic alterations, and stage. Studies indicate that 20–47 % of newly diagnosed or recurrent cancer patients had significant psychosocial concerns. However, less than half of cancer survivors experiencing psychological issues are referred for help. There are many barriers to asking for and offering psychosocial

---

D.L. Wiggins, M.D., F.A.C.O.G., F.A.C.S. (✉)
Assistant Clinical Professor of Obstetrics & Gynecology and Surgery, The Warren Alpert Medical School of Brown University, Providence, RI, USA

Director, Cancer Survivorship Program, Women's Medicine Collaborative, The Miriam Hospital, Providence, RI, USA
e-mail: doreen_wiggins@brown.edu

C. Monzon, M.D.
Assistant Clinical Professor of Psychiatry and Human Behavior, The Warren Alpert Medical School of Brown University, Providence, RI, USA

Women's Behavioral Medicine, Women's Medicine Collaborative, The Miriam Hospital, Providence, RI, USA

B.R. Hott, B.A.
Women's Medicine Collaborative, The Miriam Hospital, Providence, RI, USA

assistance to cancer patients. There is a stigma and reluctance associated with psychiatric concern acknowledgement; asking for help regarding emotional matters often embarrasses patients and family members. In 1997 the National Comprehensive Cancer Network, NCCN, created an interdisciplinary panel to develop clinical practice guidelines to address psychosocial care in oncology. The panel included members specializing in oncology, psychiatry, nursing, social work and counseling, psychology, patient advocacy, and clergy. Their first task was to recognize that there were obstacles preventing referrals for psychosocial assistance for cancer survivors. Panel members published guidelines in 1999 (National Comprehensive Cancer Network, 1999) for the management of psychosocial concerns and chose to identify patients as "distressed" rather than "psychiatric" or "social" to avoid the stigma associated with psychiatric care. The panel defined distress as a "multifactorial unpleasant emotional experience of a psychological (cognitive, behavioral, emotional), social, and/or spiritual nature that may interfere with the ability to cope effectively with cancer, its physical symptoms, and its treatment." They continue, "Distress extends along a continuum, ranging from common normal feelings of vulnerability, sadness, and fears to problems that can become disabling, such as depression, anxiety, panic, social isolation, and existential and spiritual crisis" (National Comprehensive Cancer Network, 1999). The Distress Thermometer (DT) is an effective screening tool that was developed by the NCCN panel to identify patients in need of psychosocial support. A self-report questionnaire, this screening instrument can be completed in the waiting room and measures patient distress originating from any source, cancer related or not, during the past 7 days (NCCN, 2013). The DT has been validated by many studies and has shown excellent concordance with identifying survivors in need of psychosocial support (Jacobsen, 2009; Jacobson et al., 2008; Neuss et al., 2005; Roth et al., 1998).

Impact of Diagnosis and Treatment in Relation to Age

Female reproductive cancer survivors often face not only the concerns surrounding a cancer diagnosis, treatment, and future survival but also potential repercussions regarding sexual health, fertility, motherhood, and self-fulfillment. The median age of diagnosis for cancers of the breast, cervix, ovary, uterus, and vulva is during the postmenopausal period, but a significant number (>25 % for breast and ovarian, and >50 % for cervical) will be diagnosed during reproductive adulthood (see Table 1).

Breast and gynecological cancers account for 25 % of the 21,000 young adults diagnosed with cancer annually in the USA (Bleyer, Viny, & Barr, 2006). Cancer diagnosis between the ages of 15 and 29 can have significant impact on physical and emotional well-being, reproductive potential, and personal and financial independence. A 2009 population-based National Health Interview Survey comparing cancer survivors diagnosed between ages 15 and 29 to non-cancer controls reported poorer mental health outcomes, greater prevalence of medical conditions, more

Table 1 Reproductive cancer incidence, age of diagnosis, and lifetime risk 2006–2010 [based on the NCI SEER Cancer Statistics Review (*SEER Cancer Statistics Review, 1975–2009*, 2012)]

	Breast	Cervix	Ovary	Uterus	Vulva
Median age at diagnosis	61	57	63	62	68
<20	0.0 %	0.1 %	1.3 %	0.0 %	0.2 %
20–34	1.8 %	13.8 %	3.6 %	1.6 %	2.0 %
35–44	9.6 %	25.7 %	7.2 %	5.8 %	6.7 %
45–54	22.2 %	24.2 %	18.5 %	18.7 %	15.4 %
55–64	25.2 %	17.0 %	23.7 %	33.4 %	18.9 %
65–74	20.7 %	10.7 %	20.4 %	22.8 %	18.5 %
75–84	14.8 %	5.8 %	17.2 %	13.1 %	23.1 %
85+	5.7 %	2.6 %	8.2 %	4.6 %	15.1 %
Lifetime risk	1 in 8	1 in 147	1 in 72	1 in 38	1 in 368
	12.38 %	0.68 %	1.38 %	2.64 %	0.27 %

Howlader N, Noone AM, Krapcho M, Neyman N, Aminou R, Waldron W, Altekruse SF, Kosary CL, Ruhl J, Tatalovich Z, Cho H, Mariotto A, Eisner MP, Lewis DR, Chen HS, Feuer EJ, Cronin KA (eds). SEER Cancer Statistics Review, 1975–2009 (Vintage 2009 Populations), National Cancer Institute. Bethesda, MD, http://seer.cancer.gov/csr/1975_2009_pops09/, based on November 2011 SEER data submission, posted to the SEER website, April 2012

health-related disabilities, and more psychological distress than their matched case-controlled subjects (Phillips-Salimi & Andrykowski, 2013). Extensive research on psychological adjustment to breast cancer diagnosis and treatment finds that, with a couple of exceptions (Ganz, Lee, Sim, Polinsky, & Schag, 1992; Golden-Kreutz & Andersen, 2004), a younger age at diagnosis is correlated with greater problems regarding distress and psychological adjustment following diagnosis (Avis & Deimling, 2008; Bardwell et al., 2006; Broeckel, Jacobsen, Balducci, Horton, & Lyman, 2000; Kroenke et al., 2004; Mosher & Danoff-Burg, 2005; Vinokur et al., 1990; Wenzel et al., 1999). Mor, Malin, and Allen (1994) found that younger women (<55 years) experienced the effects of their illness with greater distress and deeper emotional and financial trouble and suffered greater disruptions in daily life after chemotherapy treatment than did older women. Age-related differences persisted with negative outcomes for younger survivors, even after controlling for disease severity, social support, and demographic variables of income, education, and marital status. The authors postulated that younger cancer survivors had greater "life stage" challenges in adapting to the unexpectedness or the "off-time" diagnosis and in coping with the loss of potential future aspirations such as career goals or the threat of losing the ability to see their children grow up. Consistent with previous research, Baider et al. reported in 2003 that younger women with breast cancer experience the occurrence of severe emotional distress more often than older women (Baider et al. 2003). Younger women are considered to be less successful than older women at coping with treatment-related side effects: maintaining a positive attitude facing their diagnosis of cancer, in regulating affect, and in seeking support. Similar studies (Hoskins et al., 1996; Politi, Enright, & Weihs, 2007; Schover, 1994) support the expectation that patients with breast cancer manifest age-related differences in the psychosocial impact of their illness. Compared to older patients, younger patients diagnosed with breast cancer may require greater social support and more awareness of the need for mental health interventions that they may be receiving or requesting. In 2004, Kroenke and colleagues published a functional impact analysis, determined by age at diagnosis, in a prospective setting (Kroenke et al., 2004). They found that young women (40 years of age at therapy) who developed breast cancer experienced greater absolute and relative functional losses in physical ability, bodily pain, social function, and mental health compared to middle-aged or elderly breast cancer survivors. A 2003 study by Ganz et al. interviewed 691 women aged 65 years and older and found a significant decline in both mental and physical health during the first 15 months following breast cancer surgery (Ganz et al., 2003). Age was not a predictor of posttreatment or psychological adjustment following cancer diagnosis. Health-related quality of life in older breast cancer survivors was aligned to baseline physical functioning, psychological health, and perceived emotional support.

Physiologic Changes with Cancer Treatment and Surgery: Impact on Mental Well-Being

The diagnosis and treatment of reproductive cancers have been associated with weight gain, hair loss, and decreased functional capacity, especially in women receiving chemotherapy. Literature supports that a body mass index (BMI) of $\geq 30 \text{ kg/m}^2$ or more at breast cancer diagnosis is related to poorer prognosis (Demark-Wahnefried & Rock, 2003; Irwin et al., 2005; Lankester, Phillips, & Lawton, 2002; Saquib et al., 2007; Demark-Wahnefried et al., 2001).

Weight Change

Weight gain is more prominent in women who undergo menopause with treatment, are obese prior to treatment, or have a low level of physical activity (Goodwin et al. 1999; Yaw et al., 2011). In breast cancer survivors undergoing chemotherapy, 50 % will observe weight gain of 2.5–5.0 kg (5.5–11 lb), with 20 % observing weight gain of 10–20 kg (22–44 lb) (Aslani, Smith, Allen, Pavlakis, & Levi, 1999; Demark-Wahnefried, Rimer, & Winer, 1997; Demark-Wahnefried, Winer, & Rimer, 1993; Goodwin et al., 1999; Saquib et al., 2007). The cause of weight gain in women undergoing chemotherapy is not completely understood. Dietary intake studies have failed to support the premise that women were eating more than normal (Brownell & Rodin, 1994; Myers et al., 2011; Tremblay & Bandi, 2003). There is evidence to suggest that weight gain with chemotherapy may be related to initiation of menopause, decreased physical activity, and a reduction in lean body mass, thus lowering the resting metabolic rate (Curtis et al., 2005; Diaz, Mainous, & Everett, 2005; Tremblay & Bandi, 2003). The After Breast Cancer Pooling Project (ABCPP) is an international collaboration of prospective studies of breast cancer survivors established to examine the role of physical activity, adiposity, dietary factors, supplement use, and quality of life in breast cancer prognosis. The study evaluated 12,915 breast cancer survivors and found that women who remained weight stable had the best prognosis. Women who lost greater than 5 % of their pre-diagnosis weight were seven times more likely to die from breast cancer. The US women who lost weight with breast cancer treatments had other comorbid conditions that contributed to the increased risk of overall mortality. They were less likely to receive the standard chemotherapy treatment and more likely to be hospitalized with treatment complications. Women who were of normal weight at the time of diagnosis were at the greatest risk for weight gain with treatment and were at the highest risk of experiencing overall mortality if their weight gain was ≥10 % from pre-diagnosis measurements.

Hair Loss

One of the most visible aspects to cancer treatment is hair loss. Alopecia, secondary to chemotherapy, is a significant psychosocial stressor for women and can cause decreased self-esteem, a negative body image, and a reduced sense of well-being (Hesketh et al., 2004). The outward change of alopecia identifies women undergoing chemotherapy as a cancer patient and visibly discloses their diagnosis to others. Stressors include the awkward transition of changing a private matter to a public display. Previous studies demonstrate that 47–58 % of female chemotherapy patients report hair loss as the most traumatic aspect of cancer treatment (Munstedt, Manthey, Sachsse, & Vahrson, 1997; Trueb, 2010). Hair loss can also represent loss of identity, diminished sense of autonomy, and further impinge upon perceived femininity by decreasing sensuality and sexuality (Borsellino & Young, 2011; Freedman, 1994; Zannini et al., 2012). In 1999, Williams et al. conducted a focus group to better understand the experiences of women developing alopecia as a result of chemotherapy. The reactions commonly experienced by the group were not feeling prepared, shock, personal embarrassment, losing a sense of self, and facing the reactions of others (Williams, Wood, & Cunningham-Warburton, 1999). Anticipatory fear regarding appearance changes related to chemotherapy can be all-consuming and can impact treatment choices (Freedman, 1994; Tierney, Taylor, & Closs, 1992). Alopecia presents with acute psychological implications and physical adjustment when women are also dealing with their diagnosis of cancer. Medical providers often do not discuss the psychosocial concerns of hair loss with patients or minimize consequences (Lemieux, Maunsell, & Provencher, 2008). Oncology practitioners can serve to facilitate proactive coping interventions related to alopecia prior to chemotherapy by discussing patient concerns and providing a timeline for hair loss and anticipated regrowth and options for hair camouflaging (Borsellino & Young, 2011; Harcourt & Frith, 2008).

Fatigue

Cancer-related fatigue, CRF, is defined by the NCCN as a distressing, persistent, subjective sense of physical, emotional, and/or cognitive tiredness or exhaustion related to cancer or cancer treatment that is not proportional to recent activity and interferes with the patient's usual functioning. According to a survey of 1,569 cancer patients, CRF is experienced by 80 % of individuals who receive chemotherapy and/or radiotherapy. In patients with metastatic disease, the prevalence of CRF exceeds 75 % (Henry et al., 2008).

CRF can occur prior to diagnosis, with treatment, and well after completion of therapy, and can significantly impinge on quality of life (Ganz et al., 2003). Once fatigue is identified, a comprehensive medical evaluation, including cancer treatment regiment, medical comorbidities, baseline energy level, and psychosocial history, is indicated. Often patients experiencing severe fatigue have confounding conditions such as chronic pain, cognitive function changes, sleep disturbance, or a previous history of anxiety and depression. Curt et al. analyzed the impact of CRF on the emotional health in patients and found that fatigue had considerable bearing on daily life (Curt et al., 2000). More than 50 % of patients reported mental exhaustion, sadness, frustration, or irritability because of fatigue and decreased interest and motivation in normal activities because of fatigue (Curt et al., 2000). The NCCN has created the Cancer-Related Fatigue Clinical Practice Guidelines to help practitioners with the management of CRF and begins with education and counseling, energy conservation to prevent depletion, nutrition and exercise intervention, and pharmacologic assistance if needed.

Reproductive Consequences of Female Cancers and Psychosocial Implications

It was estimated that 75,000 women under the age of 50 will be diagnosed with a reproductive cancer in 2013 in the USA (see Table 2). Medical management of breast and gynecologic cancers often includes surgery, chemotherapy, radiation, and

Table 2 Estimated incidence of reproductive female cancers in the USA for 2013: Women <50 years old is 75,241 and total incidence is 321,180 (*SEER Cancer Statistics Review, 1975–2009*, 2012)

Age of diagnosis	Breast	Cervix	Ovary	Uterine	Vulva
Age <50	58,085	6,170	5,560	4,956	470
Any age	232,340	12,340	22,240	49,560	4,700

Howlader N, Noone AM, Krapcho M, Neyman N, Aminou R, Waldron W, Altekruse SF, Kosary CL, Ruhl J, Tatalovich Z, Cho H, Mariotto A, Eisner MP, Lewis DR, Chen HS, Feuer EJ, Cronin KA (eds). SEER Cancer Statistics Review, 1975–2009 (Vintage 2009 Populations), National Cancer Institute. Bethesda, MD, http://seer.cancer.gov/csr/1975_2009_pops09/, based on November 2011 SEER data submission, posted to the SEER website, April 2012 adjuvant anti-hormonal therapies, all of which can directly impact sexual function and future fertility. The psychological impact of cancer on young women survivors facing reproductive and sexual consequences due to treatment is often underestimated or not even addressed. Significant clinical distress related to possible loss of fertility has been reported in 77 % of premenopausal female cancer survivors (Carter et al., 2010). The National Cancer Institute estimates that 40–100 % of cancer survivors experience some form of sexual complaint, with 50–90 % of breast cancer and 30–90 % of gynecologic cancer survivors noting long-lasting problems. Studies indicate that more than 50 % of premenopausal women diagnosed with cancer do not have discussions with their physician regarding fertility concerns or sexual function assessment prior to starting treatment. Stead et al. reported that there are many barriers to sexual assessment and discussion of concerns both before and after cancer treatment (Stead, Fallowfield, Brown, & Selby, 2001). Common reasons for not discussing concerns are time constraints at office visits, patient or physician embarrassment, not wanting to overwhelm the patient with more bad news, physician concerns regarding patient's feelings, lack of sexual training, and the provider's discomfort discussing sexuality issues.

Fertility Preservation

Premenopausal women diagnosed with cancer must process the impact of a cancer diagnosis, must face decisions regarding complex treatment options, and may be overwhelmed with fears about future survival. Discussions regarding fertility impact with treatment and possible means of fertility preservation are of great importance to patients and may well affect cancer treatment decisions (Maltaris et al., 2007). In a 2004 study by Partridge et al. on breast cancer survivors, 29 % reported that the risk of infertility influenced their regimen for cancer treatment (Partridge et al., 2004). In 2006, the American Society of Clinical Oncology (ASCO) published a clinical practice guideline on fertility preservation for patients with cancer for healthcare providers caring for newly diagnosed adults and children. We have included a table listing the ASCO guidelines key recommendations and those for fertility preservation for adult females with cancer (see Table 3). The impetus for the guidelines was a response to the paucity of providers initiating discussions of fertility concerns with newly diagnosed cancer patients.

All healthcare providers caring for cancer patients should discuss the potential risks of treatment on fertility preservation at the time of diagnosis. Referral to reproductive specialists and support of a psychosocial provider can assist patients dealing with the reproductive impact of cancer treatment and the decision-making process regarding future fertility before initiation of therapy. Letourneau and colleagues conducted a retrospective survey to determine if reproductive-aged women with cancer who received fertility counseling and options for fertility preservation from a fertility specialist had improved aspects of quality of life (Letourneau et al., 2012). Results indicate that women counseled by their oncologist and fertility specialist had significantly less decision regret with regard to fertility concerns.

Table 3 Fertility preservation for patients with cancer: American Society of Clinical Oncology Clinical Practice Guideline Update (Loren et al., 2013)

Key recommendations

Discuss fertility preservation with all patients of reproductive age (and with parents or guardians of children and adolescents) if infertility is a potential risk of therapy.

Refer patients who express an interest in fertility preservation (and patients who are ambivalent) to reproductive specialists.

Address fertility preservation as early as possible, before treatment starts.

Document fertility preservation discussions in the medical chart.

Answer basic questions about whether fertility preservation options decrease the chance of successful cancer treatment.

Refer patients to psychosocial providers if they experience distress about potential infertility.

Encourage patients to participate in registries and clinical studies.

Fertility preservation for adult females with cancer

Present both embryo and oocyte cryopreservation as established fertility preservation methods.

Discuss the option of ovarian transposition (oophoropexy) when pelvic radiation therapy is performed as cancer treatment.

Inform patients of conservative gynecologic surgery and radiation therapy options.

Inform patients that there is insufficient evidence regarding the effectiveness of ovarian suppression (GnRH analogs) as a fertility preservation method and these agents should not be relied on to preserve fertility.

Inform patients that other methods (e.g., ovarian tissue cryopreservation and transplantation procedures, which do not require ovarian stimulation or sexual maturity) are still experimental.

Modified with permission Loren, A. W., Mangu, P. B., Beck, L. N., Brennan, L., Magdalinski, A. J., Partridge, A. H., ... Oktay, K. (2013). Fertility preservation for patients with cancer: American society of clinical oncology clinical practice guideline update. *Journal of Clinical Oncology, 31*(19), 2500–2510

Sexual Function

Ninety percent of female reproductive cancer survivors experience sexual difficulties with treatment, and studies indicate that 50 % will have long-term sexual dysfunction (Ganz, Rowland, Desmond, Meyerowitz, & Wyatt, 1998; Schover, Montague, & Lakin, 1997). However, the psychosocial impact of cancer treatment on sexual function, intimacy, and possible long-term expectations is rarely discussed and is frequently neglected. Psychosocial sexual concerns relating to reproductive cancer diagnosis are multifaceted with the physical alterations from surgery and radiation, hormonal adaptations to an abrupt menopause, adjuvant chemotherapy, and anti-hormonal treatments. Since cancer treatment directly involves the anatomical body parts participating in sexual activity, it is imperative the oncologist/surgeon discuss sexual function and intimacy concerns at diagnosis. A simple sexual history taken with open-ended questions, reviewing past medical history and medications, gynecologic history including any sexual assault/trauma, and inquiring if there are any concerns regarding intimacy or sexual difficulties should be part of every initial patient evaluation. Anticipated sexual changes and expectations of therapy side effects should be reviewed prior to treatment. Intermittent review of ongoing sexual and intimacy concerns by healthcare providers should continue throughout treatment and survivorship. Predictors of patients at high risk for sexual dysfunction are previous history of sexual and relationship concerns, depression, poor self-concept, weight gain, and body image concerns (Den Oudsten, Van Heck, Van der Steeg, Roukema, & De Vries, 2010; Ganz, Desmond, Belin, Meyerowitz, & Rowland, 1999; Schover, 1991; Yurek, Farrar, & Andersen, 2000). The most common sexual difficulties of women treated for reproductive cancers are loss of desire, dyspareunia, vaginal dryness, and feelings of reduced sexual attractiveness (Andersen, 1995; Bergmark, Avall-Lundqvist, Dickman, Henningsohn, & Steineck, 1999; Ganz et al., 1999). Pelvic surgery and radiation are associated with lasting negative effects including shortened vaginal length, decreased vaginal lubrication, loss of elasticity and stenosis, ovarian failure, and dyspareunia (Denton & Maher, 2003; Jensen et al., 2003; Li et al., 1999). Breast cancer survivors treated with breast conservation and radiation compared to mastectomy tend to have an improved acceptance of body image and tend to engage in breast caressing but do not differ with respect to coital frequency, ease of orgasm, or overall sexual happiness (Stead, 2003; Yurek et al., 2000).

Beyond the direct surgical interventions for reproductive cancer treatments, medical adjuvant therapies including chemotherapy and anti-hormonal medications can cause an abrupt cessation of menstrual functioning and menopausal symptoms resulting in psychosexual consequences. A report by Wilmoth focusing on sexual function, relationship quality, self-concept, and psychological self-affecting sexuality after breast cancer treatment looked at patient responses to a questionnaire focusing on sexual changes experienced with diagnosis and treatment (Wilmoth, 2001). Results revealed three stages of adjustment that a breast cancer survivor's sexual self transitioned through with diagnosis and treatment. When learning of a new cancer diagnosis, a multitude of life changes and a very real fear for survival takes over. Women must come to an understanding regarding the surgical aspects, menopausal symptoms, and loss of sexual sensations experienced in order to come to terms with their life changes and to better adjust to their altered sexual self. Intimacy, fertility, and sexual concerns should be anticipated with the treatment of reproductive cancers to help prepare patients and to minimize problems and possibly provide better sexual outcomes. Ideally, fertility and sexuality concerns should be addressed with a multidisciplinary approach beginning with the initial treating physician and supported by fertility specialists, individual and couples therapy, and pain and function rehabilitation (McKee & Schover, 2001).

Women with Reproductive Cancers and a History of Sexual or Previous Traumas

The National Child Abuse and Neglect Data System, NCANDS, recognize four major types of maltreatment: neglect, physical abuse, psychological maltreatment, and sexual abuse (US Department of Health and Human Services, 2011).

Childhood mistreatment is a common occurrence with close to 50 % of children experiencing abuse and/or neglect. Approximately 33 % of females before the age of 18 will experience sexual abuse, and the incidence has been increasing in recent years (Wyatt, Loeb, Desmond, & Ganz, 2005; Wyatt, Loeb, Solis, & Carmona, 1999). A prior history of childhood maltreatment may have significant effects on the psychological well-being and integration of personality development into adulthood (Johnson, 2004; Weaver, Chard, Mechanic, & Etzel, 2004). Childhood sexual abuse survivors have an increased risk of depression, substance abuse, delay in seeking medical treatment, and an increase in risky sexual behaviors. Abused women are also at an increased risk for worsened psychological distress when threatened with a new trauma such as a diagnosis of cancer (Brewin, Andrews, & Valentine, 2000; Fagundes, Lindgren, Shapiro, & Kiecolt-Glaser, 2012). In addition, Davis and Frawley reasoned in 1994 that childhood sexual abuse was a "betrayal trauma" when the abuser is a person of authority and trusted adult (Davies & Frawley-O'Dea, 1994). Reproductive female cancers may cause further feelings of betrayal and distress and negatively impact cancer screening and treatment (Gallo-Silver & Weiner, 2006). A study done in 2005 by Bergmark et al. and another in 2012 by Cadman and colleagues found that sexually abused women with cervical cancer were diagnosed later and attended screening programs less frequently; these findings were thought to be related to acquired hopelessness, self-neglect or destructive behaviors, avoidant control, and fear of gynecological exams (Bergmark, Avall-Lundqvist, Dickman, Steineck, & Henningsohn, 2005; Cadman, Waller, Ashdown-Barr, & Szarewski, 2012). Avoidant behaviors and need of autonomy for survivors of childhood traumas facing a new cancer diagnosis may interfere with compliance to testing and treatment regiments (Gallo-Silver & Weiner, 2006). Oncology practitioners should screen new cancer patients for a history of childhood maltreatment and should proceed with sensitivity and understanding. Fagundes and colleagues have demonstrated that breast cancer survivors with a history of childhood abuse have a significantly decreased quality of life with respect to fatigue; poorer emotional, physical, and functional well-being; and less social support (Fagundes et al., 2012). Comprehensive cancer care should be sensitive to the psychosocial needs of reproductive cancer survivors with a history of childhood maltreatment and proceed with emotional support, respect, and facilitation of a patient's autonomy throughout treatment.

Breast and Ovarian Hereditary Mutations

On May 14, 2013, actress Angelina Jolie announced to the world through *The New York Times* that she had prophylactic mastectomies and reconstruction due to her carrying a "faulty" BRCA 1 gene mutation. Female carriers of a BRCA mutation have an 87 % lifetime risk of developing breast cancer and up to a 44 % lifetime risk of developing ovarian cancer. Risk reduction strategies exist; screening and prophylactic surgical options are available. On the heels of Ms. Jolie's public revelation and her hope that women could benefit from her experience, there has been a flurry of attention on testing and inquiries surrounding BRCA genes, such as cost and other obstacles. This social media buzz spurring public medical concern has been deemed "The Angelina Effect," so named by TIME magazine in their May 27, 2013, cover story. On June 13, 2013, the US Supreme Court ruled that isolated human genes could not be patented, a defeat for Myriad Genetics, Inc., the company who was awarded patents on the BRCA genes in the 1990s. This decision will potentially lower the cost of BRCA genetic testing, promote access, and increase awareness of preventative genomics and familial inheritance (Offit et al., 2013). Gene testing, specifically BRCA testing, does have emotional consequences. Information is limited on the psychosocial impact of a BRCA mutation on the individual carrier, family members, and offspring.

Often the suggestion of BRCA testing is concurrent with facing a new cancer diagnosis. Therefore, patients are contemplating not only their own health concerns but also the implications that a genetic mutation could have on family members. At diagnosis, a patient may feel that the addition of a possible inheritable genetic mutation is overwhelming to contemplate and may choose to forego genetic counseling and testing. Physicians and providers often encourage women with breast cancer who present with high-risk indicators for a genetic mutation and women with ovarian or fallopian tube cancers to consider genetic consultation and testing at diagnosis. Often women who choose to seek genetic counseling and testing see it as their duty to protect family members, especially if they have a daughter, from developing cancer (MacDonald, Sarna, Weitzel, & Ferrell, 2010). Women who underwent genetic cancer risk assessment reported a sense of guilt and concern about their personal involvement and role in their daughters' cancer risk (MacDonald et al., 2010). Meeting with a genetic counselor did empower the patients to learn more about their cancer risk and be proactive with cancer prevention efforts (MacDonald et al., 2010). BRCA mutations are transferred to offspring in an autosomal dominant inheritance, meaning that male and female children have a 50 % chance of inheriting the gene. BRCA testing has been marketed by Myriad to be performed in physician's offices without the benefit of meeting with a genetic counselor. However, with the advent of further development of gene testing and the new generation of gene panels, it is important to have individuals meet with a genetic counselor to determine the best course for testing and to also provide the needed emotional support.

Cancer Survivors and Posttraumatic Growth

The diagnosis of cancer, especially a female reproductive cancer with wide-reaching implications, can be a traumatic event in a woman's life. The occurrence can cause disengagement where basic life assumptions need to be dramatically changed or given up. There is a breakdown and disorganization of the self-structure concept, and then the cognitive process of transformation and positive re-framing can begin. The loss of how things should be can allow the opportunity for growth and present

Table 4 Positive changes observed following trauma and adversity

Adversarial growth	Positive by-products
Flourishing	Positive changes
Perceived benefits	Positive meaning
Benefit finding	Posttraumatic growth
Heightened existential awareness	Self-renewal
Quantum change	Stress-related growth
Thriving	Transformational coping

new meaning towards becoming a richer individual functioning beyond the pre-diagnosed self (Tedeschi & Calhoun, 2004).

Posttraumatic growth is a well-known and widely utilized concept referring to the positive psychological change experienced as a result of the struggle with a highly challenging life circumstance (Tedeschi & Calhoun, 2004). The positive changes observed following trauma and adversity have various labels, and all have been used in the literature interchangeably as posttraumatic growth (Horgan, Holcombe, & Salmon, 2011) (see Table 4).

In 2004, Tedeschi and Calhoun identified five areas of personal growth that may transpire from a traumatic event: appreciation for life, perception of personal strength, altered priorities, improved spirituality, and more meaningful relationships (Tedeschi & Calhoun, 2004).

Posttraumatic growth in cancer survivors has been documented, particularly in breast cancer survivors who are the most frequently studied group in posttraumatic growth research. It is estimated that 50–83 % of breast cancer survivors experience positive life changes as a result of their cancer diagnosis (Kucukkaya, 2010; Sears, Stanton, & Danoff-Burg, 2003). A cancer diagnosis is different than a significant traumatic event or loss due to the fact that cancer is the beginning of an unknown journey with no clear ending, and it elicits anxiety and fear. Different points along the survivorship timeline can manifest psychological distress, occurring not only at diagnosis but also with treatment and associated body changes (hair loss), completion of therapy, and follow-up screening. Supportive relationships and therapeutic assistance can help facilitate healing and posttraumatic growth of cancer survivors, even if patients are not interested in intervention. A nurse navigator or a patient advocate can assist in gaining knowledge, promote participation in preventative measures by adopting healthy lifestyles, and help achieve positive growth (Silva, Crespo, & Canavarro, 2012). Cancer survivors who experience positive growth can develop a better sense of self and can foster self-assurance as a reflection of their ability to manage a cancer diagnosis and treatment. Empathy for others can surface as a positive outcome of personal suffering with cancer treatment (Horgan et al., 2011).

Cancer survivors often become obsessed with thoughts of cancer, and cognitive rumination can set in and cause negative emotional disposition. Allowing survivors the opportunity to share their environment can promote healing. With a traumatic event it is anticipated that negative emotions, such as anger, hostility, depression, and anxiety, would be elicited. However, some individuals may experience gratitude as well as other positive emotions such as humor. The ability to genuinely feel the

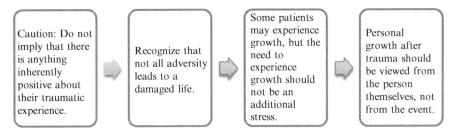

Fig. 1 Providers and post-traumatic growth

emotion of gratitude after experiencing a personal struggle has been related to resilience and growth (Ruini, 2013). The ability to see things in a positive light, dispositional optimism, the general expectation that more good things than bad will happen, can have significant positive and psychological implications (Connerty & Knott, 2013). Providers recognizing the possibility of growth and discussing growth with survivors must be cautious not to imply that there is anything inherently positive about their development of cancer. It is also important to understand as clinicians that a deep adversity does not necessarily lead to a damaged life and, for some, can lead to positive change and growth that would not have been possible without their diagnosis (Mols, Vingerhoets, Coebergh, & van de Poll-Franse, 2009). Clinicians cannot create growth for survivors, and the expectation that there should be growth should not be an added stress imposed. Fostering the realization that personal growth has come from within, and not from the struggle with the cancer diagnosis, is the key to reinforcing the inner strength of the individual (Fig. 1).

Conclusion

The impact of reproductive cancers on women's psychological well-being has widespread implications and outcomes and is as varied as the cancer itself. There are many obstacles for cancer survivors to face in obtaining psychological support for the distress and trauma a cancer diagnosis can bring to an individual and his or her family. However, the need for intervention, especially for women with reproduction cancers, is imperative yet not always addressed. Psychosocial support has been shown to improve the quality of life in survivors and to improve possible outcomes.

References

Andersen, B. L. (1995). Quality of life for women with gynecologic cancer. *Current Opinion in Obstetrics & Gynecology, 7*(1), 69–76.

Aslani, A., Smith, R. C., Allen, B. J., Pavlakis, N., & Levi, J. A. (1999). Changes in body composition during breast cancer chemotherapy with the CMF-regimen. *Breast Cancer Research and Treatment, 57*(3), 285–290.

Avis, N. E., & Deimling, G. T. (2008). Cancer survivorship and aging. *Cancer, 113*(12 Suppl), 3519–3529.

Baider, L., Andritsch, E., Uziely, B., Goldzweig, G., Ever-Hadani, P., Hofman, G., ... Samonigg, H. (2003). Effects of age on coping and psychological distress in women diagnosed with breast cancer: Review of literature and analysis of two different geographical settings. *Critical Reviews in Oncology/Hematology, 46*(1), 5–16.

Bardwell, W. A., Natarajan, L., Dimsdale, J. E., Rock, C. L., Mortimer, J. E., Hollenbach, K., & Pierce, J. P. (2006). Objective cancer-related variables are not associated with depressive symptoms in women treated for early-stage breast cancer. *Journal of Clinical Oncology, 24*(16), 2420–2427.

Bergmark, K., Avall-Lundqvist, E., Dickman, P. W., Henningsohn, L., & Steineck, G. (1999). Vaginal changes and sexuality in women with a history of cervical cancer. *The New England Journal of Medicine, 340*(18), 1383–1389.

Bergmark, K., Avall-Lundqvist, E., Dickman, P. W., Steineck, G., & Henningsohn, L. (2005). Synergy between sexual abuse and cervical cancer in causing sexual dysfunction. *Journal of Sex & Marital Therapy, 31*(5), 361–383.

Bleyer, A., Viny, A., & Barr, R. (2006). Cancer in 15- to 29-year-olds by primary site. *The Oncologist, 11*(6), 590–601.

Borsellino, M., & Young, M. M. (2011). Anticipatory coping: Taking control of hair loss. *Clinical Journal of Oncology Nursing, 15*(3), 311–315.

Brewin, C. R., Andrews, B., & Valentine, J. D. (2000). Meta-analysis of risk factors for posttraumatic stress disorder in trauma-exposed adults. *Journal of Consulting and Clinical Psychology, 68*(5), 748–766.

Broeckel, J. A., Jacobsen, P. B., Balducci, L., Horton, J., & Lyman, G. H. (2000). Quality of life after adjuvant chemotherapy for breast cancer. *Breast Cancer Research and Treatment, 62*(2), 141–150.

Brownell, K. D., & Rodin, J. (1994). Medical, metabolic, and psychological effects of weight cycling. *Archives of Internal Medicine, 154*(12), 1325–1330.

Cadman, L., Waller, J., Ashdown-Barr, L., & Szarewski, A. (2012). Barriers to cervical screening in women who have experienced sexual abuse: An exploratory study. *The Journal of Family Planning and Reproductive Health Care, 38*(4), 214–220.

Carr, D., Goudas, L., Lawrence, D., Pirl, W., Lau, J., DeVine, D., ... Miller, K. (2002, July). *Management of cancer symptoms: Pain, depression, and fatigue*. Evidence Report/Technology Assessment No. 61 (Prepared by the New England Medical Center Evidence-based Practice Center under Contract No 290-97-0019). AHRQ Publication No. 02-E032. Rockville, MD: Agency for Healthcare Research and Quality.

Carter, J., Chi, D. S., Brown, C. L., Abu-Rustum, N. R., Sonoda, Y., Aghajanian, C., ... Barakat, R. R. (2010). Cancer-related infertility in survivorship. *International Journal of Gynecological Cancer, 20*(1), 2–8.

Connerty, T. J., & Knott, V. (2013). Promoting positive change in the face of adversity: Experiences of cancer and post-traumatic growth. *European Journal of Cancer Care, 22*(3), 334–344.

Curt, G. A., Breitbart, W., Cella, D., Groopman, J. E., Horning, S. J., Itri, L. M., ... Vogelzang, N. J. (2000). Impact of cancer-related fatigue on the lives of patients: New findings from the Fatigue Coalition. *The Oncologist, 5*(5), 353–360.

Curtis, J. P., Selter, J. G., Wang, Y., Rathore, S. S., Jovin, I. S., Jadbabaie, F., ... Krumholz, H. M. (2005). The obesity paradox: Body mass index and outcomes in patients with heart failure. *Archives of Internal Medicine, 165*(1), 55–61.

Davies, J. M., & Frawley-O'Dea, M. G. (1994). *Treating the adult survivor of childhood sexual abuse: A Psychoanalytic Perspective*. New York, NY: Basic Books.

de Moor, J. S., Mariotto, A. B., Parry, C., Alfano, C. M., Padgett, L., Kent, E. E., ... Rowland, J. H. (2013). Cancer survivors in the United States: Prevalence across the survivorship trajectory and implications for care. *Cancer Epidemiology, Biomarkers & Prevention, 22*(4), 561–570.

Demark-Wahnefried, W., Peterson, B. L., Winer, E. P., Marks, L., Aziz, N., Marcom, P. K., Blackwell, K., Rimer, B. K. (2001). Changes in weight, body composition, and factors influencing energy balance among premenopausal breast cancer patients receiving adjuvant chemotherapy. *Journal of Clinical Oncology, 19*, 2381–2389.

Demark-Wahnefried, W., Rimer, B. K., & Winer, E. P. (1997). Weight gain in women diagnosed with breast cancer. *Journal of the American Dietetic Association, 97*(5), 519–526, 529; quiz 527–518.

Demark-Wahnefried, W., & Rock, C. L. (2003). Nutrition-related issues for the breast cancer survivor. *Seminars in Oncology, 30*(6), 789–798.

Demark-Wahnefried, W., Winer, E. P., & Rimer, B. K. (1993). Why women gain weight with adjuvant chemotherapy for breast cancer. *Journal of Clinical Oncology, 11*(7), 1418–1429.

Denton, A. S., & Maher, E. J. (2003). Interventions for the physical aspects of sexual dysfunction in women following pelvic radiotherapy. *The Cochrane Database of Systematic Reviews, 1*, CD003750.

Den Oudsten, B. L., Van Heck, G. L., Van der Steeg, A. F., Roukema, J. A., De Vries, J. (2010) Clinical factors are not the best predictors of quality of sexual life and sexual functioning in women with early stage breast cancer. *Psychooncology, 19*, 646–656.

Diaz, V. A., Mainous, A. G., 3rd, & Everett, C. J. (2005). The association between weight fluctuation and mortality: Results from a population-based cohort study. *Journal of Community Health, 30*(3), 153–165.

Fagundes, C. P., Lindgren, M. E., Shapiro, C. L., & Kiecolt-Glaser, J. K. (2012). Child maltreatment and breast cancer survivors: Social support makes a difference for quality of life, fatigue and cancer stress. *European Journal of Cancer, 48*(5), 728–736.

Freedman, T. G. (1994). Social and cultural dimensions of hair loss in women treated for breast cancer. *Cancer Nursing, 17*(4), 334–341.

Gallo-Silver, L., & Weiner, M. O. (2006). Survivors of childhood sexual abuse diagnosed with cancer: Managing the impact of early trauma on cancer treatment. *Journal of Psychosocial Oncology, 24*(1), 107–134.

Ganz, P. A., Desmond, K. A., Belin, T. R., Meyerowitz, B. E., & Rowland, J. H. (1999). Predictors of sexual health in women after a breast cancer diagnosis. *Journal of Clinical Oncology, 17*(8), 2371–2380.

Ganz, P. A., Guadagnoli, E., Landrum, M. B., Lash, T. L., Rakowski, W., & Silliman, R. A. (2003). Breast cancer in older women: Quality of life and psychosocial adjustment in the 15 months after diagnosis. *Journal of Clinical Oncology, 21*(21), 4027–4033.

Ganz, P. A., Lee, J. J., Sim, M. S., Polinsky, M. L., & Schag, C. A. (1992). Exploring the influence of multiple variables on the relationship of age to quality of life in women with breast cancer. *Journal of Clinical Epidemiology, 45*(5), 473–485.

Ganz, P. A., Moinpour, C. M., Pauler, D. K., Kornblith, A. B., Gaynor, E. R., Balcerzak, S. P., … Fisher, R. I. (2003). Health status and quality of life in patients with early-stage Hodgkin's disease treated on Southwest Oncology Group Study 9133. *Journal of Clinical Oncology, 21*(18), 3512–3519.

Ganz, P. A., Rowland, J. H., Desmond, K., Meyerowitz, B. E., & Wyatt, G. E. (1998). Life after breast cancer: Understanding women's health-related quality of life and sexual functioning. *Journal of Clinical Oncology, 16*(2), 501–514.

Golden-Kreutz, D. M., & Andersen, B. L. (2004). Depressive symptoms after breast cancer surgery: Relationships with global, cancer-related, and life event stress. *Psycho-Oncology, 13*(3), 211–220.

Goodwin, P. J., Ennis, M., Pritchard, K. I., McCready, D., Koo, J., Sidlofsky, S., … Redwood, S. (1999). Adjuvant treatment and onset of menopause predict weight gain after breast cancer diagnosis. *Journal of Clinical Oncology, 17*(1), 120–129.

Harcourt, D., & Frith, H. (2008). Women's experiences of an altered appearance during chemotherapy: An indication of cancer status. *Journal of Health Psychology, 13*(5), 597–606.

Henry, D. H., Viswanathan, H. N., Elkin, E. P., Traina, S., Wade, S., & Cella, D. (2008). Symptoms and treatment burden associated with cancer treatment: Results from a cross-sectional national survey in the U.S. *Supportive Care in Cancer, 16*(7), 791–801.

Hesketh, P. J., Batchelor, D., Golant, M., Lyman, G. H., Rhodes, N., & Yardley, D. (2004). Chemotherapy-induced alopecia: Psychosocial impact and therapeutic approaches. *Supportive Care in Cancer, 12*(8), 543–549.

Horgan, O., Holcombe, C., & Salmon, P. (2011). Experiencing positive change after a diagnosis of breast cancer: A grounded theory analysis. *Psycho-Oncology, 20*(10), 1116–1125.

Hoskins, C. N., Baker, S., Sherman, D., Bohlander, J., Bookbinder, M., Budin, W., ... Maislin, G. (1996). Social support and patterns of adjustment to breast cancer. *Scholarly Inquiry for Nursing Practice, 10*(2), 99–123; discussion 125–133.

Howlader, N., Noone, A., Krapcho, M., Neyman, N, Aminou, R, Waldron, W., ... Cronin, K. A. (eds). (2009). *SEER Cancer Statistics Review, 1975–2009* (Vintage 2009 Populations). National Cancer Institute. Bethesda, MD, http://seer.cancer.gov/csr/1975_2009_pops09/ based on November 2011 SEER data submission, posted to the SEER web site, April 2012.

Irwin, M. L., McTiernan, A., Baumgartner, R. N., Baumgartner, K. B., Bernstein, L., Gilliland, F. D., & Ballard-Barbash, R. (2005). Changes in body fat and weight after a breast cancer diagnosis: Influence of demographic, prognostic, and lifestyle factors. *Journal of Clinical Oncology, 23*(4), 774–782.

Jacobsen, P. B. (2009). Promoting evidence-based psychosocial care for cancer patients. *Psycho-Oncology, 18*(1), 6–13.

Jacobson, J. O., Neuss, M. N., McNiff, K. K., Kadlubek, P., Thacker, L. R., 2nd, Song, F., ... Simone, J. V. (2008). Improvement in oncology practice performance through voluntary participation in the Quality Oncology Practice Initiative. *Journal of Clinical Oncology, 26*(11), 1893–1898.

Jensen, P. T., Groenvold, M., Klee, M. C., Thranov, I., Petersen, M. A., & Machin, D. (2003). Longitudinal study of sexual function and vaginal changes after radiotherapy for cervical cancer. *International Journal of Radiation Oncology, Biology, Physics, 56*(4), 937–949.

Johnson, C. F. (2004). Child sexual abuse. *Lancet, 364*(9432), 462–470.

Kroenke, C. H., Rosner, B., Chen, W. Y., Kawachi, I., Colditz, G. A., & Holmes, M. D. (2004). Functional impact of breast cancer by age at diagnosis. *Journal of Clinical Oncology, 22*(10), 1849–1856.

Kucukkaya, P. G. (2010). An exploratory study of positive life changes in Turkish women diagnosed with breast cancer. *European Journal of Oncology Nursing, 14*(2), 166–173.

Lankester, K. J., Phillips, J. E., & Lawton, P. A. (2002). Weight gain during adjuvant and neoadjuvant chemotherapy for breast cancer: An audit of 100 women receiving FEC or CMF chemotherapy. *Clinical Oncology, 14*(1), 64–67.

Lemieux, J., Maunsell, E., & Provencher, L. (2008). Chemotherapy-induced alopecia and effects on quality of life among women with breast cancer: A literature review. *Psycho-Oncology, 17*(4), 317–328.

Letourneau, J. M., Ebbel, E. E., Katz, P. P., Katz, A., Ai, W. Z., Chien, A. J., ... Rosen, M. P. (2012). Pretreatment fertility counseling and fertility preservation improve quality of life in reproductive age women with cancer. *Cancer, 118*(6), 1710–1717.

Li, C., Wilson, P. B., Levine, E., Barber, J., Stewart, A. L., & Kumar, S. (1999). TGF-beta1 levels in pre-treatment plasma identify breast cancer patients at risk of developing post-radiotherapy fibrosis. *International Journal of Cancer, 84*(2), 155–159.

Loren, A. W., Mangu, P. B., Beck, L. N., Brennan, L., Magdalinski, A. J., Partridge, A. H., ... Oktay, K. (2013). Fertility preservation for patients with cancer: American society of clinical oncology clinical practice guideline update. *Journal of Clinical Oncology, 31*(19), 2500–2510.

MacDonald, D. J., Sarna, L., Weitzel, J. N., & Ferrell, B. (2010). Women's perceptions of the personal and family impact of genetic cancer risk assessment: Focus group findings. *Journal of Genetic Counseling, 19*(2), 148–160.

Maltaris, T., Seufert, R., Fischl, F., Schaffrath, M., Pollow, K., Koelbl, H., & Dittrich, R. (2007). The effect of cancer treatment on female fertility and strategies for preserving fertility. *European Journal of Obstetrics, Gynecology, and Reproductive Biology, 130*(2), 148–155.

McKee, A. L., Jr., & Schover, L. R. (2001). Sexuality rehabilitation. *Cancer, 92*(4 Suppl), 1008–1012.

Mols, F., Vingerhoets, A. J., Coebergh, J. W., & van de Poll-Franse, L. V. (2009). Well-being, post-traumatic growth and benefit finding in long-term breast cancer survivors. *Psychology & Health, 24*(5), 583–595.

Mor, V., Malin, M., & Allen, S. (1994). Age differences in the psychosocial problems encountered by breast cancer patients. *Journal of the National Cancer Institute. Monographs, 16*, 191–197.

Mosher, C. E., & Danoff-Burg, S. (2005). A review of age differences in psychological adjustment to breast cancer. *Journal of Psychosocial Oncology, 23*(2–3), 101–114.

Munstedt, K., Manthey, N., Sachsse, S., & Vahrson, H. (1997). Changes in self-concept and body image during alopecia induced cancer chemotherapy. *Supportive Care in Cancer, 5*(2), 139–143.

Myers, J., Lata, K., Chowdhury, S., McAuley, P., Jain, N., & Froelicher, V. (2011). The obesity paradox and weight loss. *The American Journal of Medicine, 124*(10), 924–930.

National Comprehensive Cancer Network. (1999). NCCN practice guidelines for the management of psychosocial distress. *Oncology, 13*(5A), 113–147.

National Comprehensive Cancer Network. (2013). NCCN distress thermometer for patients. http://www.nccn.org/patients/resources/life_with_cancer/pdf/nccn_distress_thermometer.pdf. Accessed October 15, 2013.

Neuss, M. N., Desch, C. E., McNiff, K. K., Eisenberg, P. D., Gesme, D. H., Jacobson, J. O., ... Simone, J. V. (2005). A process for measuring the quality of cancer care: The Quality Oncology Practice Initiative. *Journal of Clinical Oncology, 23*(25), 6233–6239.

Offit, K., Bradbury, A., Storm, C., Merz, J. F., Noonan, K. E., & Spence, R. (2013). Gene patents and personalized cancer care: Impact of the Myriad case on clinical oncology. *Journal of Clinical Oncology, 31*(21), 2743–2748.

Partridge, A. H., Gelber, S., Peppercorn, J., Sampson, E., Knudsen, K., Laufer, M., ... Winer, E. P. (2004). Web-based survey of fertility issues in young women with breast cancer. *Journal of Clinical Oncology, 22*(20), 4174–4183.

Politi, M. C., Enright, T. M., Weihs, K. L. (2007). The effects of age and emotional acceptance on distress among breast cancer patients. *Support Care Cancer, 15*, 73–9.

Phillips-Salimi, C. R., & Andrykowski, M. A. (2013). Physical and mental health status of female adolescent/young adult survivors of breast and gynecological cancer: A national, population-based, case-control study. *Supportive Care in Cancer, 21*(6), 1597–1604.

Roth, A. J., Kornblith, A. B., Batel-Copel, L., Peabody, E., Scher, H. I., & Holland, J. C. (1998). Rapid screening for psychologic distress in men with prostate carcinoma: A pilot study. *Cancer, 82*(10), 1904–1908.

Ruini, C. (2013). The role of gratitude in breast cancer: Its relationships with post-traumatic growth, psychological well-being and distress. *Journal of Happiness Studies, 14*(1), 263.

Saquib, N., Flatt, S. W., Natarajan, L., Thomson, C. A., Bardwell, W. A., Caan, B., ... Pierce, J. P. (2007). Weight gain and recovery of pre-cancer weight after breast cancer treatments: Evidence from the women's healthy eating and living (WHEL) study. *Breast Cancer Research and Treatment, 105*(2), 177–186.

Schover, L. R. (1991). The impact of breast cancer on sexuality, body image, and intimate relationships. *CA: A Cancer Journal for Clinicians, 41*(2), 112–120.

Schover, L. R. (1994). Sexuality and body image in younger women with breast cancer. *Journal of the National Cancer Institute. Monographs, 16*, 177–182.

Schover, L. R., Montague, D. K., & Lakin, M. (1997). Supportive care and the quality of life of the cancer patient: Sexual problems. In V. DeVita, S. Hellman, & S. Rosenberg (Eds.), *Cancer: Principles and practice of oncology* (5th ed., pp. 2857–2872). Philadelphia, PA: J. B. Lippincott & Co.

Sears, S. R., Stanton, A. L., & Danoff-Burg, S. (2003). The yellow brick road and the emerald city: Benefit finding, positive reappraisal coping and posttraumatic growth in women with early-stage breast cancer. *Health Psychology, 22*(5), 487–497.

Siegel, R., DeSantis, C., Virgo, K., Stein, K., Mariotto, A., Smith, T., … Ward, E. (2012). Cancer treatment and survivorship statistics, 2012. *CA: A Cancer Journal for Clinicians, 62*(4), 220–241.

Silva, S. M., Crespo, C., & Canavarro, M. C. (2012). Pathways for psychological adjustment in breast cancer: A longitudinal study on coping strategies and posttraumatic growth. *Psychology & Health, 27*(11), 1323–1341.

Stead, M. L. (2003). Sexual dysfunction after treatment for gynaecologic and breast malignancies. *Current Opinion in Obstetrics & Gynecology, 15*(1), 57–61.

Stead, M. L., Fallowfield, L., Brown, J. M., & Selby, P. (2001). Communication about sexual problems and sexual concerns in ovarian cancer: Qualitative study. *British Medical Journal, 323*(7317), 836–837.

Tedeschi, R. G., & Calhoun, L. G. (2004). Posttraumatic growth: Conceptual foundations and empirical evidence. *Psychological Inquiry, 15*(1), 1–18.

Tierney, A. J., Taylor, J., & Closs, S. J. (1992). Knowledge, expectations and experiences of patients receiving chemotherapy for breast cancer. *Scandinavian Journal of Caring Sciences, 6*(2), 75–80.

Tremblay, A., & Bandi, V. (2003). Impact of body mass index on outcomes following critical care. *Chest, 123*(4), 1202–1207.

Trueb, R. M. (2010). Chemotherapy-induced alopecia. *Current Opinion in Supportive and Palliative Care, 4*(4), 281–284.

U.S. Department of Health and Human Services, Administration for Children and Families, Administration on Children Youth and Families, & Children's Bureau. (2011). *Child maltreatment.* http://www.acf.hhs.gov/programs/cb/research-data-technology/statistics-research/child-maltreatment. Accessed on August 8, 2013.

Vinokur, A. D., Threatt, B. A., Vinokur-Kaplan, D., & Satariano, W. A. (1990). The process of recovery from breast cancer for younger and older patients: Changes during the first year. *Cancer, 65*, 1242–1254.

Weaver, T. L., Chard, K. M., Mechanic, M. B., & Etzel, J. C. (2004). Self-injurious behaviors, PTSD arousal, and general health complaints within a treatment-seeking sample of sexually abused women. *Journal of Interpersonal Violence, 19*(5), 558–575.

Wenzel, L. B., Fairclough, D. L., Brady, M. J., Cella, D., Garrett, K. M., Kluhsman, B. C., Crane, L. A., & Marcus, A. C. (1999). Age-related differences in the quality of life of breast carcinoma patients after treatment. *Cancer, 86*, 1768–1774.

Williams, J., Wood, C., & Cunningham-Warburton, P. (1999). A narrative study of chemotherapy-induced alopecia. *Oncology Nursing Forum, 26*(9), 1463–1468.

Wilmoth, M. C. (2001). The aftermath of breast cancer: An altered sexual self. *Cancer Nursing, 24*(4), 278–286.

Wyatt, G. E., Loeb, T. B., Desmond, K. A., & Ganz, P. A. (2005). Does a history of childhood sexual abuse affect sexual outcomes in breast cancer survivors? *Journal of Clinical Oncology, 23*(6), 1261–1269.

Wyatt, G. E., Loeb, T. B., Solis, B., & Carmona, J. V. (1999). The prevalence and circumstances of child sexual abuse: Changes across a decade. *Child Abuse & Neglect, 23*(1), 45–60.

Yaw, Y. H., Shariff, Z. M., Kandiah, M., Mun, C. Y., Yusof, R. M., Othman, Z., … Hashim, Z. (2011). Weight changes and lifestyle behaviors in women after breast cancer diagnosis: A cross-sectional study. *BMC Public Health, 11*, 309.

Yurek, D., Farrar, W., & Andersen, B. L. (2000). Breast cancer surgery: Comparing surgical groups and determining individual differences in postoperative sexuality and body change stress. *Journal of Consulting and Clinical Psychology, 68*(4), 697–709.

Zannini, L., Verderame, F., Cucchiara, G., Zinna, B., Alba, A., & Ferrara, M. (2012). 'My wig has been my journey's companion': Perceived effects of an aesthetic care programme for Italian women suffering from chemotherapy-induced alopecia. *European Journal of Cancer Care, 21*(5), 650–660.

The Role of Reproductive Psychiatry in Women's Mental Health

Emily C. Dossett

Introduction

Reproductive psychiatry is a medical specialty focusing on psychiatric symptoms during times of hormonal change. Worldwide, women bear a disproportionately large burden of mental illness, with rates of depression that are twice as high as those in men and elevated levels of almost all anxiety disorders (World Health Organization, 2009). This gender divide begins in puberty as young women undergo menarche, and it continues until menopause is reached. For the 30–40 years between these milestones, women experience hormonal fluctuations monthly with their menstrual cycle; significant hormonal shifts with each pregnancy and postpartum period; and erratic hormone changes during perimenopause. Many women experience infertility or pregnancy loss as well. All of these hormonal shifts can leave women vulnerable to psychiatric symptoms of mood, anxiety, and thought disorders (Brizendine, 2006).

Reproductive psychiatry is a specialized field of medicine that seeks to understand and treat such disorders. It is a relatively new discipline, since many years of stigma and lack of focused attention on female-specific health needs have prevented research and education in women's mental health (World Health Organization, 2009). This chapter describes the training, education, and research opportunities in reproductive psychiatry as well as the role of the specialist in women's health care. Evolving theories of mental illness and their connection to times of reproductive change, as well as how to assess these conditions, are reviewed. Treatment recommendations, including medications and other evidence-based interventions, are described as well as the informed consent process. The goal is for each reader to develop a stronger understanding of what reproductive psychiatrists do and what needs to be done to further our knowledge in this area.

E.C. Dossett, M.D., M.T.S. (✉)
Assistant Clinical Professor, Department of Psychiatry and Biobehavioral Sciences and Department of Obstetrics Gynecology, Keck School of Medicine, Los Angels, University of Southern California Medical Center, Pasadena, CA, USA
e-mail: edossett@gmail.com

Reproductive Psychiatry as a Clinical Specialty

The reproductive psychiatrist's role includes evaluation and diagnosis; informed consent and medication management; psychotherapy or collaboration with a therapist; and close teamwork with the patient's family and other health care providers. Understanding how psychiatric disorders may present differently during times of hormonal change is a key component of this field. The reproductive psychiatrist trains not only in the medication management of these mood-related disorders but in psychotherapeutic approaches as well. Decisions about medication are an integral part of any treatment plan but are especially important when mood, anxiety, or psychotic symptoms become so severe that a woman's ability to care for herself or others is impeded. When focused on the peripartum, reproductive psychiatry attends to treatment decisions that minimize the risk for both mother and child, often in situations with "no perfect solution" (Wisner et al., 2000; Wisner, Sit, & Moses-Kolko, 2006). These complicated decisions require careful psychiatric assessment and a fully informed conversation about risks and benefits of medication use, which is often beyond the scope of a general practitioner or even a psychiatrist without specialized training in assessment, diagnosis, and treatment during times of reproductive change.

However, this specialized training can be difficult to obtain, as the American Board of Psychiatry and Neurology does not offer any official fellowships or certifications in reproductive psychiatry. The closest match would be a subspecialty in psychosomatic medicine, "a subspecialty that involves the diagnosis and treatment of psychiatric disorders and symptoms in medically complex patients," including "high-risk pregnancies," among many other medical conditions (www.abpn.org/sub_psychmed.html). However, how much exposure to reproductive psychiatry a fellow in psychosomatic medicine receives depends on where he or she is training. Similarly, whether or not an interested medical student or psychiatric resident is able to learn about reproductive psychiatry is dependent on what educational or clinical opportunities exist where he or she is training. Anecdotally, most medical school programs offer at most one to two lectures on women's mental health, and even psychiatric residencies may offer only a few hours of teaching on the subject. Fortunately, 1-year post-residency research and/or clinical fellowships are emerging around the country at universities with a strong interest in reproductive psychiatry, such as Brigham and Women's Hospital at Harvard Medical School (http://www.brighamandwomens.org) and the University of Illinois in Chicago (http://www.psych.uic.edu).

Once formal training is complete, reproductive psychiatrists practice in a variety of settings. Many are in private practice, and most engage in medication management, psychotherapy, or both. Some work in hospital settings as consultation-liaison psychiatrists, serving as a bridge between psychiatry and obstetrics or gynecology. Increasingly, reproductive psychiatrists are working as consultants in primary care settings, as health care moves more toward providing specialty care, including mental health care, in outpatient "medical homes" (Baker-Ericzen et al., 2012; Yawn et al., 2012). Finally, reproductive psychiatrists often work in academic settings, where they perform research, teach medical trainees, and treat patients.

An up-do-date knowledge of psychiatric medications and their safety profile in general, and even more specifically during times of hormonal change, is essential. This can be accomplished in numerous ways. Several professional organizations offer yearly conferences that provide continuing medical education. The North American Society for Psychosocial Obstetrics and Gynecology, or "NASPOG," brings together psychiatrists, psychologists, obstetricians–gynecologists, and other professionals interested in the intersection of mental and reproductive health (www. NASPOG.org). NASPOG is the North American branch of the Marcé Society, an international group dedicated to women's mental health. The American Psychiatric Association offers multiple courses on reproductive psychiatry during their annual meeting. Postpartum Support International, or PSI, is the largest lay-volunteer organization dedicated to perinatal mental health, and their annual conference typically offers psychosocial and medical training.

Medical journals, such as the *Archives of Women's Health*, publish articles on the latest research on many aspects of reproductive psychiatry, including medication use, psychotherapy, and other evidence-based interventions. More and more non-specialty journals, such as the *Journal of the American Medical Association* (JAMA) or the flagship journals in both psychiatry and obstetrics–gynecology, publish papers relevant to women's mental health. Online resources, such as *Journal Watch* (www.jwatch.org), summarize these findings into quickly read and easily understood e-mails that arrive regularly and help keep practitioners up to date. Blogs, such as Massachusetts General Hospital's Center for Women's Mental Health, also offer regular updates on treatment recommendations. Staying abreast of research on psychotropic medications is particularly important for the reproductive psychiatrist, as this is where much of their practice lies. Medication management is also where some of the largest clinical, as well as social, psychological, and ethical, challenges emerge.

Mood and Anxiety: What Is the Biology Behind It?

Every woman who faces mood and anxiety symptoms during times of reproductive change wants to know *why*. What is the connection between her brain, body, and hormones that has gone awry? There are several possible theories. The longest held is the "monoamine neurotransmitter" theory of depression. This theory looks at the influence of chemical messengers, called neurotransmitters, in the brain. Serotonin, norepinephrine, and dopamine are the most well-understood neurotransmitters. For many years, researchers have looked at the connection between depression and possible dysregulation of these "brain messengers" (Stahl, 2000). In addition, there is a growing understanding of the association between depression and hormonal systems in the body, as well as outside influences, that affect gene expression and how the brain itself grows and evolves (Massart, Mongeau, & Lanfumey, 2012).

For women, it has long been suspected that there is an additional link between hormones and mood, but the relationship has remained elusive. However, research is starting to reveal a possible connection, and we are learning more and more about the variety of ways that serotonin seems to have a close relationship to estrogen (Lokuge, Frey, Foster, Soares, & Steiner, 2011). Serotonin seems to need estrogen to do its job well. Clinically, it is important to note that women seem to struggle most with psychiatric symptoms during times when estrogen levels fall most rapidly: premenstrually; in the postpartum; and off and on throughout perimenopause (Brizendine, 2006; Bromberger et al., 2010). These rapid fluctuations appear to influence how well serotonin works and, subsequently, how a woman feels. Additionally, each woman responds to the shifts in hormones differently. This is why two women may have the same hormone levels, as measured in blood tests, but very different mood or anxiety symptoms.

A third rapidly evolving theory of mental illness involves immune system activation. Immune system activation means being in a "proinflammatory" state. Inflammation plays a pivotal role in the development of depression and anxiety in general (Harrison, 2013). For women specifically, research points to immune system dysregulation as a possible factor in perinatal mood and anxiety disorders. A normal pregnancy appears to shift between both pro- and anti-inflammatory states. For instance, it has long been thought that a woman's immune system becomes more subdued in pregnancy in order to protect the developing fetus from being rejected by the very womb that holds it. New research shows even more subtle and complex immune changes during the normal course of a woman's pregnancy (Chen, Liu, & Sytwu, 2012). If that complexity is derailed and shifts toward more inflammation, perinatal mood and anxiety disorders may result (Bergink et al., 2013). Interestingly, elevated inflammation is also linked to common medical problems in pregnancy, including preeclampsia, preterm delivery, and gestational diabetes. If depression is possibly caused by abnormal changes in a woman's inflammatory state, then all these processes may, in fact, be linked. Extensive research is currently looking into the connection between both physical and mental health in pregnancy, with a possible common denominator of a dysregulated immune system (Osborne & Monk, 2013). In the future, we may be able to promote treatments for depression that target inflammation. For now, however, medications based on the monoamine hypothesis of anxiety and depression remain the mainstay of treatment.

The Psychiatric Assessment

How does this understanding of biology present in "real life," in the faces and voices of women who are suffering? The women who present with symptoms in my office are usually in the grips of raw emotion: tears that seem to come from nowhere; terror at facing another night fighting for sleep; and despair that she will ever "feel like normal" again. Sometimes there is even suicidality, brought on by intense feelings of hopelessness and helplessness. A husband, partner, or mother sometimes accompanies her; sometimes she is nursing a newborn; sometimes she is very much alone. A psychiatrist's office is often the last stop in a long line of efforts to heal, particularly if she is pregnant or nursing, and the possibility of needing medication is fraught with challenges. Women often struggle greatly with the stigma of mental illness as well as with their own guilt and shame around possibly needing psychiatric help.

Before making any decision about medication, however, a careful assessment is always needed. The first question in any assessment is what each woman is feeling and what her primary concerns may be. Is she struggling with monthly mood changes around her menstrual cycle? Is she planning a pregnancy, pregnant already, or newly postpartum? Is she caught in the ups and downs of perimenopausal hormonal shifts? In the midst of these biological realities, is she facing social and psychological transitions as momentous as moving through adolescence, becoming a mother, or watching her grown children leave home? How does she describe and experience all these changes?

Questions about safety are of utmost importance. Is she truly safe, or is suicide a real possibility? Is she having thoughts of harming others, including her own child? It is imperative that the reproductive psychiatrist talk directly and openly with a woman about any unusual thoughts she might be having and if any thoughts or images feel out of control. Studies indicate that suicide is a leading cause of death in women during the first year after delivering a child, with one study demonstrating that suicide accounts for 28 % of maternal deaths (Almond, 2009; Oats, 2003). Similarly, for women suffering from postpartum psychosis, rates of infanticide are roughly 4 %, making the diagnosis a medical emergency (Spinelli, 2009). When assessing safety in any woman, having the input of a loved one that can verify and add information, as well as provide support, is enormously helpful.

Another objective for the initial evaluation is to assess "functioning." In other words, can she sleep? Can she eat, shower, and brush her teeth? Is she able to study for school, go to work, or care for her children? Or is her illness and its accompanying symptoms so pronounced that she cannot get out of bed, keep food down, or manage the basics of her day-to-day routine?

Once her concerns have been reviewed, safety has been established, and basic functioning evaluated, symptoms need to be assessed. She should be carefully and thoroughly asked about symptoms of depression, mania, anxiety, panic attacks, obsessions, compulsions, psychosis, eating disorders, substance use, or any other upsetting or disruptive symptoms. This can be challenging, particularly in pregnancy, as many of the symptoms of a "normal" pregnancy can mimic depression. For instance, four of the nine criteria necessary for a diagnosis of major depressive disorder—sleep disruption, appetite disruption, low energy, and poor concentration—are often experienced by pregnant or postpartum women who, in fact, have no depression at all (American Psychiatric Association, 2013). In this situation, looking for other symptoms, such as profound low mood, agitation, a feeling of disconnection from the pregnancy or the infant, or excessive anxiety, can be helpful.

Other helpful tools are screening tests. The Edinburgh Postnatal Depression Screen, EPDS, has been used for years to detect depression and anxiety in perinatal women (Cox, Holden, & Sagovsky, 1987). The EPDS3, a shortened version consisting of only three questions, can pick up on excessive anxiety (Swalm, Brooks, Doherty, Nathan, & Jacques, 2010). More recently, the Patient Health Questionnaire-9, or PHQ9, has been shown to work with most adults, including pregnant or postpartum women (Davis, Pearlstein, Stuart, O'Hara, & Zlotnick, 2013; Sidebottom, Harrison, Godecker, & Kim, 2012). Asking only the first two questions of the PHQ9, a test called the "PHQ2," can be used quickly and easily done in a busy prenatal or primary care office (National Centre for Health and Clinical Excellence, 2007). Several other screening tools exist as well, such as the Postpartum Depression Screening Scale (PDSS) and the Center for Epidemiological Studies Depression Scale (CES-D).

Current guidelines from both the American College of Obstetrics and Gynecology (ACOG) and the American Academy of Pediatrics (AAP) recommend screening in each trimester and again at frequent intervals in the postpartum, including during well-child checks (ACOG National Committee for Quality Assurance, & Physician Consortium for Practice Improvement, Committee Opinion, 2012; Earls, & Committee on Psychosocial Aspects of Child and Family Health American Academy of Pediatrics, 2010). On the other hand, the US Preventive Services Task Force only recommends screening if there are referrals for women who screen positive (US Preventive Services Task Force, 2009). This debate will continue until we have enough resources for all women to receive quality mental health care; for now, however, screening tools can help distinguish between a fairly normal pregnancy and one marked by depression and anxiety.

For all women, it is also important to look more specifically at her past reproductive psychiatric history. If she is newly postpartum and struggling with depression, did she also feel this way in previous pregnancies? If she is going through perimenopause and feels tense and irritable, did she also feel this way prior to the onset of her periods? New research suggests that there may be a subset of women who are genetically predisposed to more intense psychiatric symptoms during times of hormonal change (Bath et al., 2012; Epperson & Bale, 2012). Similarly, their mothers and sisters may feel this way; consequently, taking a good family history becomes essential.

Many women also want to have their hormone levels tested, with the hope that this will explain their psychiatric symptoms. In reality, research has not yet demonstrated a link between specific hormone levels and mental illness. What seems to matter, as mentioned previously, is the rate of change of reproductive hormones (such as estrogen or progesterone) as they fluctuate up or down. However, testing for thyroid dysfunction can be helpful and should be part of any women's assessment. Thyroid dysregulation is common in women of childbearing age, and it can often present as anxiety, low mood, sluggishness, or other symptoms that mimic mood or anxiety shifts (De Groot et al., 2012). Making sure that a woman's thyroid function is good can help reduce the need for further psychiatric management, if, in fact, this is the underlying cause of her symptoms.

Additional medical work-up includes ensuring that she is not on any medications that cause or worsen psychiatric symptoms. These include beta blockers, a family of blood pressure medications that make women feel tired; opiates, which also cause lethargy; hormone-based drugs, such as oral contraceptives or infertility medications, that can trigger mood swings; or even tamoxifen, a breast cancer prevention drug that sometimes has neurocognitive symptoms as side effects (Danhauer et al., 2012). Gathering an exhaustive list of all medications a woman may be taking, including over-the-counter, herbal, and vitamin supplements, is important so that their possible interactions and safety can be assessed. In addition, assessing substance use is of critical importance: alcohol and drug use clearly affect a woman's mood, anxiety levels, and cognition.

Putting together the pieces to this puzzle provides reproductive psychiatrists with the information they need to make effective treatment decisions. Information from the assessment can be organized into "the four Ps:"

- Predisposing factors
- Precipitating factors
- Perpetuating factors
- Protective factors

Predisposing factors are long-standing issues that put a woman at higher risk for psychiatric symptoms and include family history, history of substance use, and chronic medical problems, to name a few. Precipitating factors send women "over the edge" into more severe symptoms. Examples are new-onset intimate partner violence, the death of a loved one, or even a pregnancy or a delivery itself. Perpetuating factors are aspects of her life that will cause her symptoms to continue or worsen if left unchecked; examples include lack of social support, chronic financial stress, or ongoing violence. Finally, protective factors draw on a woman's own strengths and can lessen symptoms or prevent them from developing. Protective factors can include physical health, sobriety, a strong community of support, and love of children or family members. Looking closely at "the four Ps" helps the reproductive psychiatrist organize a treatment plan into interventions that reduce chronic risk factors, ameliorate the current crisis, and build on a woman's individual resources.

In general, medications are reserved for women who have symptoms that are moderate to severe and impact functioning. They are used if a woman is so ill that she feels suicidal. Medications are often typically clinically necessary when a woman experiences psychiatric symptoms of mania, psychosis, obsessions, compulsions, or panic attacks. Therapy is essential with all of these conditions as well, and with many patients psychotherapy should be a front-line treatment; in other patients, however, medications are necessary for stability and even to save lives (Yonkers et al., 2009). When a woman is faced with needing medication while she is pregnant or nursing, treatment decisions grow even more complicated.

Why Do Medications Cause Fear?

The possibility of medication, particularly during pregnancy or lactation, strikes fear in many women. Pregnant women are often told that psychiatric medications should be stopped at all costs, regardless of which medication it is or why it was prescribed. Well-meaning physicians give this advice frequently, and the media often presents frightening information out of context. Television advertisements for class-action lawsuits blast scary messages about antidepressant use in pregnancy, urging women to call "1-800-BAD-DRUG." A Google search for "antidepressants and pregnancy" turns up a website for law firms promising "National Assistance for

Birth Defects from Antidepressant Use." Parenting websites lead with articles such as "Common Antidepressants Too Risky During Pregnancy, Researchers Say." To be fair, many articles with more positive or nuanced approaches are regularly published as well, but for a woman who is already fearful, the negative headlines prove the most eye-catching.

There are general struggles and doubts around medication use that extend beyond possible harm to a developing fetus or a breastfeeding baby. Women who use medications for any reason, are often reluctant, and understandably so, to try psychiatric medications. Many women worry about side effects. They may have had negative experiences in the past with medications, or they may be struggling with their current regimen. Other women do not like the idea of having to take a medication to address mood or anxiety. They want to be able to "do it themselves" and believe that taking medication is not addressing the root problem. They often will express the belief that taking medication feels like a moral failing or character flaw. Sometimes women worry that psychotropic medications are addictive and that if they start, they will need to take them for the rest of their life. More commonly, no matter what phase of life a women is in, she worries about being judged.

Some of these concerns are valid. Many women do have side effects, though the majority are mild and pass within a few days of taking them. However, there are rare, but serious, side effects with most drugs. Some medications are addictive and need to be carefully monitored and used for short periods of time. Aside from these more practical concerns, the underlying question is really one about what mental illness actually *is*. Is it a disease, with symptoms to be addressed with pharmaceuticals? Or is it a choice, one that if she just worked a little harder she could overcome? Does it mean that a woman has failed in some way; that she is simply not strong enough, smart enough, or savvy enough to move forward on her own? And for the woman who is pregnant or breastfeeding, the doubts and questions are even more profound. Does taking medication mean that she can also be a good mother?

From the moment of conception, if not before, the vast majority of women want to be the best mother possible. Pregnant and postpartum mothers are understandably frightened by the idea that they could harm their child by choosing to take a medication with any degree of risk. This terror comes not only from worry about the baby but also from the scary thought that the mother has somehow failed from the very beginning if she is suffering from depression or anxiety. In other words, she believes the message that "good mothers do not get depressed" and the corollary message that needing medication solidifies that failure (Los Angeles County Perinatal Mental Health Task Force, 2013). Underneath it all, many women perceive the message that should she continue an antidepressant in pregnancy or lactation, she is choosing her happiness over her baby's health, and she is somehow a "bad mother." The question that many women in this situation ask is the following: "Can I even be a good mother?"

The short answer is *yes*, she can. In fact, women who are happy and healthy are often able to be better mothers (Pearson et al., 2013; Sandman, Davis, Buss, & Glynn, 2012). Making a choice to take care of oneself is surprisingly difficult in our world, particularly for women, but is often the right one for making sure that one's baby is happy and healthy. Medications, though not without their own risks, can be one tool to accomplish this. They are not appropriate for everyone, nor are they "happy pills" that will wipe away all problems. They should only be taken after full informed consent. They should not medicate away normal emotions but instead should simply put a floor under depression and a ceiling on anxiety so that symptoms do not become devastating. They should help a woman feel more in control of her emotions. They should help her body start sleeping, eating, and concentrating again. Most importantly, they should free her from the torment and exhaustion that mental illness can cause, so that she can turn her attention to the most important task at hand: taking care of herself, her family, her work, and her life.

Classes of Medication

Antidepressants

The most commonly prescribed antidepressants are the selective serotonin reuptake inhibitors, SSRIs. The first SSRI was fluoxetine, or Prozac, which was released onto the market in 1987. Fluoxetine was relatively effective and much safer than previous antidepressants, which had burdensome side effects (such as following strict diets to avoid dangerous rises in blood pressure) or could be fatal in overdose. After fluoxetine, other SSRIs were developed in rapid succession: paroxetine (Paril), sertraline (Zalofs), fluvoxamine (Luvox), citalopram (Cerexa), and escitalopram (Lexapro). As of 2008, one in ten Americans over the age of 12 takes an antidepressant. Women are 2½ times more likely to take one than men, and 23 % of women in their forties and fifties take an antidepressant (Pratt, Brody, & Gu, 2011). The proportion of pregnancies with any antidepressant use increased from 5.7 % of pregnancies in 1999 to 13.4 % in 2007; the majority of these were prescribed an SSRI (Cooper, Willy, Pont, & Ray, 2007). SSRIs are believed to work by modulating the amount of serotonin available to neurons.

Antidepressants in other families target different neurotransmitters. For instance, the serotonin norepinephrine reuptake inhibitors, SNRIs, target both serotonin and norepinephrine. These medications include venlafaxine (Effexor), desvenlafaxine (Pristiq), and duloxetine (Cymbalta) as well as an older family of medications called tricyclic antidepressants (TCAs). Both SSRIs and SNRIs are effective for depression as well as a variety of anxiety disorders, including generalized anxiety disorder, panic disorder, and obsessive-compulsive disorder. Since many women experience anxiety and depression symptoms together, medications that treat both types of symptoms with one pill are extremely useful.

Other antidepressants work in more unique ways. Bupropion (Wellbutrin), a commonly used antidepressant that also has effectiveness for smoking cessation, seems to facilitate dopamine function. Dopamine is linked to motivation, energy, and a sense of well-being. A number of antidepressants are simply labeled "other" because they do not fit neatly into a particular class. These include mirtazapine, trazodone, and atomoxetine.

Mood Stabilizers

Mood stabilizers treat symptoms of both depression and mania. As our understanding of mood disorders grows, more people seem to suffer from both high mood as well as low mood than previously thought. Most people with bipolar disorder do not have full-blown manic episodes of euphoric mood, extreme grandiosity, or profound behavioral changes. Instead, diagnoses such as bipolar II or cyclothymia describe symptoms of mood swings, irritability, decreased need for sleep, a pressured sense of purpose, thought, speech, and impulsive behavior that can occur in varying degrees and for varying lengths of time (American Psychiatric Association, 2013). At the same time, most people with bipolar disorder spend more time depressed than "up" in their mood (Kupka et al., 2007).

Regardless of presentation, mood stabilizers are the treatment of choice for bipolar disorder, even bipolar depression. Lithium was the first mood stabilizer, and it remains the gold standard for bipolar disorder type I. However, it can be complicated to monitor and becomes toxic easily. Other well-known mood stabilizers include carbamazepine (Tegregol), valproic acid (Depakote), and lamotrigine (Lamictal). These are also used for epilepsy, and much of the safety data that we have for them comes from studies done on pregnant women with seizure disorders. Increasingly, a class of medications called atypical antipsychotics is also used to manage mood instability.

Antipsychotics

Atypical antipsychotics are the newest generation of medications targeting psychosis and, as described above, some mood symptoms. "Psychosis" is not a disorder, but a set of symptoms based on disturbed thoughts and perceptions. Hearing voices, feeling paranoid, and holding delusional beliefs are a few manifestations of psychosis and can be present in a variety of disorders, including postpartum psychosis. Atypical antipsychotics work quickly to manage these symptoms and can be very effective. The main challenge is weight gain; atypicals, as they are called, can lead to obesity as well as diabetes and cholesterol problems (McCloughen & Foster, 2011; Pramyothin & Khaodhiar, 2010). All patients want to avoid this, but particularly women who are pregnant or who are already struggling with weight.

Older antipsychotics, or "typical antipsychotics" since they were developed first, have been in use for nearly six decades. However, they are often considered "second line" to atypicals because of side effects. These side effects include neuromuscular abnormalities, tremor, and motor tics, some of which last a lifetime, as well as weight gain and sedation. Nonetheless, in reproductive psychiatry, typical antipsychotics have the advantage of years of safety data in pregnant and postpartum women. For this reason, plus the fact that atypicals can be so challenging for weight management, typical antipsychotics are still used at times, including occasionally with pregnant women who are psychotic.

Antianxiety Medications

Many antidepressants also work effectively to treat anxiety. These include most of the serotonin- or norepinephrine-based medications. Ideally this allows a woman that is suffering from both anxiety and depression to take a single drug to address both sets of symptoms. However, most of these medications can take up to 6 weeks to take effect, and many women cannot tolerate symptoms of anxiety without relief for that long. In this case, shorter acting, more temporary agents can be helpful.

Benzodiazepines work much more quickly and on an "as-needed" basis for more intense symptoms of anxiety, such as panic attacks. Common benzodiazepines include diazepam (Valium), alprazolam (Xanax), lorazepam (Ativan), and clonazepam (Klonopin). They generally take effect within a few minutes to an hour and provide relief from anxiety; in addition, they can be helpful with insomnia, particularly if it is driven by anxiety. However, they are also potentially addictive and should only be used on a short-term basis or on infrequent occasions.

Additional Psychotropic Medications

The armamentarium of psychotropic medications is much broader than that of those listed above, and medications from other branches of medicine are often used to treat psychiatric symptoms as well. Buspirone is an alternative antianxiety medication. Gabapentin is often used for anxiety, as well. Stimulants can be used to treat attention-deficit disorder, ADD. Naltrexone has some evidence for its use to treat substance-abuse disorders (Pettinati, O'Brien, & Dundon, 2013). New medications are constantly researched and often released to the market. Even as this book goes to press, new research continues to provide glimpses into potential medications that work in novel ways and may be even more effective.

Evidence-Based Interventions

Psychotherapy

Medications are certainly not the only type of treatment available and, in fact, are most effective when used in conjunction with psychotherapy (Yonkers et al., 2009). For many women, psychotherapy is much preferred. Interpersonal psychotherapy, whether individual or group, works well for perinatal women as they transition into motherhood and for perimenopausal women as they are often navigating changes in their own family status during the same time of life (Sockol, Epperson, & Barber, 2011). In addition, cognitive-behavioral therapy can be effective for symptoms of anxiety and depression (O'Mahen, Himle, Gedock, Henshaw, & Flynn, 2013). In general, if a patient needs to take medication, ideally she should be in therapy as well.

Omega-3 Fatty Acids

Omega-3 fatty acids, often referred to as "fish oils," decrease inflammation in a variety of ways. As mental health has increasingly been linked to increased inflammation, research into omega-3 fatty acids as a possible treatment has increased (Deligiannidis & Freeman, 2010). Modest efficacy has been shown for doses upwards of 3,000 mg a day for general depression and anxiety (Dennis & Dowswell, 2013; Luberto, White, Sears, & Cotton, 2013). Data is sparse for treatment of premenstrual or perimenopausal mood symptoms with omega-3s, though one study did show a decrease in hot flashes (Lucas, Asselin, Merette et al., 2009). For perinatal mood and anxiety disorders, data are mixed. Studies showing the most efficacy tend to use docosahexaenoic acid, DHA, and eicosapentaenoic acid, EPA, in a ratio of roughly 1:2. For women taking prenatal vitamins, DHA is often already included; taking a supplement may be necessary to reach the recommended doses. In addition, pregnant or nursing women should choose a form of fish oil that is low in mercury in order to avoid toxicity.

Folate

Folate is a B vitamin that is important for a variety of reasons, including healthy cell division and metabolism of amino acids. Folate is naturally present in some foods, and folic acid is the form of folate used in supplements. Recent research into the use of folate to help treat depression has been encouraging. Folate itself is not an antidepressant, but individuals with higher folate levels seem to respond better to antidepressants. Current recommendations suggest adding 15 mg of L-methyl folate a day to one's antidepressant dose (Papakostas et al., 2012). For pregnant women, prenatal vitamins typically contain 400 μg (or 0.4 mg) of folic acid to prevent two common central nervous system malformations, spina bifida and anencephaly. Folate supplementation may then achieve two goals: reducing the risk of birth defects as well as increasing the efficacy of antidepressants.

Calcium Carbonate

Calcium carbonate, 1,200 mg a day, can be effective for treating premenstrual mood and anxiety symptoms, though data is sparse. While not as effective as an antidepressant, some studies have shown effectiveness with premenstrual tiredness, appetite changes, and depressive symptoms (Ghanbari, Haghollahi, Shariat, Foroshani, & Ashrafi, 2009; Yonkers, Pearlstein, & Gotman, 2013). For women who would like a non-psychotropic approach to premenstrual symptoms, calcium carbonate is an option.

Exercise

Exercise is a well-established way to improve mood, anxiety, and physical health. For premenstrual symptoms, exercise reduces personal stress, anxiety, tension, and depression as well as breast tenderness, fluid retention, and cramps (Deligiannidis & Freeman, 2010). The ACOG recommends 30 min of moderate exercise most days for pregnant women, unless there is a clear medical reason not to do so (American College of Obstetrics and Gynecology, 2002, reaffirmed 2009). For perimenopausal women, moderate aerobic exercise three times a week improves sleep quality, insomnia, and depression; however, it does not seem to have an effect on hot flashes or other vasomotor symptoms (Sternfeld et al., 2014).

Acupuncture

Increasingly, women seek acupuncture for a variety of symptoms, including anxiety, depression, and infertility. Acupuncture consists of the placement of needles throughout the bodies' channels, or "meridians," to facilitate the flow of *qi* and relieve symptoms. Along with herbal medications, acupuncture is an essential modality in traditional Chinese medicine. While it is extremely difficult to study using Western methods of randomized, controlled trials, anecdotally some women report relief from symptoms with acupuncture (Luberto et al., 2013). One consideration for the reproductive psychiatrist is any potential interaction between Chinese herbal medicine and psychotropic medications. Very little data is available on possible changes in drug metabolism or serum levels when these two approaches are used together. This is not to say that the two approaches are incompatible, but rather close symptom control and, when necessary, serum level monitoring of psychotropics are important.

Bright Light Therapy

Bright light therapy was initially evaluated in the treatment of seasonal affective disorder, and it has shown some effectiveness in treating depression as well. Bright light therapy consists of spending a set amount of time each day, often half an hour, in front of a "light box" that provides 10,000 lx white light. For premenstrual disorders, small studies have shown reduction in depression as well as irritability and physical symptoms (Lam et al., 1999; Parry, Mahan, Mostofi, Lew, & Gillin, 1993). Small trials have also been modestly effective for perinatal depression; at this point larger studies are needed as well as guidelines regarding use in women with bipolar depression (Dennis & Dowswell, 2013). To date, there are no available data on bright light therapy in depressed perimenopausal women.

Brain Stimulation Therapies

Brain stimulation therapies involve activating the brain through electricity, magnets, or implants in order to treat mood symptoms. The oldest, best researched is electroconvulsive therapy, ECT. Since the late 1930s, this technique has been used to treat severe, seemingly intractable cases of mood and psychotic disorders. ECT consists of inducing a seizure in a patient under a controlled setting. ECT is not contraindicated in pregnancy, and rates of success are often higher than for pharmacotherapy (Anderson, 2009; Dierckx, Heijnen, van den Broek, & Birkenhager, 2012). However, side effects of headache and short-term memory loss, as well as the stigma attached to ECT, prevent its more widespread use.

Newer brain stimulation therapies include repetitive transcranial magnetic stimulation, or rTMS; vagus nerve stimulation; magnetic seizure therapy; and deep brain stimulation. Many of these are still considered experimental, but rTMS is gaining traction as a treatment option (Hovington, McGirr, Lepage, & Berlim, 2013). It also induces electrical activity in the brain, similar to ECT, but in a much more targeted way with fewer side effects. Data thus far have been somewhat mixed, but increasingly more positive as the technique is refined. A series of case studies in pregnant women demonstrate safety and efficacy; the next step is more large-scale studies (Zhang, Liu, Sun, & Zheng, 2010). This is a particularly attractive option because it might reduce the need for medication and therefore creates less of an exposure for the developing fetus.

Hormonal Therapies

A logical treatment option for psychiatric symptoms around times of hormonal fluctuation is to use hormones themselves. Despite the rationality of this, data remains mixed for most studies examining this approach. For premenstrual mood symptoms, the oral contraceptive pill may benefit some women; for others, however, it seems to make depression or irritability worse (Rapkin & Winer, 2008). Trials of estrogen for postpartum women have been promising in reducing depression symptoms, based on the theory that adding estrogen immediately after delivery lessens the significant drop in reproductive hormones that occurs within hours after birth and may be responsible for postpartum depression. However, these have not been explored in larger trials and are not currently standard practice (Moses-Kolko, Berga, Kairo, Sit, & Wisner, 2009). Using hormone replacement therapy provides relief to many, but not all, women undergoing the menopausal transition. This approach can be used alone or with serotonergic and noradrenergic antidepressants as well as psychological supports (Soares, 2013). However, there can be health concerns with hormone replacement therapy that make collaboration with a gynecologist important.

The Decision-Making Process

Since many treatment options exist, sorting through which ones are potentially most helpful requires careful assessment and a clear sense of what the goal of treatment is for each woman. If medications do seem appropriate, a few simple rules can help determine which ones to use. If a woman has tried medication in the past, it is helpful to look and see how she responded. If a particular medication worked, then it may be worth trying it, or a medicine in the same family, again. Another guideline is monotherapy or the idea that one medication is preferable to multiple. The principle of monotherapy is particularly important to consider for pregnant or nursing women in order to minimize the number of drug exposures to the fetus or the infant. However, this may not suffice for all women, and current psychiatric guidelines often suggest adding in a second medicine to augment one that may only be partially effective (Gaynes et al., 2012). When choosing doses, one maxim is "start low, go slow, but go!" This teaches to start at a low dose and increase slowly to try and find the lowest possible effective dose. However, it is important to "go," in other words, to treat until the medication is effective.

For many women, a pre-pregnancy consultation can be enormously helpful in educating a woman and her family about the risks and benefits of medication use so that she can plan ahead for the safest possible perinatal period. A thorough treatment plan is based on the biopsychosocial model. Biological recommendations may include whether or not to use medications or supplements, check thyroid function, or address other medical conditions. Psychological support through individual or group therapy should be strongly considered. Finally, social aspects of care need to be included, such as how to increase social support or connect with other new mothers. A written summary of this information ensures that the potential mother is clear on her options and the risks and benefits they involve. In addition, this written report can be shared with her obstetrician and her child's pediatrician after delivery.

Vignettes

What do these treatment choices look like in real life? The following vignettes describe common situations seen in reproductive psychiatry.

Vignette 1
Sarah is a 23-year-old woman who comes in to your office because she feels "crazy" right before her period. For five days before her period starts, she becomes full of rage and weepy, to the point that she must take time off work and her boyfriend has threatened to leave her. The rest of the month, she feels well. She is stable in her mood, with no profound anxiety or tension. She sleeps, eats, and concentrates well, and has no suicidal thoughts or other concerning symptoms. However, she is worried that her premenstrual symptoms are causing serious damage to her life. She wants you to check her hormone levels and help her in any way you can.

Many women have questions about their hormone levels and whether or not they are "off." However, there is little evidence to support checking hormone levels in order to explain psychiatric symptoms. What matters is an individual woman's response to her hormone fluctuations. Many women like Sarah feel mood and anxiety symptoms acutely during these times of flux, but there is no lab value that corresponds with this. The more important questions focus on symptoms and, in the case of premenstrual disorders, on whether she truly feels these symptoms just during the luteal phase (the time in her menstrual cycle directly before her period actually starts) or whether she actually feels them to some degree all month.

The best way to determine this is by tracking her moods as well as when her period starts and stops. In order to have a true diagnosis of premenstrual dysphoric disorder, such tracking must happen for 2 months and demonstrate that symptoms are isolated to the luteal phase (American Psychiatric Association, 2013). This is important because it determines the course of treatment. If symptoms are solely in the luteal phase, then many women benefit from intermittent dosing of SSRI medications (Rapkin & Winer, 2008). This means that she can take an SSRI from the time immediately before her symptoms typically start until they end, usually right after her period begins. She does not need them the rest of the month, and she typically does not have side effects associated with starting or stopping the medication. On the other hand, if she is having symptoms all month, with a worsening before her period, she needs "continuous dosing" of an SSRI. This means taking the medication all month. Some women do well with the same dose all month. Other women find that they are stable on a lower dose for most of the month but require a temporary increase in dose during the luteal phase in order to best contain symptoms.

SSRIs are not the only option for women with premenstrual mood and anxiety symptoms. Some women benefit from oral contraceptive pills. If they do, this is a streamlined way to control symptoms as well as to provide birth control, if desired. Other women feel poorly on OCPs, and prefer the antidepressant route. Which one to try first depends mostly on patient preference, on past experience with the types of medications, and on how effective the two different treatments are for the individual woman.

For women with milder symptoms, the ACOG recommends moderate exercise, a complex-carbohydrate diet, and reducing alcohol and caffeine use (American College of Obstetricians and Gynecologists, 2011). Calcium carbonate can also be effective in alleviating milder symptoms.

For the patient described above, however, her symptoms are more severe. Tracking reveals that they are isolated to the 5 days before the onset of her period and she opted for intermittent dosing with fluoxetine. She also began taking calcium supplements and trying to implement diet and exercise changes, though these were challenging during a time of the month when she did not feel well physically. However, her efforts paid off. She responded well, and her work life and relationship both improved.

Vignette 2
Melinda is a 28-year-old woman who calls for an appointment because she is three months pregnant. She was previously taking an antidepressant, but tapered off because she wanted to become pregnant and her obstetrician told her that antidepressants were harmful to the baby. She was only off the medication a few weeks before she became pregnant. Melinda did well initially, but over the past month she has become increasingly more sad, anxious,

and fearful. She thinks constantly about possible negative outcomes with the baby. She ruminates on this at night and finds herself unable to sleep. She feels as if she has "knots in her stomach," and her weight has dropped to the point that her obstetrician is worried. She began seeing her therapist again, who advised that she seek care from a reproductive psychiatrist as well.

Melinda's situation is common: well-intentioned advice from care providers often guides women to stop their medications. Unfortunately, rates of relapse are high; one study showed that nearly 70 % of women who were doing well on antidepressants but stopped because of pregnancy relapsed. Over half of these women relapsed early, in the first trimester (Cohen et al., 2006). This is the case with Melinda.

At this point, the decision of whether or not to restart medications should be based on an evidence-based, well-thought-out risk–benefit analysis. This should include the risks of untreated illness as well as the risks of medications themselves. It is this risk of untreated illness that is often left out of the equation: women are usually told of risks of medication use but not of poor outcomes that are associated with untreated mood and anxiety disorders in pregnancy.

Melinda's visit with a reproductive psychiatrist began with a careful assessment of her symptoms and her current history. She relapsed before when tapering off antidepressants, and many of the symptoms she is feeling now are consistent with how she has felt in the past. This is significant because the risks of untreated depression and anxiety are well documented, and research on this topic continues to grow. Untreated depression makes it much harder for pregnant or postpartum women to take care of themselves, even with such basics as eating, sleeping, or getting good medical care. Women with depression in pregnancy are at risk for delivering prematurely (Grigoriadis et al., 2013; Straub, Adams, Kim, & Silver, 2012) as well as for having small-for-gestational-age babies (Grote et al., 2010; Hosseini et al., 2009). In addition, an expectant mother's depression and anxiety in pregnancy may impact the developing fetus' own stress management system, and infants are born with more irritability, jitteriness, and a higher likelihood of experiencing anxiety themselves (Sandman et al., 2012; van der Wal, van Eijsden, & Bonsel, 2007). Finally, untreated depression in pregnancy is one of the biggest risk factors for postpartum anxiety and depression, with research indicating that women with antenatal depression are 5 times more likely to develop postpartum depression (Milgrom et al., 2008; Topiwala, Hothi, & Ebmeier, 2012). Postpartum mood and anxiety disorders are serious illnesses, leading to poor bonding between mother and child, less breastfeeding (Ystrom, 2012), and even high rates of suicide (Almond, 2009; Oats, 2003).

However, these risks of untreated illness need to be weighed against the risk of medication use (Byatt, Deligiannidis, & Freeman, 2013; Koren & Nordeng, 2012). It is notoriously difficult to assess data in this field, as ethical constraints prevent testing drugs on pregnant or nursing women (Einarson, Kennedy, & Einarson, 2012; Palmsten & Hernandez-Diaz, 2012). As a result, all the data we have tends to emerge after the fact, i.e., once a medication has already been on the market for many years. In addition, it is very difficult to tease out the risks of medication use versus all the risks of untreated depression. These include both the biological effects of depression on the body as well as behavioral risks such as poor appetite, disrupted sleep, and possible alcohol or drug use. Even with these challenges, however, new research continues to change the way reproductive psychiatry is practiced, making any recommendations on medication use obsolete before this book goes to press.

However, while specific recommendations are beyond the scope of this chapter, the basic framework on how to weigh the risks or the benefits of medications in pregnancy remains the same. While we have more information on SSRIs than other drug classes (and thus, the information below focuses on SSRIs), this framework applies to any medication. There are four major areas to consider. First are concerns concentrated mostly in the first trimester, namely, birth defects or pregnancy loss. For SSRIs specifically, data is mixed on these topics, but most articles are more reassuring, with the risks of medication not appearing to exceed the standard risks of pregnancy (Ross et al., 2013; United States Food and Drug Administration, 2013). However, there are other studies that do show patterns of elevated risk for various birth defects (Malm, Artama, Gissler, & Ritvanen, 2011), though these are different in design and the results are hard to generalize.

The second set of concerns centers on any medical issues for either mother or infant closer to the time of delivery. A well-described "poor neonatal adaptation syndrome" affects roughly 5–10 % of all babies, but that number increases to 10–30 % in babies exposed to SSRIs in utero. Common symptoms include respiratory distress, jitteriness, irritability, alterations in blood glucose, and, very rarely, seizures; these are transient, with no known long-lasting effects, and usually resolve with observation or symptomatic management (Maschi et al., 2008). Preterm delivery is a concern with SSRIs as well (Suri et al., 2011; Yonkers et al., 2012), though some studies show rates fairly equivalent to those seen with untreated depression (Wisner et al., 2009). Another potential medical issue, though again with some studies showing an association and others not, is persistent pulmonary hypertension of the newborn (PPHN). This more serious respiratory illness is linked to a variety of risk factors, and exposure to SSRIs in pregnancy appears to increase the risk from roughly 1/1,000 to 2/1,000 (Kieler et al., 2012). Third are questions about more long-term developmental issues, such as whether in utero exposure affects intelligence, language, or behavior. The majority of these studies with SSRIs are reassuring, with no differences between infants exposed to antidepressants in utero versus unexposed.

Finally, the possibility of breastfeeding should be considered from the very beginning. Ideally, if medications are indicated, she should be on the same agent in pregnancy through delivery, and into the postpartum. The first few days and weeks postpartum, when breastfeeding is established, are of the most high risk for mood and anxiety symptoms, and a woman should move into this time period without having to change medications for drug safety reasons during lactation. This minimizes her risk of relapse, plus decreases the number of exposures for the infant. For many women, a pre-pregnancy consultation can be enormously helpful in educating her and her family about the risks and benefits of medication use so that she can plan ahead for the safest possible perinatal period.

In Melinda's case, no pre-pregnancy consultation was available; she is already pregnant and needing to make treatment decisions. She knows from past experience that her symptoms will continue unless she treats them with antidepressants. She is worried about taking any sort of medication during pregnancy, but she is also worried about her weight loss, anxiety, and inability to sleep. After much thought, she decides to restart the antidepressant. This time, her obstetrician is supportive, as she has seen firsthand how ill Melinda becomes when untreated.

Melinda does not want to rely on medication alone, however, and she inquires into other treatments that might help keep her healthy and stable in pregnancy. Her reproductive psychiatrist advises her that there are measures that pregnant and postpartum women can take to address anxiety and depression. Melinda talks further to her obstetrician, and she begins a supplemental fish oil capsule along with her prenatal vitamins. She starts prenatal yoga as well as half-hour walks in her neighborhood several times a week. Most importantly, she finds a therapist trained in perinatal mood and anxiety disorders, and she starts seeing her on a regular basis. After a few weeks of these efforts, along with antidepressant use, her mood is brighter, her anxiety lower, and her weight gain and sleep are back on track. She plans on continuing the medication throughout pregnancy and into the postpartum, and she is already talking to her psychiatrist about making sure that her medication choice will be safe while breastfeeding.

Vignette 3
Tracy is a 32-year-old woman who gave birth to her second child three weeks ago. She felt happy and grounded after her first baby was born, with no anxiety or depression at all. However, this time, she is frantic with worry. She wakes up in the night with "cold sweats" and feeling as if, "I have electrical currents running through my body." She has frequent diarrhea and can barely eat. She is trying to nurse her baby, however, and feels pressure to breastfeed exclusively, "because I did it the first time around." She does not want to take medication, but she is desperate. Her therapist advised her to come in for a consultation.

Tracy arrives at your office slightly disheveled and exhausted appearing, with dark circles under her eyes. She continually jiggles her foot up and down, and she is struggling to sit still long enough to nurse her baby, who is crying. Tracy herself begins crying when she describes her symptoms. Her appetite has plunged; she is up hours every night, even after her children are asleep; and she cannot focus on simple tasks. She feels anxious constantly, with spikes upward into panic several times daily.

You carefully assess for manic symptoms, particularly given her agitation and inability to sleep. The practitioner should always ask about elevated or irritable mood, impulsive behavior, racing thoughts, or feelings of grandiosity. She says that while her mind is "spinning"—a common symptom with anxiety—she does not have these other experiences. She denies hearing voices, feeling paranoid, or other signs of paranoia. She also clearly denies thoughts or plans of suicide. She also denies any plan or intention to harm or kill her infant, though at times she has unbidden "images" of this that cause her even more anxiety.

Tracy had read about the "Baby Blues" online and was hoping for the first 2 weeks that this was causing her feelings. However, now that 3 weeks have passed and her symptoms are getting worse, not better, she is worried about more serious illness. Her therapist, who is trained in perinatal mood and anxiety disorders, has diagnosed her with postpartum depression and anxiety, and you concur. In addition, you are worried about panic attacks and possible OCD given the intrusive and upsetting images that she is describing. Because of your thorough screen of symptoms, you are able to rule out mania and psychosis as possible diagnoses. Tracy is also very clear that she is not using alcohol or illicit drugs.

Tracy initially declined medication when her therapist had recommended it, but today in your office, she is ready to discuss it further. Her main concern is breastfeeding: she really feels committed to continuing but is worried about transfer of any medication to the baby. You discuss at length the available medications that are known to have minimal transfer to the infant (Lanza di Scalea, 2009). One such medication in particular is helpful for sleep and appetite, as well as anxiety and depression, and this is the one you agree on together. You also discuss flexibility in breastfeeding, and she acknowledges that the pressure she feels to nurse exclusively is worsened by her anxiety and vice versa.

You recommend ongoing therapy to address this dilemma as well as work on her relationship with her new baby and how to incorporate him into her life. Other supportive measures include omega-3 fatty acids, and you give Tracy a handout on which ones are the most reliably safe and effective. You also discuss at length ways to ensure that she have a break from childcare so that she can rest, engage in moderate exercise, and allow time to heal. She agrees to discuss this with her husband and gives you permission to speak to him as well.

When you see her again for a follow-up appointment in 2 weeks' time, she is already showing signs of improvement, and you continue the current treatment plan.

Vignette 4
Janet is a 51-year-old woman who comes into your office at the advice of her therapist, who she just started seeing recently. She sought care because her own mother had a psychotic break at age 50, and she is worried this will happen to her. She herself has experienced no psychosis, and has no other psychiatric history. However, she has had times filled with rage and profound irritability for the past three years. During this time, she has also had weight gain, insomnia, poor concentration, and difficulty with short-term memory and word-finding. She initiated therapy because she is "normally happy," but has found it increasingly hard to get out of the bed in the morning.

Janet begins the session describing the intense irritability that seems to be worsening; she cannot stand how guilty she feels after she lashes out at her husband or daughter. She feels as if "I have PMS all the time." Her period is very erratic; the last time was 6 months ago. She tried to use black cohosh, a herbal medication often recommended for perimenopause (Deligiannidis & Freeman, 2010). She felt as if it helped initially, but her symptoms have worsened to the point that the herb is no longer effective. She wants to discuss different treatment options for how she is feeling.

You begin with a conversation about whether she is more interested in addressing her symptoms through hormone replacement therapy or through psychotropic medication. Because of a history of blood clots with one of her pregnancies, she is wary of any hormonal treatment. In addition, because of her family's mental health history, she is more interested in a psychiatric approach. She has never tried any sort of psychotropic medication before.

Given her mother's mood and psychotic symptoms, you screen carefully for bipolar disorder and psychosis in Janet. Antidepressants can sometimes make these symptoms worse, and a mood stabilizer or an antipsychotic would be more appropriate if any such symptoms were present. However, she denies any such symptoms. Her main complaints remain irritability, insomnia, weight gain, and poor concentration. Janet is pleased to hear that certain antidepressants have also been approved for hot flashes associated with perimenopause, as she is also suffering from these multiple times daily.

Together you decide on a trial of a serotonergic-based medication. She tries it for roughly 2 weeks but found herself feeling sedated and gaining even more weight. After more discussion, you agree to switch to a different family of medications, one that acts on both serotonin and norepinephrine. This family of medicine also has good evidence for containing mood and anxiety symptoms associated with perimenopause (Soares, 2013). Fortunately, she responds well this time, with the more tolerable side effect of a slight headache that resolves after a few days. She starts to feel better within a month, with much reduced irritability, better sleep, and improved concentration.

However, once her main symptoms are better contained, she also starts to mourn the loss of her own mother's mental health as well as the fact that her only daughter is about to leave for college. She and her husband are arguing more as well, after nearly 25 years of marriage. You recommend individual as well as family therapy, and she readily agrees. Six months later, she is much more stable in terms of her relationships as well as perimenopausal symptoms.

Conclusion

An emerging awareness of the scope and depth of reproductive mental illness has led to a dramatic increase in research, education, and clinical resources; however, there is much more to do, and we have a long way to go. To date, there are very few training programs specifically for reproductive psychiatry, and there is no officially recognized subspecialty in this field within psychiatry. Mental health care remains difficult to access for most people, but the specialized care of a reproductive psychiatrist can feel unattainable. The media, and even the medical establishment itself, continues to endorse the idea that psychiatric medications, regardless of the type of medication or the severity of illness that they are treating, should be stopped without question in pregnancy or postpartum. Stigma, financial and insurance constraints, and lack of education still prevent many women from seeking help. Despite these challenges, reproductive psychiatrists can provide the much-needed care to vulnerable and suffering women, and this exciting field is becoming more acceptable and available with each passing year.

Resources

- http://www.brighamandwomens.org—The teaching hospital for Harvard Medical School.
- www.jwatch.org—An online resource provided by the New England Journal of Medicine. Journal Watch reviews a broad base of scientific research to present important clinical findings and commentary.
- www.marcesociety.com—The Marcé Society is a research organization dedicated to increasing awareness, understanding, prevention, and treatment of mental illness related to childbearing.
- www.motherisk.org—Motherisk is a clinical research and teaching program at the Hospital for Sick Children in Toronto, Ontario, Canada, that provides information and guidance to pregnant or breastfeeding women and to health care professionals regarding risks to the fetus from exposure to drugs, chemicals, diseases, radiation, and environmental agents.
- www.NASPOG.org—The NASPOG was formed as a collaboration among obstetrician–gynecologists, psychiatrists, and psychologists with the mission of fostering scholarly scientific and clinical study of the biopsychosocial aspects of obstetric and gynecologic medicine.
- www.postpartum.net—Postpartum Support International brings together families, communities, and professionals working to support families during pregnancy, pregnancy loss, and the postpartum period in an effort to increase awareness about perinatal illness.
- www.psych.org—The American Psychiatric Association is a medical specialty organization representing more than 33,000 psychiatric physicians from the USA and around the world with the goal of insuring effective and appropriate treatment for all individuals with mental disorders.
- http://www.womenandinfants.org—Women and Infants Hospital is the teaching hospital of the Warren Alpert Medical School of Brown University. Their Center for Women's Behavioral Health specializes in outpatient care for a wide range of behavioral health issues, including mood and anxiety disorders during pregnancy and the postpartum period, substance abuse, psychiatric complications from medical disorders, crisis management and anxiety and depression stemming from pregnancy loss, infertility, a cancer diagnosis, trauma, or other crises.
- www.womensmentalhealth.org—The Massachusetts General Hospital Center for Women's Mental Health is a perinatal and reproductive psychiatry information center. The website provides a range of current information that includes new research findings in women's mental health and how these studies inform current clinical practice.

References

ACOG National Committee for Quality Assurance, Physician Consortium for Practice Improvement. Committee Opinion. (2012). Maternity care: Performance Measurement Set Measure #3: Behavioral health risk assessment.

Almond, P. (2009). Postnatal depression: A global public health perspective. *Perspectives in Public Health, 129*(5), 221–227.

American College of Obstetricians and Gynecologists. (2011). FAQ057: Premenstrual syndrome.

American College of Obstetrics and Gynecology. (2002). *Exercise during pregnancy and the postpartum period*. Washington, DC: Committee on Obstetric Practice. Reaffirmed 2009.

American Psychiatric Association. (2013). *Diagnostic and statistical manual of mental disorders* (5th ed.). Retrieved from http://dx.doi.org/10.1176/appi.books.9780890425596.910646

Anderson, E. L. (2009). ECT in pregnancy: A review of the literature from 1941-2007. *Psychosomatic Medicine, 71*, 235–242.

Baker-Ericzen, M. J., Duenas, C., Landsverk, J. A., Connelly, C. D., Hazen, L., & Horwitz, S. M. (2012). A collaborative care telemedicine intervention to overcome treatment barriers for Latina women with depression during the perinatal period. *Families, Systems & Health, 30*(3), 224–240.

Bath, K. G., Chuang, J., Spencer-Segal, J. L., Amso, D., Altemus, M., McEwen, B. S., & Lee, F. S. (2012). Variant brain-derived neurotrophic factor (Valine66Methionine) polymorphism contributes to developmental and estrous stage-specific expression of anxiety-like behavior in female mice. *Biological Psychiatry, 72*, 499–504.

Bergink, V., Burgerhout, K. M., Weigelt, K., Pop, V. J., de Wit, H., Drexhage, R. C., ... Drexhage, H. A. (2013). Immune system dysregulation in first-onset postpartum psychosis. *Biological Psychiatry, 73*(10), 1000–1007.

Brizendine, L. (2006). *The female brain*. New York, NY: Broadway Books.

Bromberger, J. T., Schott, L. L., Kravitz, H. M., Sowers, M., Avis, N. E., Gold, E. B., ... Matthews, K. A. (2010). Longitudinal change in reproductive hormones and depressive symptoms across the menopausal transition: Results from the Study of Women's Health Across the Nation (SWAN). *Archives of General Psychiatry, 67*(6), 598–607.

Byatt, N., Deligiannidis, K. M., & Freeman, M. P. (2013). Antidepressant use in pregnancy: A critical review focused on risks and controversies. *Acta Psychiatrica Scandinavica, 127*(2), 94–114.

Chen, S.-J., Liu, Y.-L., & Sytwu, H.-K. (2012). Immunologic regulation in pregnancy: From mechanism to therapeutic strategy for immunomodulation. *Clinical & Developmental Immunology, 2012*, 1–10. Article ID:258391.

Coern, L. A., Grether, J. K., Yoshida, C. K., Odouli, R., & Hendrick, V. (2011). Antidepressant use during pregnancy and childhood autism spectrum disorders. *Archives of General Psychiatry, 68*(11), 1104–1112.

Cohen, L. S., Altshuler, L. L., Harlow, B. L., Nonacs, R., Newport, D. J., Viguera, A. C., ... Stowe, Z. N. (2006). Relapse of major depression during pregnancy in women who maintain or discontinue antidepressant treatment. *Journal of the American Medical Association, 295*(5), 499–507.

Cooper, W. O., Willy, M. E., Pont, S. J., & Ray, W. A. (2007). Increasing use of antidepressants in pregnancy. *American Journal of Obstetrics & Gynecology, 196*, 544.e1–544.e5.

Cox, J. L., Holden, J. M., & Sagovsky, R. (1987). Detection of postnatal depression: Development of the 10-item Edinburgh Postnatal Depression Scale. *British Journal of Psychiatry, 150*, 782–786.

Danhauer, S. C., Legault, C., Bandos, H., Kidwell, K., Constantino, J., Vaughan, L., ... Shumaker, S. (2012). Positive and negative affect, depression, and cognitive processes in the cognition in the Study of Tamoxifen and Raloxifene (Co-STAR) trial. *Neuropsychology Development and Cognitive Section B. Aging Neuropsychology and Cognition, 20*(5), 532–552.

Davis, K., Pearlstein, T., Stuart, S., O'Hara, M., & Zlotnick, C. (2013). Analysis of brief screening tools for the detection of postpartum depression: Comparisons of the PRAMS 6-item instrument, PHQ-9, and structured interviews. *Archives of Women's Mental Health, 16*(4), 271–277.

De Groot, L., Abalovich, M., Alexander, E. K., Amino, N., Barbour, L., Cobin, R. H., ... Stagnaro-Green, A. (2012). Management of thyroid dysfunction during pregnancy and postpartum: An Endocrine Society clinical guideline. *Journal of Clinical and Endocrinology Metabolism, 97*(8), 2543–2565.

Deligiannidis, K., & Freeman, M. (2010). Complementary and alternative medicine for the treatment of depressive disorders in women. *Psychiatry Clinics of North America, 33*(2), 441–463.

Dennis, C. L., Dowswell, T. (2013). Interventions (other than pharmacological, psychosocial or psychological) for treating antenatal depression. *Cochrane Database Systematic Reviews,* (4), CD006795. doi: 10.1002/14651858.CD006795.pub3.

Dierckx, B., Heijnen, W. T., van den Broek, W. W., & Birkenhager, T. K. (2012). Efficacy of electroconvulsive therapy in bipolar versus unipolar major depression. *Bipolar Disorder, 14*(2), 146–150.

Earls, M. F., & Committee on Psychosocial Aspects of Child and Family Health American Academy of Pediatrics. (2010). Incorporating recognition and management of perinatal and postpartum depression into pediatric practice. *Pediatrics, 126*(5), 1032–1039.

Einarson, T. R., Kennedy, D., & Einarson, A. (2012). Do findings differ across research design? The case of antidepressant use in pregnancy and malformations. *Journal of Popular Therapy Clinical Pharmacology, 19*(2), e334–e348.

Epperson, C. N., & Bale, T. L. (2012). *BDNF Val66Met* polymorphism and brain-derived neurotrophic factor levels across the female life span: Implications for the sex bias in affective disorders. *Biological Psychiatry, 72,* 434–436.

Gaynes, B. N., Dusetzina, S. B., Ellis, A. R., Hansen, R. A., Farley, J. F., Miller, W. C., & Sturmer, T. (2012). Treating depression after initial treatment failure: Directly comparing switch and augmenting strategies in STAR*D. *Journal of Clinical Psychopharmacology, 32*(1), 114–119.

Ghanbari, Z., Haghollahi, F., Shariat, M., Foroshani, R., & Ashrafi, M. (2009). Effects of calcium supplement therapy in women with premenstrual syndrome. *Taiwan Journal of Obstetrics & Gynecology, 48*(2), 124–129.

Grigoriadis, S., VonderPorten, E. H., Mamisashvili, L., Tomlinson, G., Dennis, C. -L., Koren, G., ... Ross, L. E. (2013). The impact of maternal depression during pregnancy on perinatal outcomes: A systematic review and meta-analysis. *Journal of Clinical Psychiatry, 74*(4), e321–e341.

Grote, N. K., Bridge, J. A., Gavin, A. R., Melville, J. L., Iyengar, S., & Katon, W. J. (2010). A meta-analysis of depression during pregnancy and the risk of preterm birth, low birth weight, and intrauterine growth restriction. *Archives of General Psychiatry, 67*(10), 1012–1024.

Harrison, N. (2013). Inflammation and mental illness. *Journal of Neurological Neurosurgical Psychiatry, 84*(9), e1.

Hosseini, S. M., Bigian, M. W., Larkby, C., Brooks, M. M., Gorin, M. B., & Day, N. L. (2009). Trait anxiety in pregnant women predicts offspring birth outcomes. *Paediatric Perinatal Epidemiology, 23*(6), 557–566.

Hovington, C. L., McGirr, A., Lepage, M., & Berlim, M. T. (2013). Repetitive transcranial magnetic stimulation (rTMS) for treating major depression and schizophrenia: A systematic review of recent meta-analyses. *Annals of Medicine, 45*(4), 308–321.

Kieler, H., Artama, M., Engeland, A., Ericsoon, O., Furu, K., Gissler, M., ... Haglund, B. (2012). Selective serotonin reuptake inhibitors during pregnancy and risk of persistent pulmonary hypertension of the newborn: A population based cohort study from the five Nordic countries. *British Medical Journal, 344,* d8012.

Koren, G., & Nordeng, H. (2012). Antidepressant use during pregnancy: The risk-benefit ratio. *American Journal of Obstetrics & Gynecology, 207*(3), 157–163.

Kupka, R. W., Altshuler, L. L., Nolen, W. A., Suppes, T., Luckenbaugh, D. A., Leverich, G. S., ... Post, R. M. (2007). Three times more days depressed than manic or hypomanic in both bipolar I and bipolar II disorder. *Bipolar Disorder, 9*(5), 531–535.

Lam, R. W., Carter, D., Misri, S., Kuan, A. J., Yatham, L. N., & Zis, A. P. (1999). A controlled study of light therapy in women with late luteal phase dysphoric disorder. *Psychiatry Research, 86*(3), 185–192.

Lanza di Scalea, T. (2009). Antidepressant medication use during breastfeeding. *Clinical OBGYN, 52*(3), 483–497.

Lokuge, S., Frey, B. N., Foster, J. A., Soares, C. N., & Steiner, M. (2011). Depression in women: Windows of vulnerability and new insights into the link between estrogen and serotonin. *Journal of Clinical Psychiatry, 72*(11), 1563–1569.

Los Angeles County Perinatal Mental Health Task Force. (2013). *Bringing light to motherhood: Community provider perinatal mental health toolkit* (2nd ed.). Los Angeles, CA: Los Angeles County Perinatal Mental Health Task Force.

Luberto, C. M., White, C., Sears, R. W., & Cotton, S. (2013). Integrative medicine for treating depression: An update on the latest evidence. *Current Psychiatry Reports, 15*(9), 391. doi:10.1007/s11920-031-0391-2.

Lucas, M., Asselin, G., Merette, C., et al. (2009). Effects of ethyl-eicosapentaenoic acid omega-3 fatty acid supplementation on hot flashes and quality of life among middle-aged women: A double-blind, placebo-controlled, randomized clinical trial. *Menopause, 16*(2), 357–366.

Malm, H., Artama, M., Gissler, M., & Ritvanen, A. (2011). Selective serotonin reuptake inhibitors and risk for major congenital abnormalities. *Obstetrics & Gynecology, 118*(1), 111–120.

Maschi, S., Clavenna, A., Campi, R., Schiavetti, B., Bernat, M., & Bonati, M. (2008). Neonatal outcome following pregnancy exposure to antidepressants: A prospective controlled cohort study. *British Journal of Obstetrics & Gynecology, 115*, 283–289.

Massart, R., Mongeau, R., & Lanfumey, L. (2012). Beyond the monoaminergic hypothesis: Neuroplasticity and epigenetic changes in a transgenic mouse model of depression. *Philosophical Transactions of the Royal Society B, 367*, 2485–2494.

McCloughen, A., & Foster, K. (2011). Weight gain associated with taking psychotropic medication: An integrative review. *International Journal of Mental Health Nursing, 20*(3), 202–222.

Milgrom, J., Gemmill, A. W., Bilszta, J. L., Hayes, B., Barnett, B., ... Buist, A. (2008). Antenatal risk factors for postpartum depression: A large prospective study. *Journal of Affective Disorders, 108*, 147–157.

Moses-Kolko, E. L., Berga, S. L., Kairo, B., Sit, D. K., & Wisner, K. L. (2009). Transdermal estradiol for postpartum depression: A promising treatment option. *Clinical Obstetrics & Gynecology, 52*(3), 516–529.

National Centre for Health and Clinical Excellence. (2007). *Antenatal and postnatal mental health: Clinical management and service guidance (CG)*. London: NICE.

O'Mahen, H., Himle, J. A., Gedock, G., Henshaw, E., & Flynn, H. (2013). A pilot randomized controlled trial of cognitive behavioral therapy for perinatal depression adapted for women with low incomes. *Depression and Anxiety, 30*, 679–687.

Oats, M. P. (2003). Perinatal psychiatric disorders: A leading cause of maternal morbidity and mortality. *British Medical Bulletin, 67*, 219–229.

Osborne, L. M., & Monk, C. (2013). Perinatal depression - The fourth inflammatory morbidity of pregnancy?: Theory and literature review. *Psychoneuroendocrinology, 38*(10), 1929–1952. doi:10.1016/j.psychneuen.2013.03.019.

Palmsten, K., & Hernandez-Diaz, S. (2012). Can non-randomized studies on the safety of antidepressants during pregnancy convincingly beat confounding, chance, and prior beliefs? *Epidemiology, 23*(5), 686–688.

Papakostas, G. I., Shelton, R. C., Zajecka, J. M., Etamad, B., Rickels, K., Clain, A., ... Bottiglieri, T. (2012). L-Methylfolate as adjunctive therapy for SSRI-resistant major depression: Results of two randomized, double-blind, parallel-sequential trials. *American Journal of Psychiatry, 169*, 1267–1274.

Parry, B. L., Mahan, A. M., Mostofi, N., Lew, G. S., & Gillin, J. C. (1993). Light therapy of late luteal phase dysphoric disorder: An extended study. *American Journal of Psychiatry, 150*(9), 1417–1419.

Pearson, R. M., Fernyhough, C., Bentall, R., Evans, J., Heron, J., & Joinson, C. (2013). Association between maternal depressogenic cognitive style during pregnancy and offspring cognitive style 18 years later. *American Journal of Psychiatry, 170*(4), 434–441.

Pettinati, H. M., O'Brien, C. P., & Dundon, W. D. (2013). Current status of co-occurring mood and substance use disorders: A new therapeutic target. *American Journal of Psychiatry, 170*, 23–30.

Pramyothin, P., & Khaodhiar, L. (2010). Metabolic syndrome with the atypical antipsychotics. *Curent Opinions in Endocrinology, Diabetes & Obesity, 17*(5), 460–466.

Pratt, L. A., Brody, D. J., & Gu, Q. (2011). *Antidepressant use in persons aged 12 and over: United States, 2005–2008. NCHS data brief, no 76*. Hyattsville, MD: National Center for Health Statistics.

Rai, D., Lee, B. K., Dalman, C., Golding, J., Lewis, G., & Manusson, C. (2013). Parental depression, paternal antidepressant use during pregnancy, and risk of autism spectrum disorders. *British Medical Journal, 346*, f2059.

Rapkin, A. J., & Winer, S. A. (2008). The pharmacologic management of premenstrual dysphoric disorder. *Expert Opinions in Pharmacotherapy, 9*(3), 429–445.

Ross, L. E., Grigoriadis, S., Mamishashvili, L., Vonderporten, E. H., Roerecke, M., Rehm, J., … Chueng, A. (2013) Selected pregnancy and delivery outcomes after exposure to antidepressant medication: A systematic review and metaanalysis. *Journal of the American Medical Association Psychiatry, 70*(4), 436–443.

Sandman, C. A., Davis, E. P., Buss, C., & Glynn, L. M. (2012). Exposure to prenatal psychobiological stress exerts programming influences on the mother and her fetus. *Neuroendocrinology, 95*, 8–21.

Sidebottom, A. C., Harrison, P. A., Godecker, A., & Kim, H. (2012). Validation of the Patient Health Questionnaire (PHQ)-9 for prenatal depression screening. *Archives of Women's Mental Health, 15*(5), 367–374.

Soares, C. N. (2013). Depression in peri- and postmenopausal women: Prevalence, pathophysiology and pharmacological management. *Drugs & Aging, 30*(9), 677–685.

Sockol, L. E., Epperson, C. N., & Barber, J. P. (2011). A meta-analysis of treatment for perinatal depression. *Clinical Psychology Review, 31*(5), 839–849.

Spinelli, M. G. (2009). Postpartum psychosis: Detection of risk and management. *American Journal of Psychiatry, 166*(4), 405–408.

Stahl, S. M. (2000). *Essential psychopharmacology: Neuroscientific basis and practical applications* (2nd ed.). Cambridge: Cambridge University Press.

Sternfeld, B., Guthrie, K. A., Ensrud, K. E., Lacroix, A. Z., Larson, J. C., Dunn, A. L., … Caan, B. J. (2014). Efficacy of exercise of menopausal symptoms: A randomized controlled trial. *Menopause, 21*(4), 330–338.

Straub, H., Adams, M., Kim, J. J., & Silver, R. K. (2012). Antenatal depressive symptoms increase the likelihood of preterm birth. *American Journal of Obstetrics & Gynecology, 207*(329), e1–e4.

Suri, R., Hellemann, G., Stowe, Z. N., Cohen, L. S., Aquino, A., & Altshuler, L. L. (2011). A prospective, naturalistic, blinded study of early neurobehavioral outcomes for infant following prenatal antidepressant exposure. *Journal of Clinical Psychiatry, 72*(7), 1002–1007.

Swalm, D., Brooks, J., Doherty, D., Nathan, E., & Jacques, A. (2010). Using the Edinburgh postnatal depression scale to screen for perinatal anxiety. *Archives of Women's Mental Health, 13*, 515–522.

Topiwala, A., Hothi, G., & Ebmeier, K. P. (2012). Identifying patients at risk of perinatal mood disorders. *Practitioner, 256*(1751), 15–18. 2.

United States Food and Drug Administration. (2013). Use of selective serotonin reuptake inhibitors in pregnancy and cardiac malformations: A propensity-score matched cohort in CPRD. *Pharmacoepidemiology and Drug Safety, 22*(9), 942–951.

USA Preventive Services Task Force. (2009). Screening for depression in adults: U.S. Preventive Services Task Force Recommendations Statement. *Annals of Internal Medicine, 151*, 784–792.

van der Wal, M. F., van Eijsden, M., & Bonsel, J. G. (2007). Stress and emotional programs during pregnancy and excessive infant crying. *Journal of Developmental Behavioral Pediatrics, 28*(6), 431–437.

Wisner, K. L., Sit, K. K., Hanusa, B. H., Moses-Kolko, E. L., Bogen, D. L., Hunker, D. F., … Singer, L. T. (2009). Major depression and antidepressant treatment: Impact on pregnancy and neonatal outcomes. *American Journal of Psychiatry, 166*, 557–566.

Wisner, K. L., Sit, D. K. Y., & Moses-Kolko, E. L. (2006). Antipsychotic treatment during pregnancy: A model for decision-making. *Advances in Schizophrenia and Clinical Psychiatry, 3*(1), 48–55.

Wisner, K. L., Zarin, D. A., Holmboe, E. S., Appelbaum, P. S., Gelenberg, A. J., Leonard, H. L., & Frank, E. (2000). Risk-benefit decision making for treatment of depression during pregnancy. *American Journal of Psychiatry, 157*(12), 1933–1940.

World Health Organization. (2009). *Mental health aspects of women's reproductive health: A review of the literature*. Geneva: WHO Press.

Yawn, B. P., Dietrich, A. J., Wollan, P., Bertram, S., Graham, D., Huff, J., … Pace, W. D. (2012) TRIPPD: A practice-based network effectiveness study of postpartum depression screening and management. *Annals of Family Medicine, 10,* 320–329.

Yonkers, K. A., Norwitz, E. R., Smith, M. V., Lockwood, C. J., Gotman, N., Luchansky, E., … Belanger, K. (2012). Depression and serotonin reuptake inhibitor treatment as risk factors for preterm birth. *Epidemiology, 23*(5), 677–685.

Yonkers, K. A., Pearlstein, T. B., & Gotman, N. (2013). A pilot study to compare fluoxetine, calcium, and placebo in the treatment of premenstrual syndrome. *Journal of Clinical Psychopharmacology, 33*(5), 614–620.

Yonkers, K. A., Wisner, K. L., Stewart, D. E., Oberlander, T. F., Dell, D. L., Stotland, N., … Lockwood, C. (2009). The management of depression during pregnancy: A report from the American Psychiatric Association and the American College of Obstetrics and Gynecology. *General Hospital Psychiatry, 31*(5), 403–413.

Ystrom, E. (2012). Breastfeeding cessation and symptoms of anxiety and depression: A longitudinal cohort study. *BMC Pregnancy Childbirth, 12*(1), 36.

Zhang, X., Liu, K., Sun, J., & Zheng, Z. (2010). Safety and feasibility of repetitive transcranial magnetic stimulation (rTMS) as a treatment for major depression during pregnancy. *Archives of Women's Mental Health, 13*(4), 369–370.

Index

A
Acupuncture, 114, 150, 151, 313
Adenocorticotropin-releasing hormone (ACTH), 7
Adolescence, 8, 29, 32, 34, 38, 39, 42, 102, 237, 239, 249, 251, 305
Affective disorders, 5–7, 52
African American teens, 33
Ainsworth, M., 82
Amenorrhea, 237, 240–243, 250, 264
American Academy of Pediatrics, 96, 133, 248, 306
American College of Obstetrics and Gynecology (ACOG), 51, 52, 60, 62, 94, 306, 313, 316
American Psychiatric Association (APA), 33, 35, 40, 42, 51, 92, 111, 114–116, 123, 124, 130, 165, 238, 303, 305, 310, 316, 322
American Society of Clinical Oncology (ASCO), 289, 290
American Society of Reproductive Medicine (ASRM), 141, 142, 144, 148, 149, 153, 195, 196, 208, 209
Anhedonia, 54, 180, 216
Anorexia nervosa (AN), 11, 14, 147, 237, 238, 253
Anorexia tardive, 250
Antenatal Psychosocial Health Assessment (ALPHA), 95
Antenatal screening, 95
Antianxiety medications, 311
Antidepressants, 60, 92, 93, 102, 114, 118, 119, 149, 150, 172, 307–309, 311, 312, 314, 316–319, 321
Anti-Mullerian hormone (AMH) level, 202

Antipsychotics, 124, 128–129, 132, 133, 277, 310, 321
Antral follicle count, 200, 202–203
Anxiety, 6, 27, 51, 76, 98, 109, 142, 159, 178, 203, 218, 238, 263, 283, 301
  and depression related to fertility, 218
Archives of Women's Mental Health, 303
Attachment
  styles, 12, 86, 180
  theory, 82, 162
Auditory hallucinations, 124, 131, 135
Autism, 8, 11, 92, 318

B
Baby blues, 110–112, 320
Beck depression inventory (BDI), 98, 100, 101
Binge eating disorder (BED), 237–241, 243, 244, 246, 247
Biological clock, 195–210
Biopsychosocial theory, 31
Bipolar I, 124
Bipolar II, 124, 275, 310
Bipolar affective disorder, 52, 123–125, 130, 135
Bipolar disorder, 8, 91–94, 103, 112, 123–127, 129, 131–134, 136, 263, 274–277, 310, 321
Birth trauma, 177–189
Bisexual teens, 30
Body
  dissatisfaction, 27, 31, 32, 38
  image, 168, 247, 249, 250, 287, 291
  satisfaction, 33, 37
Bowlby, J., 12, 82
Brain stimulation, 314

Breast cancer, 225, 226, 285–287, 289, 291–294, 306
Breastfeeding, 91, 92, 110, 114, 115, 119, 129, 132, 133, 183–184, 188, 246–248, 269, 308, 317–320, 322
  and medications, 92, 114, 129, 320
Bright light therapy, 313
Bulimia, 237, 238

C

Caesarean section, 109, 115, 198
Cancer and hair loss, 286, 287, 294
CBT. *See* Cognitive-behavioral therapy (CBT)
Center for Epidemiological Studies Depression Scale (CES-D), 98, 99, 101, 102, 216, 306
Childbirth, 4, 10, 75, 77, 87, 91, 119, 123, 125, 130, 131, 177–189
Chronic mental illness, 123–136
Cigarette smoking, 60, 224
Clomid, 204, 205
Cognitive-behavioral therapy (CBT), 62, 118, 129, 134, 150, 153, 311
Contraception, 92, 141, 144, 196, 243, 263–278
Contraceptive options, 264, 266–269, 271
Corticotropin-releasing hormone (CRH), 7, 8, 57
Cortisol response, 57, 63

D

Delusions, 117, 124, 126, 131, 135, 310
Depression, 6, 27, 50, 80, 91, 109, 123, 142, 159, 177, 203, 215, 238, 263, 283, 303
Diagnostic and Statistical Manual of Mental Disorders, 5th Edition (DSM-V), 130, 178, 180
Dissociative disorders, 14
Distress thermometer (DT), 284
Domino Theory, 219
Donor egg, 153, 208
Dysphoria, 218
Dysthymia, 50, 52, 264

E

Eating disorders, 38, 238–241
  and fertility, 242
  and postpartum, 246–248
  and pregnancy, 240–248, 251, 253
  and risk factors, 239–240
  and sexual functioning, 241–242
Ectopic pregnancy, 160, 170, 200
Edinburgh Postnatal Depression Scale (EPDS), 94–103, 111, 305

Egg donation, 208–209
Electroconvulsive therapy (ECT), 129, 134, 314
Emotional regulation, 37, 240
EPDS. *See* Edinburgh Postnatal Depression Scale (EPDS)
Epigenetic, 8–9, 56, 252–254, 266
Estradiol, 59, 61, 200–202, 217, 239, 267, 268, 272, 275
Estrogen, 50, 53–55, 110, 113, 132, 201, 204, 205, 217, 219, 221, 265–267, 273–275, 277, 278, 304, 306, 314
Estrogen replacement therapy (ERT), 219, 225
Exercise and depression, 152, 224–225, 313

F

Fertility
  and acupuncture, 150–151
  and miscarriage, 148–149, 198
  outcomes, 141–155, 242
  preservation, 208, 289–290
  treatment, 143, 144, 148, 196, 198, 200, 201, 203–210, 242
  and yoga, 151–152
Fetal programming hypothesis, 4
Folate, 312
Follicle stimulating hormone (FSH), 50, 200–202, 205, 217

G

Generalized anxiety disorder, 53, 114, 115, 309
Gestation, 5, 6, 75–88, 94, 151, 160, 161, 165, 197, 209–210, 242
Glucocorticoids, 5, 266
Gonadotropin control ovarian stimulation (COH), 204, 205
"Good mother", 77–83, 87, 136, 308

H

Hays, S., 79, 82
Hormonal changes, 49, 110, 112, 217, 270, 302, 303, 306
Hormonal contraception, 263–278
Hormonal fluctuations, 53–58, 226, 275, 301, 314, 316
Hormonal treatment, 61–62, 199, 321
Hormone replacement therapy (HRT), 225–226, 314, 321
Hyperemesis gravidarum, 245
Hypothalamic–pituitary–adrenal (HPA) axis, 7–8, 12, 19, 117, 264, 265

Index

I

Identity work, 27, 28
Infertility, 141–150, 152–154, 159, 161, 163, 165, 195, 196, 200, 203–206, 208, 210, 250, 289, 301, 306, 313, 322
Intensive mothering, 79, 82
Internal working models, 13
Interpersonal psychotherapy, 113–114, 150, 311
Intracytoplasmic sperm injection (ICSI), 146, 147
Intrusive thoughts, 117, 160, 166, 171
In vitro fertilization (IVF), 144–147, 150–154, 161, 164–166, 196, 200–202, 204, 206, 207

J

Journal of the American Medical Association (JAMA), 303
Journal Watch, 303

K

Kessler 10 Scale, 99

L

Lactogenesis II, 184, 188
Lesbian teens, 31
Lesbian women, 168
Lipton, B., 4
Lithium, 92, 93, 124, 128, 133, 310
Lupron, 264

M

Major depressive disorder (MDD), 14, 52, 62, 100, 111, 126, 130, 166, 216, 246, 265, 305
Malattachment, 14, 15, 17–19
Mania, 92, 123–125, 127–135, 305, 307, 310, 320
Manic episodes, 123–125, 131, 310
Marcé Society, 303, 322
Mask of motherhood, 79
Maternal ambivalence, 86–87
Maternal role, 77, 80, 85, 86
Maternal stress, 5–8, 16
Menopause, 58, 59, 62, 112, 197, 202, 207, 215, 217, 221–223, 237–254, 277, 286, 290, 301, 321
Menstrual cycle, 31, 49–52, 54, 57, 58, 61, 110, 148, 197, 201, 202, 205, 206, 215, 218, 220, 221, 240, 241, 263, 264, 270, 271, 275, 276, 278, 301, 305, 316

Mindfulness, 33, 37, 41, 63
Mood
 disorders, 8, 38, 60, 86, 87, 91–103, 130, 131, 142, 203, 218, 220–221, 227, 237, 263, 265, 266, 270–278, 310
 lability, 51, 52, 110, 131, 216
 stabilizers, 92, 93, 124, 128, 132, 133, 276, 310, 321
 symptoms, 50, 51, 59, 111, 112, 226, 271, 273, 310, 312, 314
Motherhood
 constellation, 85
 crisis, 80
 identity, 81–82
 mandate, 87

N

National Comprehensive Cancer Network (NCCN), 284, 288
Neonatal death, 160, 161
Neonaticide, 135
Neurotransmitters, 152, 217, 263, 303, 309
North American Society for Psychosocial Obstetrics and Gynecology (NASPOG), 303, 322

O

Obsessive-compulsive disorder (OCD), 14, 114, 116–118, 160, 309, 320
Odent, M., 10
Oligomenorrhea, 237, 240–243, 250
Omega-3 fatty acids, 114, 312, 320
Oocytes, 146, 147, 196–209
Orenstein, P., 28
Ovarian reserve, 153, 200–203, 206–208
Ovulation, 50, 53, 58, 60, 204–206, 267
Oxytocin, 10–12, 113, 263, 265, 266

P

Panic disorder, 53, 114–116, 118, 120, 309
Patient Health Questionnaire-9 (PHQ-9), 98, 100, 101
Perimenopausal depression, 215–216, 218–220, 222, 223, 225, 226, 264, 313
Perimenopause, 59, 113, 215–227, 301, 304, 306, 308, 320, 321
Perimenstrual period, 50
Perinatal demise, 150–174
 Perinatal grief, 162–163, 172
 Perinatal loss, 160–163, 165–169, 171–174, 185
Perry, B., 9

Persistent complex bereavement disorder (PCBD), 165–166
Pipher, M., 28
Polycystic ovarian syndrome (PCOS), 205, 241
Postmenopause, 58, 221
Postpartum, 10–12, 109–136, 246–248
  psychosis, 117, 130–135, 305, 310
  relapse, 131
  screening, 94–96
Postpartum depression (PPD), 59, 91–93, 95–99, 101–103, 111–115, 117, 184, 187, 189, 220, 245–247, 251, 263–265, 274, 275, 314, 317, 320
Postpartum Depression Predictors Inventory (PDPI), 95
Postpartum Depression Screening Scale (PDSS), 96–98, 100–102, 306
Postpartum mood and anxiety disorders (PMADs), 35, 43, 182, 317
Postpartum Support International (PSI), 303, 322
Posttraumatic growth, 187, 293–295
Post-traumatic stress disorder (PTSD), 39, 56, 126, 160, 165, 170, 172, 173, 177–189, 263
Preconception care, 92–93
Pregnancy, 4, 35, 84, 93, 123–136, 160, 170, 172–173, 200, 240–248, 251, 253
  loss, 160, 161, 165, 167–169, 200, 301, 318, 322
Pregnancy risk questionnaire (PRQ), 95
Premenstrual disorders (PMDs), 49–53, 313, 316
Premenstrual dysphoric disorder (PMDD), 32, 49–63, 218, 271, 272, 316
Premenstrual exacerbation (PME), 50, 52–53
Premenstrual symptoms, 49–53, 55, 56, 58, 59, 61, 62, 271, 312, 313, 315
Premenstrual syndrome (PMS), 32, 38, 50–62, 110, 112, 218, 220, 221, 263, 271, 272, 320
Premenstruum, 49, 52, 53, 56–59
Prenatal experience, 4, 5
Primary infertility, 141–142
Primary maternal pre-occupation, 82
Progesterone, 50, 53, 54, 57, 58, 60, 61, 110, 132, 215, 225, 263–265, 272, 273, 306
Proinflammatory state, 304
Prolonged grief disorder (PGD), 165
Psychological gestation, 75–88
Psychosis, 94, 117, 126–135, 221, 305, 307, 310, 320, 321
Psychosocial adaptation to pregnancy, 84
Psychotherapy, 62, 113, 114, 127, 129, 134, 150, 172, 188, 302, 303, 307, 311
Psychotic denial of pregnancy, 126, 135
Psychotic symptoms, 117, 126, 128, 130–132, 135, 221, 277, 302, 321
PTSD. *See* Post-traumatic stress disorder (PTSD)
Puberty, 30–32, 38, 239, 301
Purging disorder, 237, 238

R
Relational-cultural theory (RCT), 28–29
Relational resilience, 29, 30, 37, 39–40, 42
Repetitive transcranial magnetic stimulation (rTMS), 314
Reproductive cancer, 200, 283–295
Reproductive loss, 159, 161, 163–165, 167, 170
Reproductive mental health, 18, 42, 237, 238, 240, 253
Reproductive psychiatry, 301–322
Reproductive story, 159–174
Rich, A., 77, 82, 86

S
Schizoaffective disorder, 126, 130
Schizophrenia, 5, 6, 8, 94, 123, 124, 126, 127, 129–131, 134, 136, 221, 276–277
Schore, A., 14, 19
Screening, 91–103, 111, 209, 210, 250–252, 254, 283, 284, 292, 294, 305, 306
  instruments, 95, 97, 98, 102, 284
Selective serotonin reuptake inhibitors (SSRIs), 54, 60–62, 149–150, 225, 226, 309, 316, 318
Self-differentiation, 14, 16–19
Self-injury, 18, 27, 39
Self-objectification, 18, 32, 33, 35, 37, 38
Self-regulation, 12, 14, 16
Serotonin norepinephrine reuptake inhibitors (SNRIs), 61, 309
Sexual abuse, 18, 56, 185, 291, 292
Sexual dysfunction and infertility, 203–204
Sexuality, 27–30, 34–36, 40–43, 143, 203, 287, 289, 291
Sexualization, 34, 35, 41, 42
Sexual trauma, 182, 185
Simkin, P., 177
Single-embryo transfer (SET), 161
Sleep disturbance, 111, 131, 151, 218, 288
Social construction of motherhood, 78–80
Social support, 85, 101, 113, 118, 129, 146, 172, 222, 223, 227, 247, 285, 286, 292, 307, 315
Spock, B., 78

SSRIs. *See* Selective serotonin reuptake inhibitors (SSRIs)
Stages of reproductive aging workshop (STRAW), 215, 226
Stern, D., 18, 85
Stillbirth, 159–174
Substance abuse, 27, 127, 292, 311, 322
Suicidal ideation, 27, 103, 172
Suicide, 10, 11, 17, 103, 112, 113, 124, 128, 132, 135, 150, 305, 317, 319

T
Tamoxifen, 306
Teen pregnancy, 35
Telephone screening, 101
Thyroid dysregulation, 306
Transition to motherhood, 75, 76, 84, 85, 243
Trauma, 10, 14–16, 18, 19, 27, 29, 31, 35, 39, 56, 118, 130, 159, 164, 167–169, 171–173, 177–189, 239, 290, 292, 294, 295, 322

and breastfeeding, 183–184
Traumatic birth, 179–184, 186, 187, 189
Traumatic stress, 56, 186

U
Unipolar depression, 91
Uterine polyps, 199

V
Vanishing twin syndrome, 17
Vasomotor symptoms, 218, 313
Visual analogue scale (VAS), 100–101

W
Winnicott, D.W., 82
World Health Organization (WHO), 34, 51, 264, 267–269, 274–276, 301

Made in the USA
Las Vegas, NV
09 September 2021